Neuroradiology of Brain Tumors

Fabio Maria Triulzi

Neuroradiology of Brain Tumors

Practical Guide based on the 5th Edition of WHO Classification

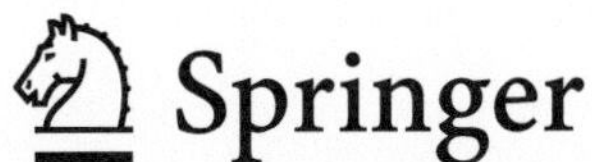

Fabio Maria Triulzi
Neuroradiology Unit
Università degli Studi, Milan, and Fondazione IRCCS Ca' Granda Ospedale
Maggiore Policlinico
Milan, Italy

ISBN 978-3-031-38155-3   ISBN 978-3-031-38153-9   (eBook)
https://doi.org/10.1007/978-3-031-38153-9

This Springer imprint is published by the registered company Springer Nature Switzerland AG
The registered company address is: Gewerbestrasse 11, 6330 Cham, Switzerland

This book is dedicated to my family, and to the memory of my parents.

Vivre sans lecture c'est dangereux, il faut se contenter de la vie, ça peut amener à prendre des risques.

—Michel Houellebecq, *Plateforme*

Preface

This book is inspired by a simple consideration.

After many years of practicing this profession, what seemed to me once a matter of course in diagnostic imaging of brain tumors has progressively come under scrutiny. Furthermore, numerous new diagnostic categories have been introduced alongside the previously established ones.

We could summarize those thoughts in the simple paradoxical observation that the increase of knowledge always increases ignorance.

In the last 30 years, imaging, particularly magnetic resonance imaging (MRI), has enormously developed, and alongside those first acquisition sequences many others have been developed, often with the promise of being more accurate than the previous ones. But as we have clearly learned, there are no acquisition methods that alone allow us to make truly accurate diagnoses. Indeed, even today it often seems difficult to simply be able to tell whether a tumor is highly aggressive or not.

I believe that the most correct approach to the diagnosis of a brain tumor with neuroimaging techniques is to put together as much information as possible that comes first of all from the basic morpho-structural MRI sequences: the T1- and T2-weighted images and the FLAIR images, and to these add those sequences which have proved to be more effective over time such as first of all diffusion and spectroscopy, and more recently the SWI and perfusion techniques, without forgetting the CT scan and in any case the use of the contrast medium which remains of fundamental importance in the differential diagnosis of brain tumors.

The evaluation of a brain tumor therefore becomes the composition of a mosaic made up of different tiles, each of which can provide a small, but still important part of the information that leads to composing the definitive picture of the diagnosis.

Surely over the next few years, artificial intelligence will be able to analyze the information already available today from the mosaic tiles in a much more effective way, but at the state of the art, the cultural and clinical synthesis role of the neuroradiologist is still fundamental in formulating a diagnostic hypothesis. I still believe that what we can call diagnostic "gestalt" is an exquisitely human procedure and as such not to be abandoned but rather to be cultivated and made to grow.

Therefore, to facilitate this approach to the matter, the simple idea of the book is to produce a series of summarized pictures of the different aspects of brain tumor imaging through the synthesis of the different pieces of the mosaic.

In our times, the diagnosis of a brain tumor cannot be separated from the study of its molecular profile and based on this, new therapies have been developed to improve the prognosis of this disease which remains one of the most complex and difficult to treat.

The question may therefore be whether and how much imaging can be of real help in the diagnosis and in the perspective of treatment of a brain tumor. The answer is in this book which faithfully follows the latest classification proposed by WHO in 2021, showing for each neoplasm the mosaic of images that characterize it, trying at least to put together a series of clues that can guide the diagnosis. If it is true that the diagnosis of a brain tumor is increasingly difficult, learning to consider all the mosaic tiles that make up an image can help us better understand its nature and make our work more useful and effective.

Milan, Italy
February 2023

The original version of this book has been revised. The unit name in the author affiliation was initially published with an error as 'Nueoradiololgy', which has now been corrected. The correction to this book can be found at https://doi.org/10.1007/978-3-031-38153-9_12

Acknowledgments

As in any work by a single author, there are many people to thank.

First of all my neuroradiologist colleagues with whom I have shared an incredibly intense clinical experience over the last 12 years, so I want to remind: Clara Sina, Antonella Costa, Claudia Cinnate, Sabrina Avignone, Giorgio Conte, Aldo Paolucci, Chiara Gaudino, Elisa Scola, Silvia Casale, Valentina Genovese, Giulia Platania, Luca Caschera, and Francesco Lo Russo. Together with the doctors, however, I do not want to forget to mention the fantastic radiographers and nursing staff of our group and our administrative staff without whom nothing could be done.

Pathologists and neurosurgeons were then fundamental colleagues in being able to bring this work to a close and I would like to mention here among pathologists: Stefano Ferrero and Letterio Runza; and neurosurgeons: Paolo Rampini, Marco Locatelli, Manuela Caroli, Mauro Pluderi, and Giulio Bertani. Neurologists are another essential components of the team and I would remind the colleagues: Nereo Bresolin, Giacomo Comi, Elio Scarpini, and Andrea Arighi. Among the people who have inspired me most in recent years by their profound culture and professionalism, I would also like to mention the director of the neurointensive care unit Prof Nino Stocchetti.

As mentioned above, this work owes much to fellow Italian neuroradiologists who have helped me by providing me with their cases; I would like to mention with special thanks Dr. Stefania Colafati of the Bambino Gesù Pediatric Hospital in Rome who has an incredible series of rare pediatric tumor cases.

Below is the list of colleagues who have kindly contributed their cases and the reference to the image provided:

Figure Credits:

- Dr. Stefania Colafati. Children's Hospital Bambino Gesù, Rome (Figs. 3.1, 3.5, 3.12, 3.15, 3.29, 4.6, 4.12, 6.17, 8.13, 8.14, and 8.15)
- Dr. Cristina Baldoli. San Raffaele Hospital, Milan (Figs. 6.14, 9.17, and 9.18)
- Prof Giovanni Morana. Children's Hospital Regina Margherita, Turin (Figs. 3.13, 3.14, and 5.2)
- Dr. Luisa Chiapparini. San Matteo Hospital, Pavia (Figs. 5.1 and 6.7)
- Dr. Nadia Colombo, Center for the Epilepsy Surgery, Niguarda Hospital, Milan (Figs. 3.3 and 3.4)
- Dr. Lorenzo Pinelli. Spedali Civili, Brescia (Figs. 3.2 and 4.16)
- Dr. Roberto Liserre. Spedali Civili, Brescia (Fig. 2.29)
- Dr. Andrea Righini, Children's Hospital Vittore Buzzi, Milan (Fig. 3.27)

Contents

Introduction

The idea of this book is to provide a schematic overview of tumor imaging by faithfully following the latest WHO classification of the central nervous system tumors, which will henceforth simply be referred to as "WHO 2021."

Being an incredibly vast topic, this work is necessarily the result of a great simplification and is limited to giving a schematic and essential view of those aspects of imaging that I believe are most important for characterizing that type of neoplasm.

Most likely this is therefore not a book for expert neuroradiologists, but above all for the younger ones who are approaching this magnificent profession or for those radiologists who can only occasionally deal with neuroradiology, it is certainly a book that can be useful to neurologists and neurosurgeons and to those who in various capacities deal with neuro-oncology.

The book is divided into 11 chapters. The first chapter is an introductory one providing general notes on the epidemiology, clinic, and history of tumor classification, as well as the different imaging techniques and the more general aspects of the differential diagnosis.

In the following 10 chapters the various tumors are considered, following the order foreseen by the WHO classification, and inevitably the longest and most complex chapter is the one dedicated to gliomas being by far the most frequent tumors of the central nervous system.

For each type of tumor, it will be briefly described:

(a) the definition given by WHO,
(b) epidemiology,
(c) location,
(d) the clinical features,
(e) the prognosis.

All these information will be obtained directly from the last two WHO classifications or from large databases such as the American CBTRUS.

The part dedicated to imaging will then follow, in which all the characteristics of the tumor under examination will be described from the basic to the advanced sequences with reference images.

Finally, for each tumor all the main imaging characteristics will be summarized in a table.

Most of the images come directly from the experience gained at our center over the last 12 years, obviously it is very difficult for a single center to have such a vast series of cases that it can cover the entire variety of brain tumors, and, as reported in the acknowledgments, this work was possible thanks to the generosity of many colleagues who contributed with their cases to fill the missing boxes.

This unfortunately does not mean that this text can present images of "all" brain tumors, there are empty boxes of rare tumors where I have limited myself to describing the characteristics as reported in the literature, but there are no reference images, and it could be a stimulus for an otherwise tentative second edition as the classification of brain tumors is continuously updated and revised.

The bibliographic references are limited and essential, and they refer to fundamental texts or articles or to references on what is currently known in the field of imaging in the case of particularly rare tumors or new acquisition techniques. I have taken for granted what has been established in the last 40 years by the literature and by my personal experience of more frequent tumors.

General Overview

1.1 Epidemiology

1.1.1 Incidence

The Central Brain Tumor Registry of the United States (CBTRUS) is, up to date, the most accurate, large, and robust epidemiological database available on brain tumors. No comparable data are available from other countries and, even though with some caution, it can be considered as a general reference for brain tumor epidemiology.

According to the last CBTRUS report [1] brain and other CNS tumors were the most common cancer in both males and females aged **0–14 years** *(pediatric group),* with an average annual age-adjusted incidence rate of **5.65 per 100,000** population.

Brain and other CNS tumors had an average annual age-adjusted incidence of **11.20 per 100,000** population among those aged **15–39 years** *(adolescent young adult group).* These tumors were the second most common cancer in males in this age group and the third most common cancer in females in this age group.

Finally brain and other CNS tumors were the eighth most common cancer among males and the fifth most common cancer among females among persons aged 40+ years *(adult group)* with an average annual age-adjusted incidence of **44.47 per 100,000 population** (Table 1.1).

In Table 1.2 the incidence rate of different types of brain tumor is summarized. The total incidence of the most frequent 7 types covers approximately **90%** of all tumors.

Table 1.1 Most common tumors in the three different group of age

	0–14 years	15–39 years	+ 40 years
1	**Brain and CNS**	Breast (female only)	Breast (female only)
2	Leukemia	Thyroid	Prostate (male only)
3	Soft tissue	**Brain and CNS**	Lung and bronchus
4	Non-Hodgkin lymphoma	Testis (male only)	Colon and rectum
5	Kidney and renal pelvis	Melanoma of the skin	Corpus and uterus (female)
6	Bones and joints	Cervix uteri (female only)	Urinary bladder
7	Endocrine (incl. Thymus)	Colon and rectum	Melanoma of the skin
8	Hodgkin lymphoma	Non-Hodgkin lymphoma	**Brain and CNS**

F. M. Triulzi, *Neuroradiology of Brain Tumors*, https://doi.org/10.1007/978-3-031-38153-9_1

Table 1.2 Summary of incidence rate (cases for 100,000 populations)

Metastasis	14
All meningiomas	8.13
Glioblastoma	3.5
Pituitary adenomas	3.49
All tumors of the cranial and paraspinal nerves	1.76
Pilocytic astrocytoma	0.84
Diffuse astrocytoma	0.75
Total 1–7	32.47
Langerhans cells histiocytosis	0.50
All mesenchymal non-meningoendothelial tumors	0.50
All lymphomas	0.46
Ependymoma/anaplastic ependymoma	0.43
Anaplastic astrocytoma	0.35
Pleomorphic astrocytoma	0.30
Oligodendroglioma	0.28
All neuronal and mixed neuronal-glial tumor	0.28
All embryonal tumor	0.26
Craniopharyngioma	0.18
Anaplastic oligodendroglioma	0.11
All germ cell tumor	0.10
Hemangiopericytoma	0.08
Myxopapillary ependymoma	0.05
Choroid plexus papilloma	0.05
All pineal tumor	0.04
Total 8–23	3.97

1.1.2 Mortality Rate

According to CBTRUS [1] malignant brain tumors and other CNS tumors among pediatric group had an average annual age-adjusted mortality rate of **0.72 per 100,000** and were the eighth most common cause of death in this age group but the **most common cause of cancer death.**

Malignant brain and other CNS tumors among adolescent and young adult group had an average annual age-adjusted mortality rate of **0.96 per 100,000** and were the thirteenth most common cause of death in this age group and the **second most common cause of cancer death**, together with leukemia.

Among the adult group malignant brain and other CNS tumors had an average annual age-adjusted mortality rate of **9.01 per 100,000** and were the twenty-ninth most common cause of death and the **fourteenth most common cause of cancer death** (Table 1.3).

Table 1.3 Most common cause of death in the three different group of age

	0–14 years	15–39 years	+ 40 years
1	Perinatal conditions	Accident, adverse effects	Disease of heart
2	Congenital anomalies	Suicide, self-inflicted injury	Other causes
3	Accident, adverse effects	Other causes	Lung and bronchus tumors
4	**Brain and other CNS tumors**	Breast cancer	Prostate (male only) cancer
5	Leukemia	**Brain and other CNS tumors**	Colon and rectum cancer
6	Endocrine (excl. Thyroid)	Leukemia	Miscellaneous cancer
7	Soft tissue tumors	Cervix uteri (female only) cancer	Breast cancer
8	Bones and joints tumors	Colon and rectum cancer	**Brain and other CNS tumors**

1.2 **Clinical Presentation**

Clinical symptoms and signs associated with brain tumors can be subdivided into general symptoms associated or not to raised intracranial pressure and in focal symptoms due to direct focal damage of the brain [2].

1.2.1 **General Symptoms**

1. *Headache.* According to [2] the prevalence of brain imaging abnormalities on magnetic resonance imaging (MRI) is low in patients without headache. Headache is rare as the only symptom on presentation (8%), but about 2/3 of patients with a brain tumor complained of headache at diagnosis.
2. *Nausea and vomiting.* They usually occurred under stimulation of the chemotactic trigger of the area postrema and are usually related to raised intracranial pressure, but in case of posterior fossa tumor they can occur by direct compression of the tumor.
3. *Papilledema.* It is usually directly related to a raised intracranial pressure and it is more easily seen in children even though due to the diffusion of neuroimaging it is now rarely seen in patients at the diagnosis.
4. *Seizures.* They are a frequent symptom in patients with a brain tumor with a variable incidence from 30% to 100% depending on the tumor type. Slow growing tumors are usually most epileptogenic.
5. *Herniation syndromes.* They are rare as clinical presentation, but in someway their incidence progressively increases with the course of the disease. They are typically subdivided into five different syndromes: (a) *Subfalcine herniation.* The cingulate gyrus is pushed under the falx cerebri with compression of anterior cerebral arteries and frontomesial infarction. (b) *Uncal herniation.* The uncus herniated through the tentorium causes ipsilateral oculomotor palsy and controlateral hemiparesis, a compression of posterior cerebral arteries with occipital infarction is also possible. (c) *Central herniation.* The mass

effect starts from a diencephalic mass causing coma and brainstem compression. (d) *Tonsillar herniation.* The cerebellar tonsils herniate through the foramen magnum with possible compression of the medulla and death. (e) *Upward brainstem herniation.* It is caused by posterior fossa tumors compressing and displacing upward superior vermis and midbrain with possible aqueductal obstruction.

1.2.2 **Focal Symptoms**

1. *Frontal-lobe tumors.* Symptoms may be subtle and generic, however with the progression of the disease personality changes and cognitive dysfunctions may be present, eventually with a complete apathetic state. Gait instability or gait apraxia may be present. According to the disease growth speech or motor disturbances can be noted.
2. *Temporal-lobe tumors.* The predisposition to seizures is a typical feature of temporal lobe masses, typically they may have a partial onset. Visual disturbances can ensue due to the involvement of optic radiation. Expressive speech deficits may also be seen as well as cognitive and memory deficits.
3. *Parietal-lobe tumors.* Seizures are relatively frequent also in case of parietal tumor. Sensory abnormalities even sometimes particularly complex may be typically related to this location. Dyspraxia and dysphasia can occur as well.
4. *Occipital-lobe tumor.* Visual disturbance is obviously related to this location together with disfunction of oculomotor tracking or more complex symptoms such as color and visual anomia.
5. *Diencephalic tumors.* They are associated with obstruction of the foramen of Monro and hydrocephalus.
6. *Pineal region tumors.* Their growth can lead to aqueductal occlusion as hydrocephalus and the compression of the mesencephalic tectum can be associated with Parinaud's syndrome with vertical-gaze paresis.

7. *Mesencephalic tumors.* They are very frequently associated with aqueductal obstruction and hydrocephalus. Oculomotor disturbances are typically associated with mesencephalic mass as well.

8. *Pontine tumors.* Pontine mass such as diffuse intrinsic pontine glioma (DIPG) can reach great volumes without symptoms, a possible clinical presentation, other than the signs and symptoms of intracranial hypertension, could be a mono or bilateral abducens palsy.

9. *Cerebellar tumors.* Compression of the fourth ventricle with progressive hydrocephalus is frequently associated with cerebellar tumors. Lateral lesions could be associated with limb ataxia and disrupted coordination.

10. *Cerebellopontine angle tumors.* Vertigo, tinnitus, or hearing loss is the classical presentation of tumor of the VIII cranial nerve. Other cranial nerves such as VII and more rarely V can be involved by these tumors.

11. *Medullary tumors.* Lower cranial nerve deficits and motor deficits can be associated with these tumors.

1.3 Classification, Grading, and Prognosis

1.3.1 WHO Classification of Tumor of the Central Nervous System and Histological Grading

The first internationally accepted classification of brain tumor was published in 1979 under the patronage of the World Health Organization (WHO) [3]. After the first edition the WHO published other 3 editions in 1993 [4], 2000 [5], and 2007 [6], including different new subtypes of CNS tumors.

The WHO classification is based on the histological and microstructural appearance of brain tumors, but together with the histological classification the WHO introduced since the first 1979 classification the concept of *tumor grading*. Brain tumor grading is a malignancy scale rather than a strict histological grading system and it is a main guide to disease prognosis.

In summary the four grades are defined as follows:

Grade I: Low proliferative potential and possibility of cure after surgical resection.

Grade II: Infiltrative and potentially recurent tumor that tends to progress to higher grade.

Grade III: Clear histological evidence of malignancy including nuclear atypia.

Grade IV: Cytologically malignant, mitotically active, necrosis prone neoplasm associated with rapid disease evolution and fatal outcome.

1.3.2 WHO Classification of Brain Tumors 2016

In 2016 the WHO published a "revised 4th edition" [7] which, more than a simple revised version of the 2007 classification, was in fact a real new classification which introduces for the first time, alongside the traditional histological classification, a classification of brain tumors based on molecular genetics [8].

From a practical point of view greatest changes are related to a different view of disease prognosis and patient survival according to genetic profile more than to the traditional histological grading.

Thanks to this new classification some tumors with and histological grading compatible with a high mitotic index and with and apparent very rapid growth (grade IV), if associated to a particular genetic profile can have a better prognosis of some other brain tumors with an apparent less aggressive grading, but more unfavorable molecular genetis.

1.3.3 Grading and Prognostic Evaluation

Even still the most important the grading system is however only one of the criteria that lead to the prognosis and final outcome. Other important criteria should take into account the following:

- Patients age and clinical status.
- Tumor location and complete vs. partial resectability.

- Proliferation index value.
- Radiological features.
- Genetic profile.

As previously mentioned genetic profile has progressively grown in importance because some genetic characteristics can dramatically change the prognosis such the presence of IDH mutation in gliomas or some other mutations in medulloblastoma an aggressive tumor of grade IV that can reach some genetic subgroup a 95% survival rate at 5 years.

1.3.4 The Fifth Edition of WHO Classification of Brain Tumor

The latest revision is the fifth edition of the WHO Classification of Tumors of the Central Nervous System, which was released in 2021 [9, 10]. Some of the major differences between the 2016 revised fourth version and the new 2021 fifth edition are as follows:

1. Terminology: The 2021 WHO classification uses a more uniform and simplified terminology than the 2016 version. The new classification system uses the term "neuroepithelial tumors" to describe tumors that originate from cells within the brain or spinal cord, while the 2016 classification used several different terms such as "astrocytic tumors," "oligodendroglial tumors," and "gliomas." Glioblastoma is now by definition only IDH-wildtype tumors.
2. Tumor entities: The 2021 WHO classification adds several new tumor entities and modifies the diagnostic criteria for existing entities. For example, the new classification recognizes "diffuse midline glioma with H3 K27M mutation" as a distinct tumor entity, which was not present in the 2016 version. The new classification also reclassifies some tumors, such as "dysembryoplastic neuroepithelial tumor," which was previously considered a low-grade glioma but is now recognized as a distinct entity.
3. Molecular markers: The 2021 WHO classification places a greater emphasis on molecular markers in the diagnosis and classification of brain tumors. For example, the new classification recognizes "NTRK-fusion gliomas" as a distinct tumor entity, which is defined by the presence of a fusion between the NTRK gene and another gene. The new classification also incorporates other molecular markers such as "BRAF V600E mutation" and "TERT promoter mutation" into the diagnostic criteria for certain tumor entities.
4. Grading system: The 2021 WHO classification introduces a new grading system for certain tumor entities, which incorporates both histological features and molecular markers. For example, the new grading system for diffuse gliomas incorporates the IDH mutation status, 1p/19q codeletion status, and the presence of certain histological features, such as microvascular proliferation and necrosis, to classify tumors into different grades. The new grading system is designed to provide a more accurate prognosis and guide treatment decisions. Traditionally, CNS WHO tumor grades were written as Roman numerals. However, the fifth edition WHO Blue Books have emphasized more uniform approaches to tumor classification and grading and have favored the use of Arabic numerals for grading, as is currently done for all the other organ systems.

1.3.5 Classification Scheme

For the purpose of this book, we present below the simplified classification of the fifth edition of the WHO classification of brain tumors that we will use as a guide for the description of each individual tumor in the next 10 chapters (Table 1.4).

Table 1.4 Simplified classification of CNS tumors according to the fifth edition of WHO CNS tumor classification

1. Gliomas, glioneuronal tumors, and neuronal tumors		
1.1 Adult-type diffuse gliomas		
1.1.1	Astrocytoma, IDH-mutant	
	1.1.1.1	Astrocytoma, IDH-mutant, grade 2
	1.1.1.2	Astrocytoma, IDH-mutant, grade 3
	1.1.1.3	Astrocytoma, IDH-mutant, grade 4
1.1.2	Oligodendroglioma, IDH-mutant and 1p/19q-codeleted	
	1.1.2.1	Oligodendroglioma, IDH-mutant and 1p/19q-codeleted, grade 2
	1.1.2.2	Oligodendroglioma, IDH-mutant and 1p/19q-codeleted, grade 3
1.1.3	Glioblastoma, IDH-wildtype	
1.1.4	Gliosarcoma	
1.2 Pediatric-type diffuse low-grade gliomas		
1.2.1	Diffuse astrocytoma *MYB-* or *MYBL1*-altered	
1.2.2	Angiocentric glioma	
1.2.3	Polymorphous low-grade neuroepithelial tumor of the young	
1.2.4	Diffuse low-grade glioma, MAPK pathway altered	
1.3 Pediatric-type diffuse high-grade gliomas		
1.3.1	Diffuse midline glioma H3 K27-altered	
1.3.2	Diffuse hemispheric glioma H3 G34-mutant	
1.3.3	Diffuse pediatric-type high-grade glioma, H3-wildtype and IDH-wildtype	
1.3.4	Infant-type hemispheric glioma	
1.4 Circumscribed astrocytic gliomas		
1.4.1	Pilocytic astrocytoma	
1.4.2	High-grade astrocytoma with piloid features	
1.4.3	Pleomorphic xanthoastrocytoma	
1.4.4	Subependymal giant cell astrocytoma	
1.4.5	Chordoid glioma	
1.4.6	Astroblastoma *MN1*-altered	
1.5 Glioneuronal and neuronal tumors		
1.5.1	Ganglioglioma	
1.5.2	Gangliocytoma	
1.5.3	Desmoplastic infantile ganglioglioma	
1.5.4	Desmoplastic infantile astrocytoma	
1.5.5	Dysembryoplastic neuroepithelial tumor	
1.5.6	Diffuse glioneuronal tumor with oligodendroglioma-like features and nuclear clusters	
1.5.7	Papillary glioneuronal tumor	
1.5.8	Rosette-forming glioneuronal tumor	
1.5.9	Myxoid glioneuronal tumor	
1.5.10	Diffuse leptomeningeal glioneuronal tumor	
1.5.11	Multinodular and vacuolating neuronal tumor	
1.5.12	Dysplastic cerebellar gangliocytoma (Lhermitte-Duclos disease)	
1.5.13	Central neurocytoma	
1.5.14	Extraventricular neurocytoma	
1.5.15	Cerebellar liponeurocytoma	
1.6 Ependymal tumors		
1.6.1	Supratentorial ependymoma, NOS	

Table 1.4 (continued)

1.6.2	Supratentorial ependymoma, *ZFTA* fusion positive
1.6.3	Supratentorial ependymoma, *YAP1* fusion positive
1.6.4	Posterior fossa ependymoma, NOS
1.6.5	Posterior fossa group A (PFA) ependymoma
1.6.6	Posterior fossa group B (PFB) ependymoma
1.6.7	Spinal ependymoma, NOS
1.6.8	Spinal ependymoma, *MYCN*-amplified
1.6.9	Myxopapillary ependymoma
1.6.10	Subependymoma
2. Choroid plexus tumors	
2.1	Choroid plexus papilloma
2.2	Atypical choroid plexus papilloma
2.3	Choroid plexus carcinoma
3. Embryonal tumors	
3.1 Medulloblastomas molecularly defined	
3.1.1	Medulloblastoma, WNT-activated
3.1.2	Medulloblastoma, SHH-activated and *TP53*-wildtype
3.1.3	Medulloblastoma, SHH-activated and *TP53*-mutant
3.1.4	Medulloblastoma, non-WNT/non-SHH
3.2 Other CNS embryonal tumors	
3.2.1	Atypical teratoid/rhabdoid tumor
3.2.2	Embryonal tumor with multilayered rosettes
3.2.3	CNS neuroblastoma, *FOXR2*-activated
3.2.4	CNS tumor with *BCOR* internal tandem duplication
3.2.5	CNS embryonal tumor NEC/NOS
4. Pineal tumors	
4.1	Pineocytoma
4.2	Pineal parenchymal tumor of intermediate differentiation
4.3	Pineoblastoma
4.4	Papillary tumor of the pineal region
4.5	Desmoplastic myxoid tumor of the pineal region, *SMARCB1*-mutant
5. Cranial and paraspinal nerve tumors	
5.1	Schwannoma
5.2	Neurofibroma, plexiform neurofibroma
5.3	Rare nerve sheath tumors
5.4	Malignant peripheral nerve sheath tumor
5.5	Cauda equina neuroendocrine tumor (previously paraganglioma)
6. Meningioma	
6.1	Meningioma
7. Mesenchymal, nonmeningothelial tumors involving the CNS	
7.1 Fibroblastic and myofibroblastic tumors	
7.1.1	Solitary fibrous tumor
7.2 Vascular tumors	
7.2.1	Hemangiomas and vascular malformations
7.2.2	Hemangioblastoma
7.3 Skeletal muscle tumors	
7.3.1	Rhabdomyosarcoma
7.4 Tumors of uncertain differentiation	
7.4.1	Intracranial mesenchymal tumor, FET::CREB fusion positive

(continued)

Table 1.4 (continued)

7.4.2	*CIC*-rearranged sarcoma
7.4.3	Primary intracranial sarcoma, *DICER1*-mutant
7.4.4	Ewing sarcoma
7.5 Chondrogenic tumors	
7.5.1	Mesenchymal chondrosarcoma
7.5.2	Chondrosarcoma
7.6 Notochordal tumors	
7.6.1	Chordoma
8. Melanocytic tumors	
8.1 Diffuse meningeal melanocytic neoplasm	
8.1.1	Meningeal melanocytosis and melanomatosis
8.2 Circumscribed meningeal melanocytic neoplasm	
8.2.1	Meningeal melanocytoma and melanoma
9. Hematolymphoid tumors involving the CNS	
9.1 CNS lymphomas	
9.1.1	Primary diffuse large B-cell lymphoma of the CNS
9.1.2	Immunodeficiency-associated CNS lymphomas
9.1.3	Lymphomatoid granulomatosis
9.2 Miscellaneous rare lymphomas of the CNS	
9.3 Secondary CNS lymphomas	
9.4 Histiocytic tumors	
9.4.1	Langherans cell histiocytosis
9.4.2	Rare histiocytic tumors
10. Germ cell tumors	
10.1.4	Germinoma
11. Tumors of the sellar region	
11.1.1	Adamantinomatous craniopharyngioma
11.1.2	Papillary craniopharyngioma
11.1.3	Pituicytoma, granular cell tumor of the sellar region, spindle cell oncocytoma
11.1.4	Pituitary adenoma/pituitary neuroendocrine tumor (PitNET)
12. Metastases to the CNS	

1.4 Neuroradiology Features: Imaging Techniques

1.4.1 Computerized Tomography (CT)

CT still remains an important diagnostic technique in the assessment of intracranial brain tumors. In many cases it represents the first imaging technique available through the course of the disease and its features frequently represent a significant step in the final diagnosis.

The main CT features mostly contributing to achieving a general idea of the lesion can be summarized as follows:

(a) Lesion density. A highly cellulated lesion tends to be iso to slightly hyperdense, typical examples are lymphomas or germinomas or in the differential diagnosis between a medulloblastoma and a pilocytic astrocytoma the parenchymal component of the latter is usually isodense, whereas the medulloblastoma is more typically iso to slightly hyperdense (Fig. 1.1).

(b) Lesion structure. CT in particular after the administration of contrast media can provide at least a first description of the internal structure of the tumor and consequently of its homogeneity. It can depict necrosis, but overall CT can clearly identify hemorrhagic

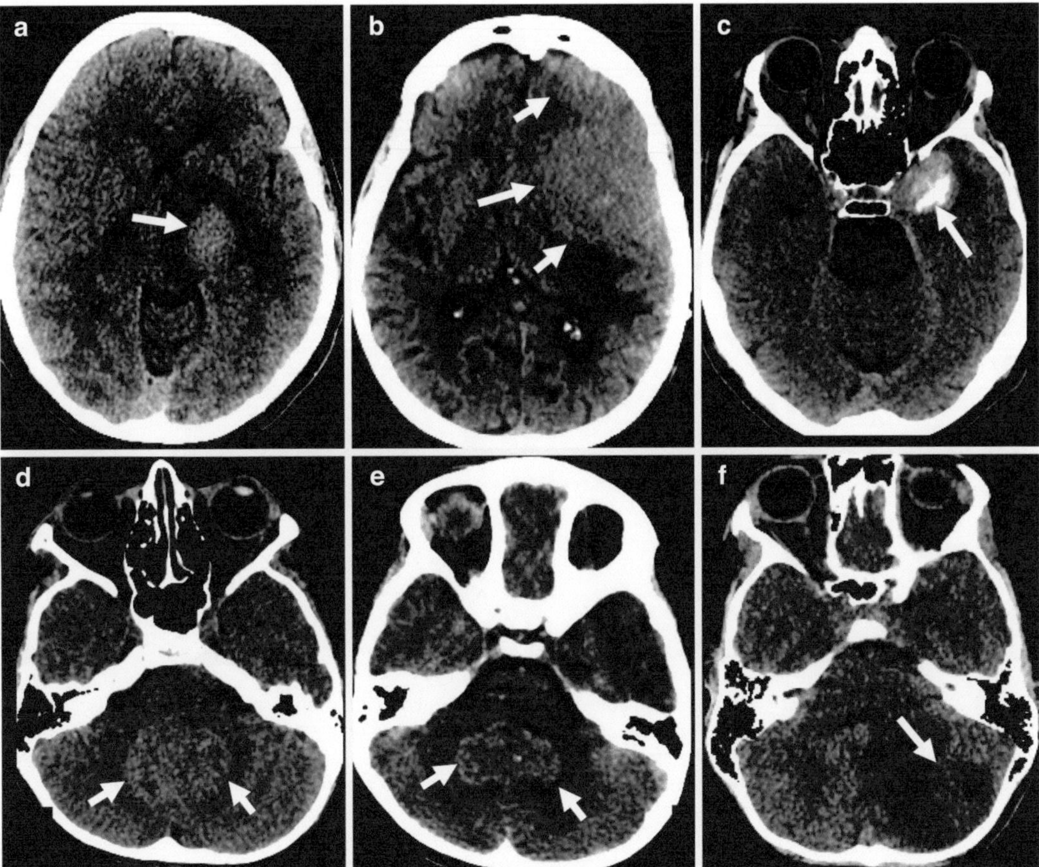

Fig. 1.1 Different tumor density on CT. Lymphoma (**a**), meningiomas (**b**, **c**), medulloblastomas (**d**, **e**), pilocytic astrocytoma (**f**). Lymphomas, meningiomas, and medulloblastomas may appear with variable hyperdensity on CT (arrows **a**–**e**). The spontaneous hyperdensity of medulloblastoma is an important diagnostic clue in the differential diagnosis of pilocytic astrocytoma, where the mural nodule of the tumor is iso to hypodense (arrow **f**)

component and in particular calcification. Even though MR is now capable thanks to susceptibility weighted sequence to identify calcification, CT still remains the most effective diagnostic technique in detecting calcified lesions within the brain (Fig. 1.2).

(c) Brain tumor and the relationship with cranial structures. Due to its sensitivity to bone structures CT is the technique of choice in the evaluation of skull. Any skull involvement in intracranial tumor can be easily evaluated by means of CT (Fig. 1.3).

1.4.2   Magnetic Resonance Imaging (MRI), Conventional Techniques, Susceptibility Weighted Imaging (SWI), and Balanced Steady-State Free Processing (bSSFP) Sequences

In the MRI evaluation of a CNS tumor conventional sequences and the use of paramagnetic contrast agent (gadolinium-based contrast agent, GBCA) are still the pillars of the diagnostic pro-

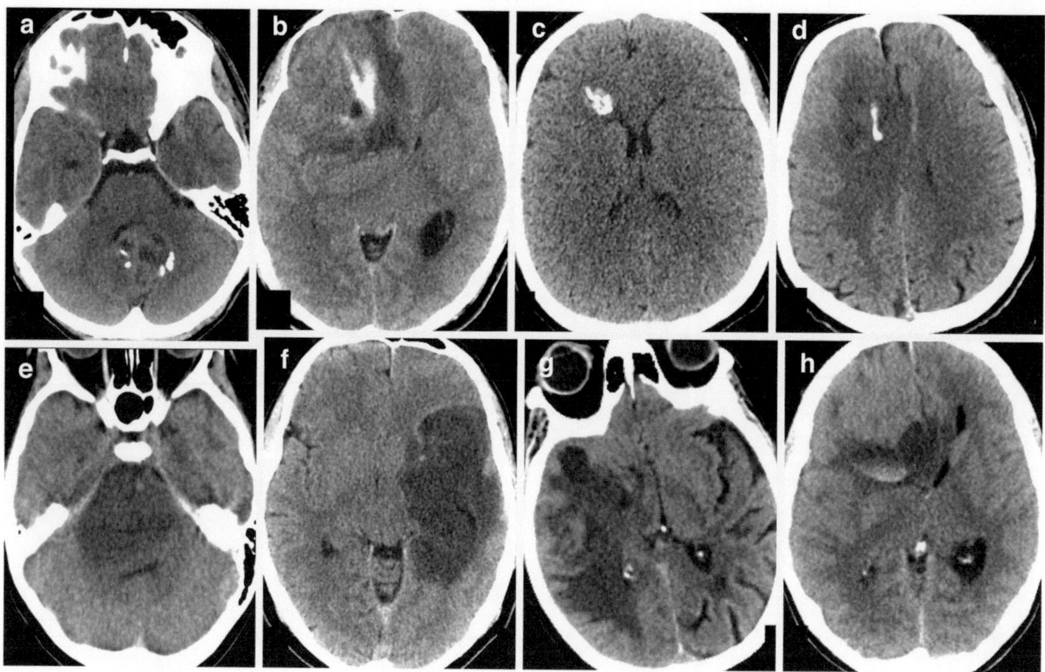

Fig. 1.2 Different tumor internal structure on CT. Superior row: different brain tumors with calcifications: cerebellar ganglioglioma (**a**), oligodendrogliomas (**b**, **d**), extraventricular neurocytoma (**c**). Inferior row: homogeneous infiltrative structure in a diffuse intrinsic pontine glioma (**e**) and in large astrocytoma (**f**), vs. highly heterogeneous structure in brain metastases (**g**) and glioblastoma with a hemorrhagic component (**h**)

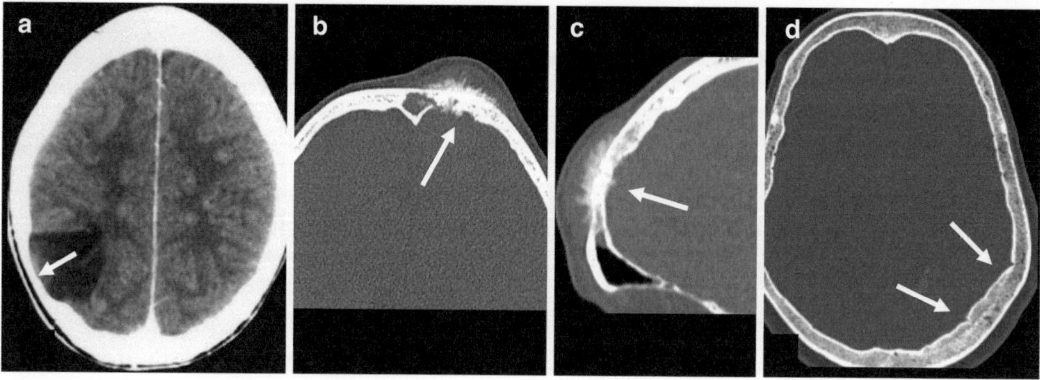

Fig. 1.3 Skull involvement in brain tumors on CT. A superficial DNT with parietal bone scalloping (arrow **a**), an intra-osseous meningioma (arrows **b**, **c**), a bone scle- rotic reaction in correspondence with a large parietal meningioma (arrows **d**)

cess (Fig. 1.4). The lesion's features on T1WI, T2WI, and FLAIR are the basis for any semeiotic process. All these three sequences are mainly influenced by the water content of the lesion, but the cellularity, the ratio nucleus/cytoplasm, the presence of hemorrhage or calcifications can largely modify the signal intensity of the lesion.

Contrast media contributes to characterize the lesion as well. In a general view the presence of contrast enhancement is related to a more aggres-

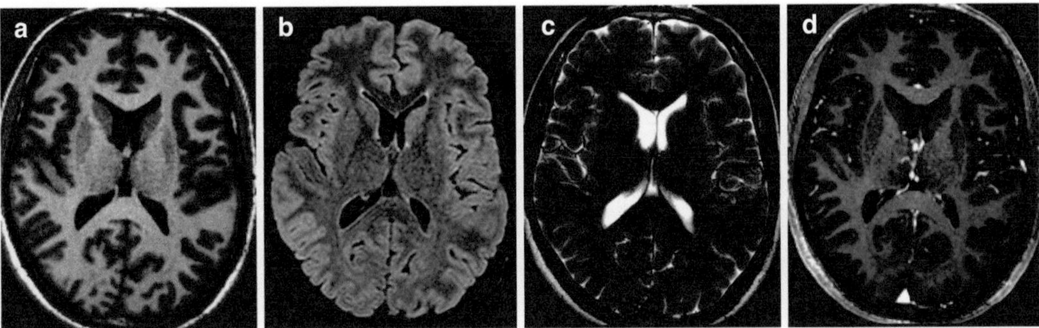

Fig. 1.4 The "pillars" of MRI. T1WI (**a**), FLAIR (**b**), T2WI (**c**), and post-contrast T1WI are still the first step sequences for any MRI evaluation of the brain looking for a brain tumor. Today T1WI and FLAIR images are usually performed with a 3D technique such as in this example, whereas T2WI is still preferable with a 2D acquisition technique for a better spatial, but also contrast resolution

sive lesion, but there are many grade 1 tumors such as pilocytic astrocytoma or glioneural tumors that can regularly show lesion enhancement after contrast (Fig. 1.5).

In the last years susceptibility weighted imaging (SWI) technique has progressively become a sequence regularly used in a standard clinical setting [11]. This sequence has a extraordinary conspicuity for any paramagnetic and even diamagnetic substance and results to be highly useful in detecting small hemorrhagic foci, increased vascularization within a lesion or even the presence of calcification thanks to the possibility of the phase image to shift the signal intensity of a calcification from hypointense to hyperintense (Fig. 1.6).

Another group of acquisition sequences has proved to be extremely useful in recent years due to the exceptional 3D spatial resolution it can achieve, with the consequent possibility of demonstrating details with surprising anatomical precision. The limitation of this sequence is that the contrast is substantially flattened between what is liquid (hyperintense) and everything else that is homogeneously hypointense. This is the large family of steady-state gradient echo sequences that can be classified into several groups: spoiled (or incoherent) steady-state sequences (FLASH, SPGR, T1-FFE), post-excitation refocused steady-state sequences (FISP, GRASS, FFE), preexcitation refocused steady-state sequences (PSIF, SSFP, T2-FFE), and fully refocused steady-state sequences (true-FISP, FIESTA, balanced-FFE). This latter group is also called balanced SSFP (b-SSFP), because only in this group are the gradients in all three axes fully balanced, so that there is not a net gradient-induced dephasing of magnetization in each TR. [12, 13].

Figure 1.7 exemplifies the advantages of the bSSFP sequence in defining the anatomical relationship of a large meningioma to the floor of the third ventricle. Its usefulness is maximum when it has to delimit structures that are in direct contact with the CSF

1.4.3 MRI Diffusion and Diffusion Tensor Imaging (DTI)

Another sequence now regularly used in the clinical setting is the diffusion weighted image (DWI) sequence and the parametric counterpart the apparent diffusion coefficient (ADC) image. These sequences allow to represent in an image the molecular water diffusion. The random movement of water molecule is known as Brownian movement. Brownian motion describes the natural motion of particles suspended in a fluid when they are randomly distributed in space in a way in which there is no preferred direction of flow. The mean velocity of the particles is related to the temperature and the water velocity is null for the temperature of 0 °C and maximum at 100 °C.

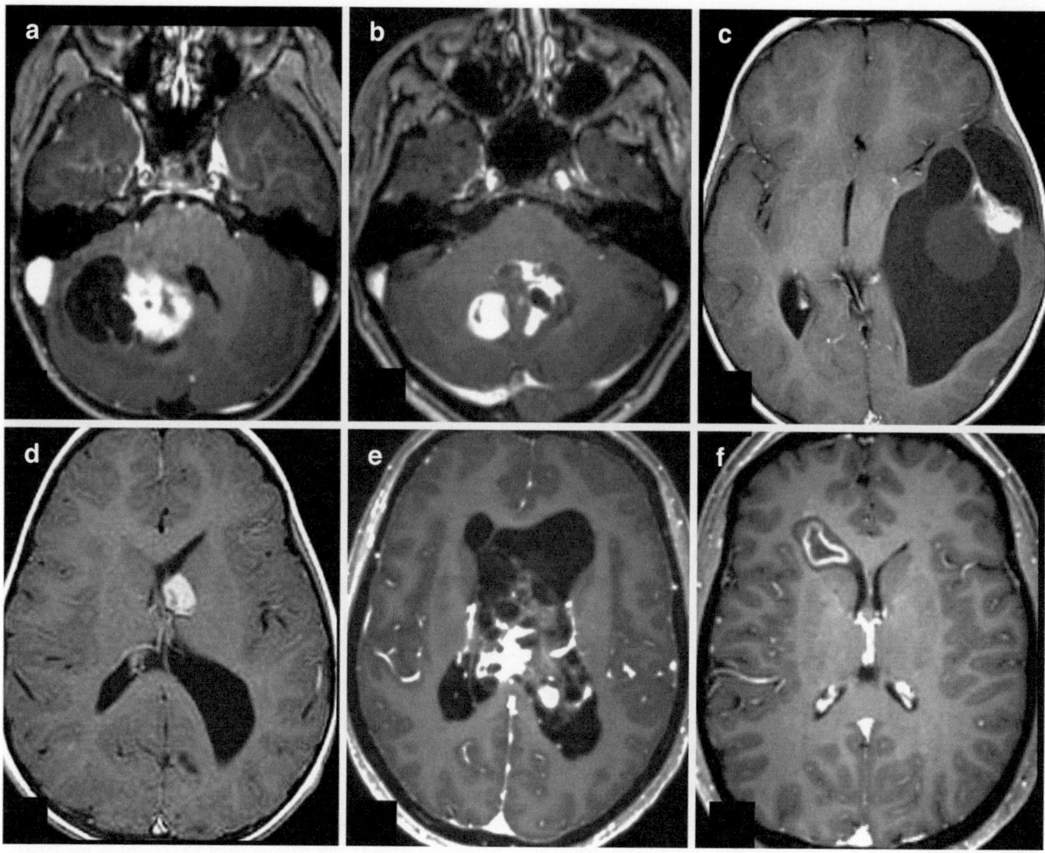

Fig. 1.5 Grade 1 brain tumor with enhancement on T1WI after contrast administration. Pilocytic astrocytoma (**a**), cerebellar ganglioglioma (**b**), desmoplastic infantile ganglioglioma (**c**), subependymal giant cell astrocytoma (**d**), central neurocytoma (**e**), extraventricular neurocytoma (**f**)

Within the brain the water molecular diffusion is maximum within the ventricles and the sub-arachnoid spaces where the water molecules do not find any obstacle to their movement, the movements are on the contrary variably reduced within the brain parenchyma. In the ADC image any pixel value corresponded to the apparent diffusion coefficient so that the value is higher within CSF and variably reduced within brain parenchyma. In DWI the image is only "weighted" for the diffusion and in the intensity of the signal other components such as T1 and T2 relaxation are present (Fig. 1.7). From a practical point of view the image results in something opposite to the ADC image, most importantly from a radiological point of view a diffusion restriction will be detected as hyperintense on DWI and hypointense on ADC, on the contrary a diffusion increase will result in hypointense on DWI and hyperintense on ADC (Figs. 1.8 and 1.9) [14].

With diffusion tensor imaging (DTI) it is possible not only to obtain the mean diffusivity of certain tissue, but also to achieve information on diffusion isotropy/anisotropy. As previously stated in an ideal fluid there is no preferential direction. That is what happened in the CSF where the isotropy is at the highest and the anisotropy was null, similarly within gray matter the anisotropy is zero even the mean diffusivity is much shorter than in CSF. That is because in gray matter the many different obstacles to the water movement are randomly distributed with no prevalent direction. On the contrary within the white matter the anisotropy is high because the direction parallel to the axons is clearly prevalent with respect to the directions perpendicular to the

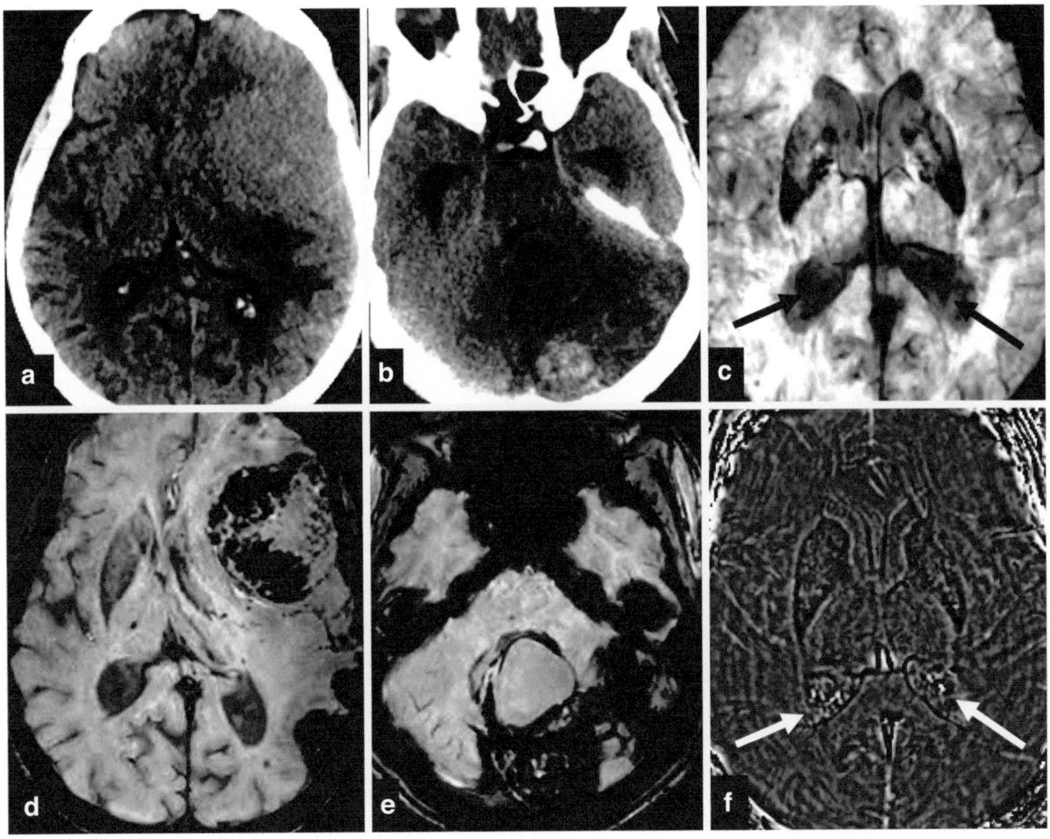

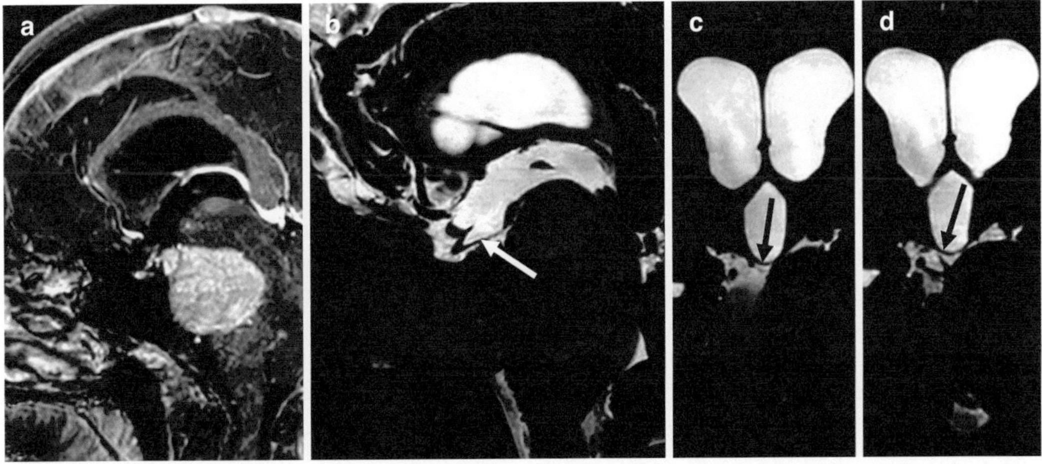

Fig. 1.6 Calcifications and hemorrhages on SWI. Diffuse microcalcification in a huge meningioma on CT (**a**) and SWI (**d**), hemorrhage in pilocytic astrocytoma on CT (**b**) and SWI (**e**). Differences between the module (**c**) and phase (**f**): SWI images allow us to differentiate the paramagnetic effect of basal ganglia iron deposit and diamagnetic effect of choroid plexus calcifications. On module image (**c**) both basal ganglia iron deposit and choroid plexus calcifications are hypointense (black arrows), whereas on phase image (**f**) the diamagnetic calcifications become predominatly hyperintense (white arrows)

Fig. 1.7 Usefulness of bSSFP sequence. MRI post-contrast T1WI (**a**), bSSFP (**b–d**). The evaluation of the anatomical relationships between this huge meningioma of the clivus and the floor of the third ventricle is important to define the possibilities of a third ventriculostomy. With the bSSFP sequence the floor of the third ventricle is demonstrated with remarkable anatomical precision (arrows **b–d**)

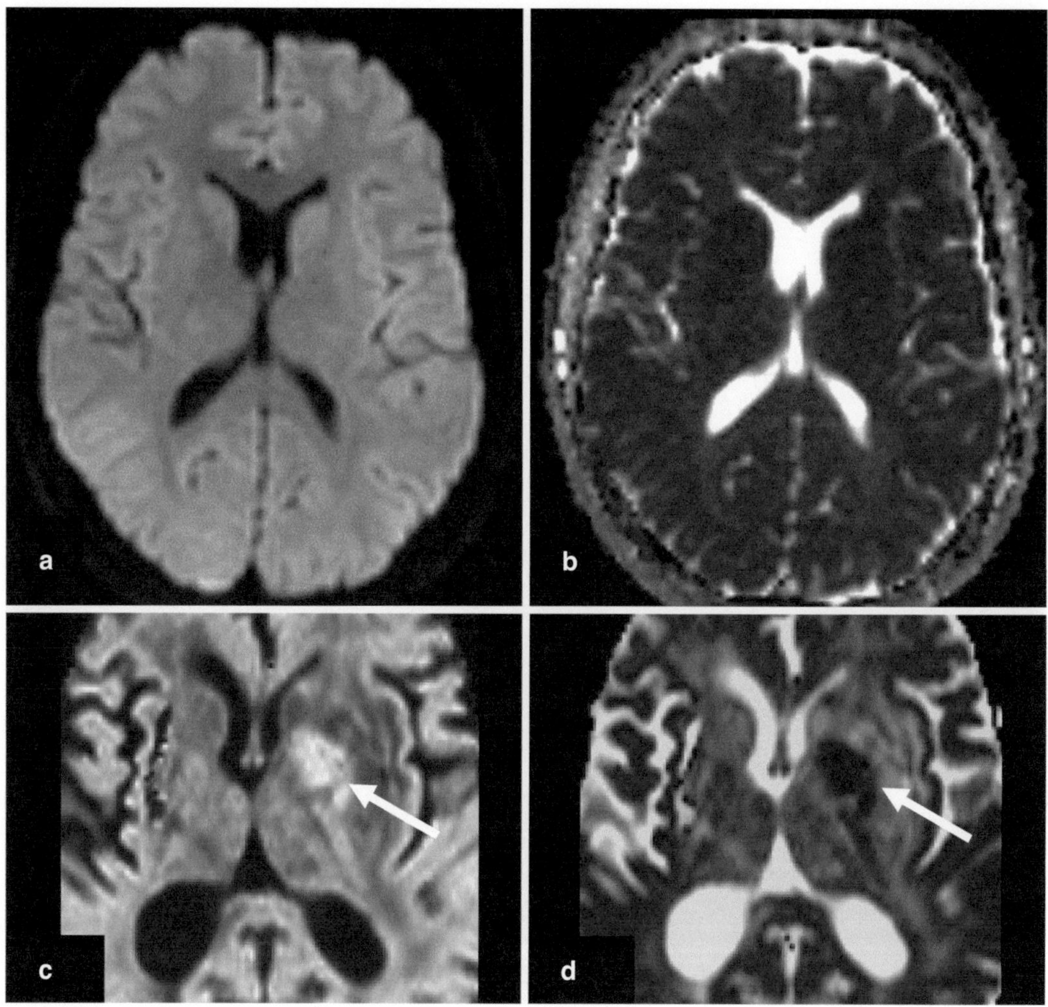

Fig. 1.8 DWI (**a**, **c**) and ADC (**b**, **d**) in a normal subject (**a**, **b**) and in a patient with primary lymphoma (**c**, **d**). In the ADC image the signal intensity corresponds to the apparent diffusion coefficient so that the highest value is within the CSF. Consequently, a diffusion restriction corresponds to a low signal on the ADC image but on a high signal on DWI, such as in the lymphoma case (arrows **c**, **d**)

axon. The fractional anisotropy map is an image in which the signal intensity is directly proportional to the anisotropy within the voxel from 1 (maximum) to 0 (minimum). Lowest values are within CSF and gray matter and highest values are within white matter. To this map a color map in red, green, and blue (RGB) can be superimposed giving direct visual information on the direction of the fibers. Red from right to left (or vice versa), green from anterior to posterior, and blue from cranial to caudal (Fig. 1.10).

Finally, a DTI data can be used to perform tractography within white matter. A particular algorithm can be used to track a fiber along its whole length reproducing a particular fiber pathway.

DWI and ADC are now widely used in the MRI assessment of brain tumors. They provide essential information on the cellularity of the tumor and consequently on its aggressiveness. Even though a linear relationship between tumor malignancy and ADC restriction cannot be

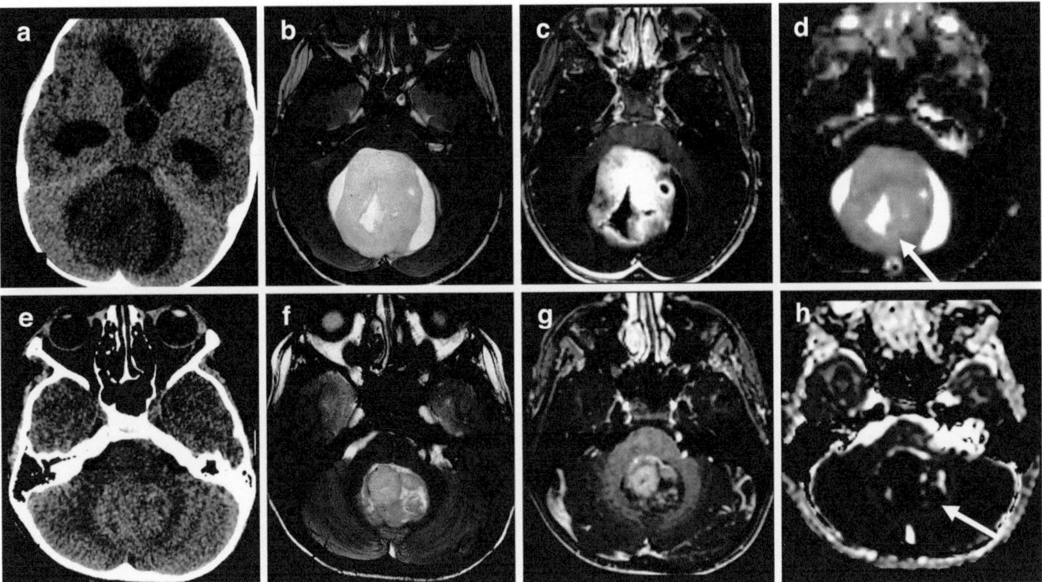

Fig. 1.9 In the upper row a pilocytic atrocytoma: CT (**a**), T2WI (**b**), post-contrast T1WI (**c**), and ADC (**d**). In the lower row a medulloblastoma: CT (**e**), T2WI (**f**), post-contrast (**g**) and ADC (**h**). The location of the tumor is similar but the increased cellularity of the medulloblas-toma results in a diffusion restriction (arrow **h**), whereas the diffusion is increased in the pilocytic astrocytoma (arrow **d**). The increased cellularity of the medulloblas-toma causes a light hyperdensity on the CT as well

drawn, a general relationship between cellularity and malignancy can be driven (Fig. 1.9).

Less immediate and practically used the DTI techniques offer some insight on the relationship between tumor and normal brain parenchyma, with DTI it is possible to determine if a tumor causes a destruction/interruption of a white matter pathway instead of a dislocation.

These aspects are particularly useful in the presurgical assessment of the lesion, it is of great help for the surgeon to understand the presence of dislocation of a crucial white matter pathway such as the cortico-spinal tract or the uncinate fasciculus before to operate on [15, 16].

1.4.4 MRI Perfusion and Permeability Techniques

Perfusion techniques are becoming widely available even in a clinical setting in the last 10 years and they largely contribute to a better evaluation and diagnosis of brain tumors.

There are many perfusion techniques available, namely dynamic susceptibility contrast (DSC) technique, dynamic contrast-enhanced (DCE) image, and arterial spin labeling (ASL) technique, the first two need the injection of a GBCA, whereas the latter does not [17].

- **DSC.** After the injection of a GBCA multiple very rapid T2 weighted sequences were repeated in order to evaluate the temporal modification of susceptibility on T2 relaxation time caused by the first pass of GBCA. Due to its paramagnetic properties gadolinium creates a local magnetic field distortion around vessels with T2 dephasing and shortening. Imaging acquisition time is around 2 min.
- **DCE.** After the injection of GBCA multiple T1-weighted images were rapidly repeated to evaluate the shortening of T1 relaxation time caused by GBCA over an approximately 5–10 min time interval.
- **ASL.** In this sequence the blood spins were labeled before entering the brain and after a

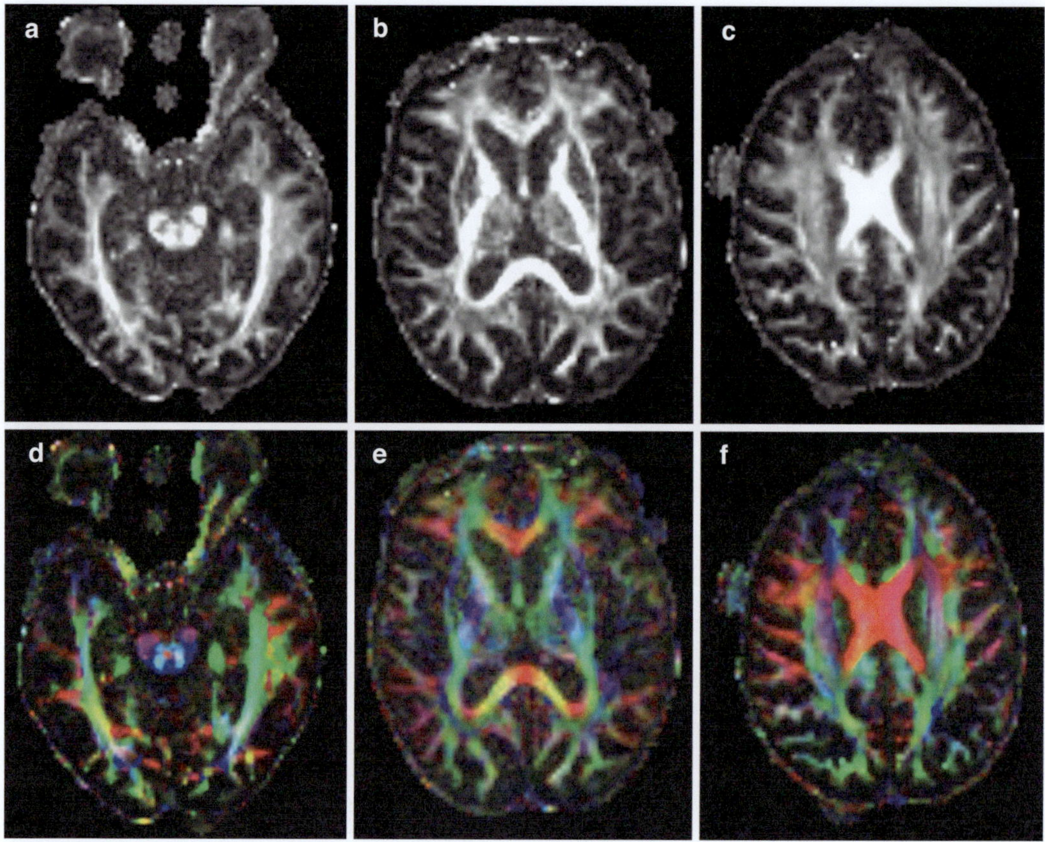

Fig. 1.10 Diffusion tensor imaging, upper row (**a–c**): fractional anisotropy (FA) images, lower row (**d–f**): correspondent RGB images. In the FA images the signal intensity value is directly proportional to the fractional anisotropy. In RGB images the color indicates the fibers direction: red, right to left; green, anterior to posterior; blue cranial to caudal

delay time they are acquired during their pass through the brain according to the different perfusion. Images are acquired both with and without labeling pulse and then subtracted. The signal-to-noise ratio is extremely low and multiple signal averages have to be acquired for a total acquisition time of approximately 3–5 min. Due to the low signal-to-noise ratio ASL performs better at 3.0T than at 1.5T.

DSC can provide information on cerebral blood flow (CBF), cerebral blood volume (CBV), mean transit time (MTT), and time to peak (TTP), whereas DCE can offer information on permeability too through some parameters such as the K-trans. ASL maps CBF but cannot measure relative CBV.

In a general view DSC is considered more straightforward in CBV measurement, whereas ASL is more straightforward in CBF measurement and DCE is useful in determining tumor permeability and overcoming the susceptibility artifacts affecting DSC that can be present in different anatomical conditions (tumors near bone structures, calcifications, metallic implants, etc.).

Malignancy is associated with an increase in neovascularization within the tumor. As a general rule, the higher the aggressiveness of the tumor, the greater the vascularization, consequently leading to increased Cerebral Blood Flow (CBF) and Cerebral Blood Volume (CBV), as depicted in Fig. 1.11. Moreover, CBF can also prove valuable in distinguishing tumor progression from radionecrosis. Radionecrosis typically exhibits normal or decreased perfusion, whereas CBF is expected to increase with tumor progression, as illustrated in Fig. 1.12.

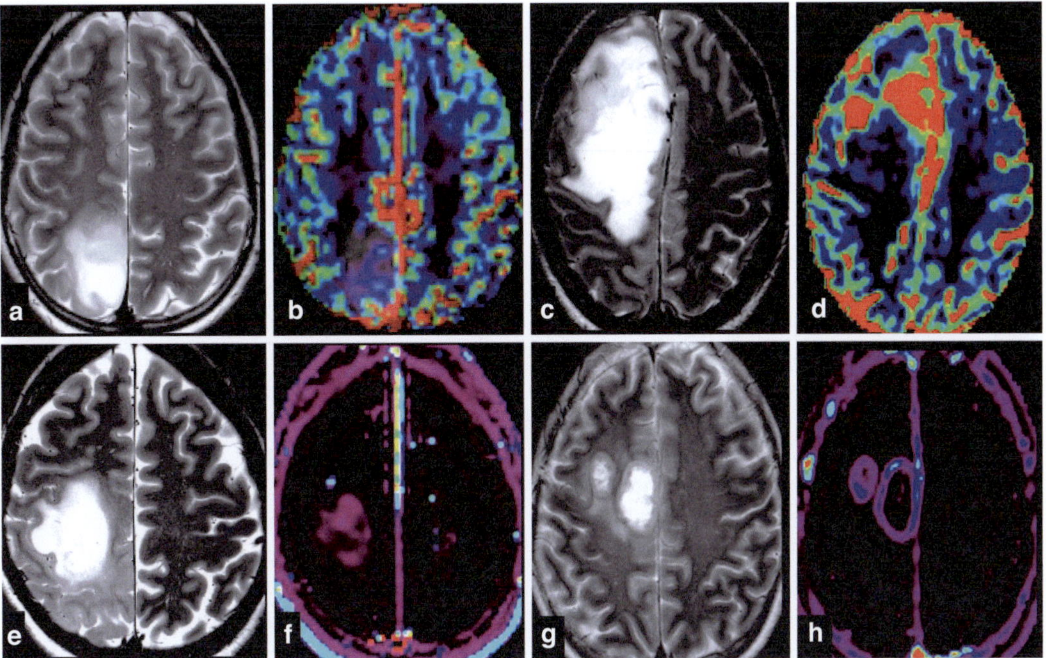

Fig. 1.11 Increased tumor vascularization with grading in different astrocytomas. Astrocytoma grade 2 MRI T2WI (**a**), CBV (**b**). Astrocytoma grade 3 MRI T2WI (**c**), CBV (**d**). Astrocytoma grade 3 MRI T2WI (**e**), k-trans (**f**). Astrocytoma grade 4 MRI T2WI (**g**), k-trans (**h**). Both blood volume and permeability are clearly increased in grade 3 and 4 astrocytomas in comparison with grade 2 astrocytoma where CBV is slightly reduced

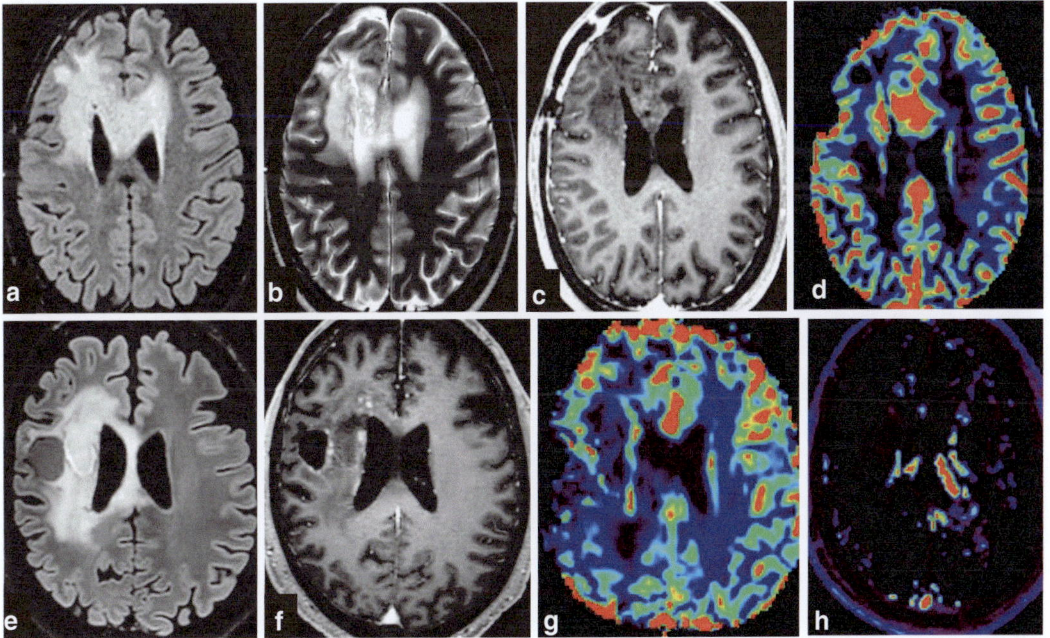

Fig. 1.12 Upper row astrocytoma grade 3 recurrence after radio-chemotherapy. MRI FLAIR (**a**), T2WI (**b**), post-contrast T1WI (**c**), CBV (**d**). Lower row radionecrosis after radiotherapy in a glioblastoma. MRI FLAIR (**e**), post-contrast T1WI (**f**), CBV (**g**), k-trans (**h**). Radionecrosis does not show any significant increase in perfusion or permeability

1.4.5 MR Amide Proton Transfer (APT) Imaging

Like magnetization transfer imaging, unfortunately not clearly useful in the diagnosis of brain tumors, amide proton transfer (APT) imaging is part of a class of imaging methods called chemical exchange saturation techniques (CEST).

In MRI at least two types of water molecules, free (bulk) and bound (hydration), are present, in CEST the signal of the bulk water is observed to decrease when the hydration population is saturated. General magnetization transfer effects are however broad and nonspecific, but it is possible to selectively stimulate a group of mobile proteins and peptides known as amides. APT effect (suppression) is calculated using subtraction pixel-by-pixel with a mask and the resulting values typically range between 0 and 5% and can be displayed as color maps overlaid conventional images [18].

Higher-grade gliomas are characterized by more actively proliferating tumor cells, and the concentrations of mobile macromolecules (such as proteins and peptides) increase with the tumor cell density and glioma grades, consequently ATP values would be different in high-grade versus low-grade gliomas. Differently from high-grade tumors, radionecrosis should be not associated with an APT increase, allowing after treatment a potential differential diagnosis between tumor progression vs. the effects of tumor chemo-radiotherapy (Fig. 1.13) [19].

1.4.6 Magnetic Resonance Spectroscopy

In vivo magnetic resonance spectroscopy (MRS) of the brain has developed rapidly since its first observation in the 1980s and proton spectroscopy (^{1}H MRS) became more prevalent in the 1990s because of its higher sensitivity and greater convenience.

In ^{1}H magnetic resonance spectroscopy each proton can be visualized at a specific chemical

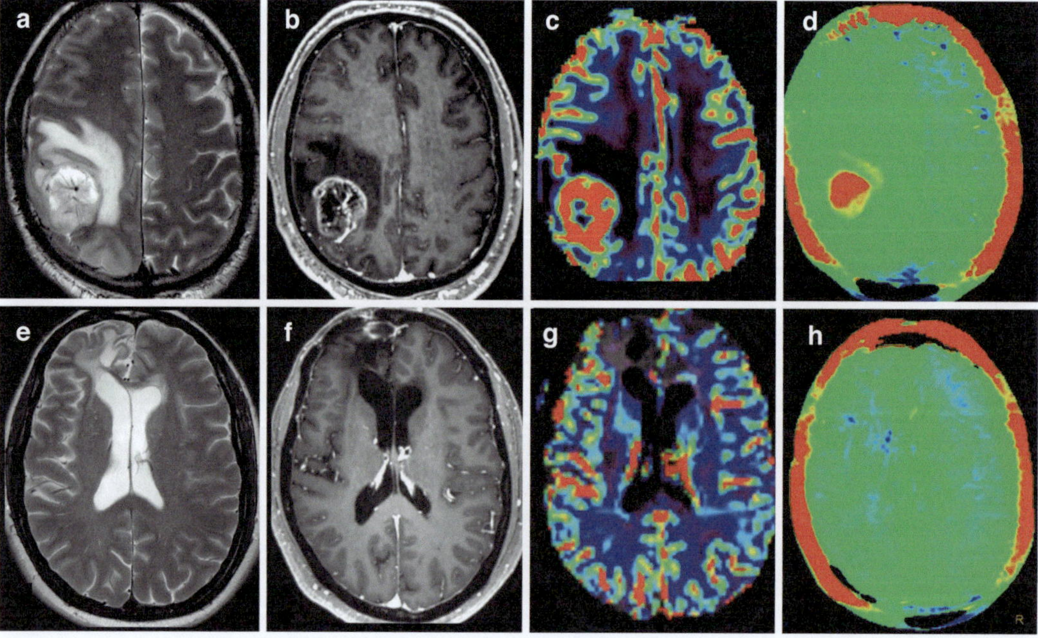

Fig. 1.13 Upper row: APT in a glioblastoma. MRI T2WI (**a**), post-contrast T1WI (**b**), CBV (**c**), APT (**d**). In the area of the neoplasm there is a great increase in APT. Lower row APT in the post-therapy assessment of a glioblas-toma. MRI T2WI (**e**), post-contrast T1WI (**f**), CBV (**g**), APT (**h**). After surgery and radio-chemotherapy a subtle area of enhancement is still visible in the area of intervention, but CBV is decreased and APT is normal

shift (peak position along *X*-axis) depending on its chemical environment. This chemical shift is dictated by neighboring protons within the molecule. Therefore, metabolites can be characterized by their unique set of ^{1}H chemical shifts [20]. The main metabolites observable in vivo and which may undergo modifications in the presence of brain tumors are the following:

1. N-acetyl-aspartate (NAA): with its major resonance peak at 2.02 ppm, decrease in levels of NAA indicates loss or damage to neuronal tissue, which results from many types of insults to the brain. Its presence in normal conditions indicates neuronal and axonal integrity.
2. Choline (Cho): with its major peak at 3.2 ppm, choline is known to be associated with membrane turnover, or increase in cell division. Increased choline indicates increase in cell production or membrane breakdown, which can suggest demyelination or presence of malignant tumors.
3. Creatine (Cr): with its major peak at 3.0 ppm, creatine marks metabolism of brain energy. Gradual loss of creatine in conjunction with other major metabolites indicates tissue death or major cell death resulting from disease, injury, or lack of blood supply. Increase in creatine concentration could be a response to cranial cerebral trauma. Absence of creatine may be indicative of a rare congenital disease.
4. Lipids (Lip): with their major aliphatic peaks located in the 0.9–1.5 ppm range, increase in lipids is seen which is also indicative of necrosis. These spectra are easily contaminated, as lipids are not only present in the brain, but also in other biological tissue such as the fat in the scalp and area between the scalp and skull.
5. Lactate (Lac): it results in a doublet (two symmetric peaks) centered about 1.31 ppm. In healthy subjects lactate is not visible, for its concentration is lower than the detection limit of MRS; however, it becomes evident in different types of aggressive tumors, in particular in the presence of necrosis. In the short TE spectrum, it can be confounded with lipid peak whereas in intermediate TE spectrum the doublet peak is reverse and can be easily detected.
6. Myoinositol (mI): with its major peak at 3.56 ppm, an increase in myoinositol has been seen in patients with pilocytic astrocytoma and a decrease of mI/Cr ratio has been reported with the increase in tumor grading [21].

In the diagnosis of brain tumors, single volume techniques are mainly used, which allow for a greater signal with both short and intermediate echo acquisitions (Fig. 1.14). However, spectroscopic imaging techniques with several small volumes that form a coarse section in the area affected by the tumor can be used. In this case, long-echo acquisition techniques are used to maximize the signal-to-noise ratio, but only the three main peaks can be analyzed.

In the presence of brain tumor, the major change in the spectrum is the increase in the Cho/NAA ratio which is roughly proportional to tumor grading. In the presence of aggressive tumors with necrosis, a lactate or lipid peak may appear (Fig. 1.15). In general we can say that the specificity of MRS remains low, but it represents an important element in the overall diagnostic evaluation of a brain tumor [22].

1.4.7 MR Functional Technique in the Presurgical Assessment

Although fMRI has not been shown to be of clinical utility in diagnosing brain tumors it is currently one of the most commonly used non-invasive neuroimaging modalities for surgical planning and has proven effective in guiding epilepsy and tumor surgery.

The most common approach in the presurgical assessment of brain tumors is task-based fMRI, which involves asking the patient to perform a specific task (such as moving a limb or speaking) while being scanned. The resulting fMRI data can then be analyzed to identify the regions of the brain that are activated during the task and to determine how close these regions are to the tumor.

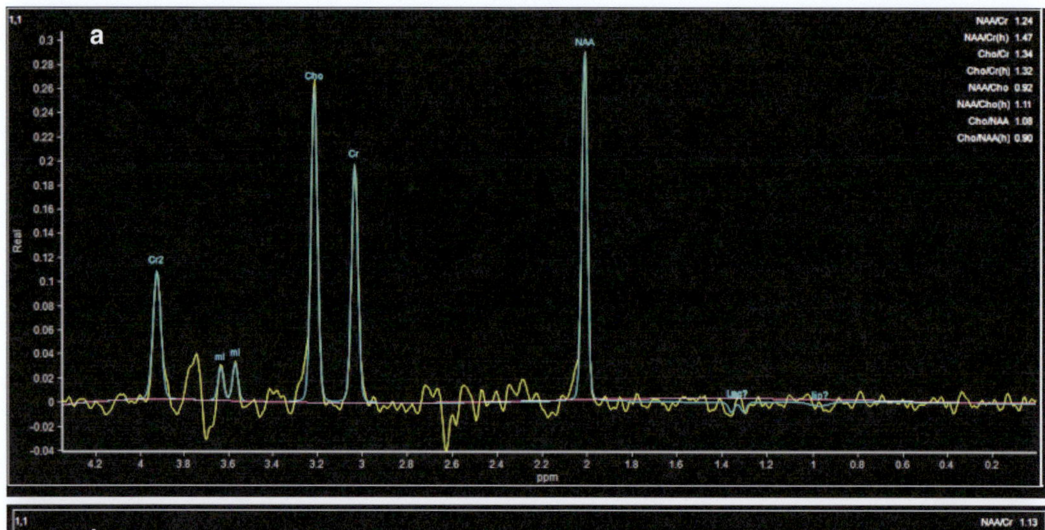

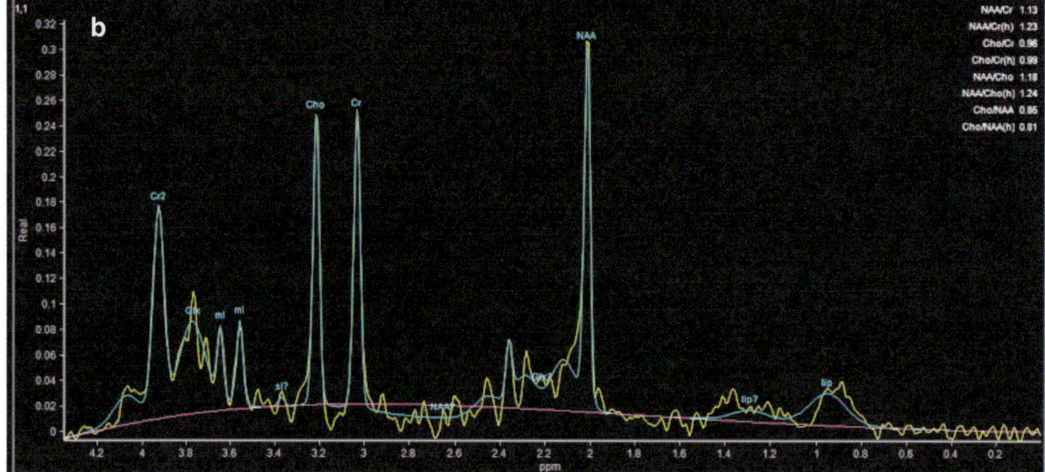

Fig. 1.14 Brain MR spectra obtained with single volume technique with intermediate TE (**a**) and short TE (**b**). With short TE technique a greater number of peaks, such as myo-inosytol can be clearly visible

Another fMRI technique that is used in the presurgical assessment of brain tumors is resting-state fMRI. This technique involves measuring the spontaneous fluctuations in blood flow that occur when the patient is at rest. By analyzing these fluctuations, clinicians can identify patterns of functional connectivity between different regions of the brain. This information can be used to identify regions that are functionally connected to the tumor and to assess the potential impact of removing the tumor on the brain's overall functional connectivity.

Despite its many benefits, there are also some limitations to the use of fMRI in the presurgical assessment of brain tumors. For example, fMRI data can be affected by artifacts such as motion, which can make it difficult to accurately localize functional regions of the brain. In addition, fMRI

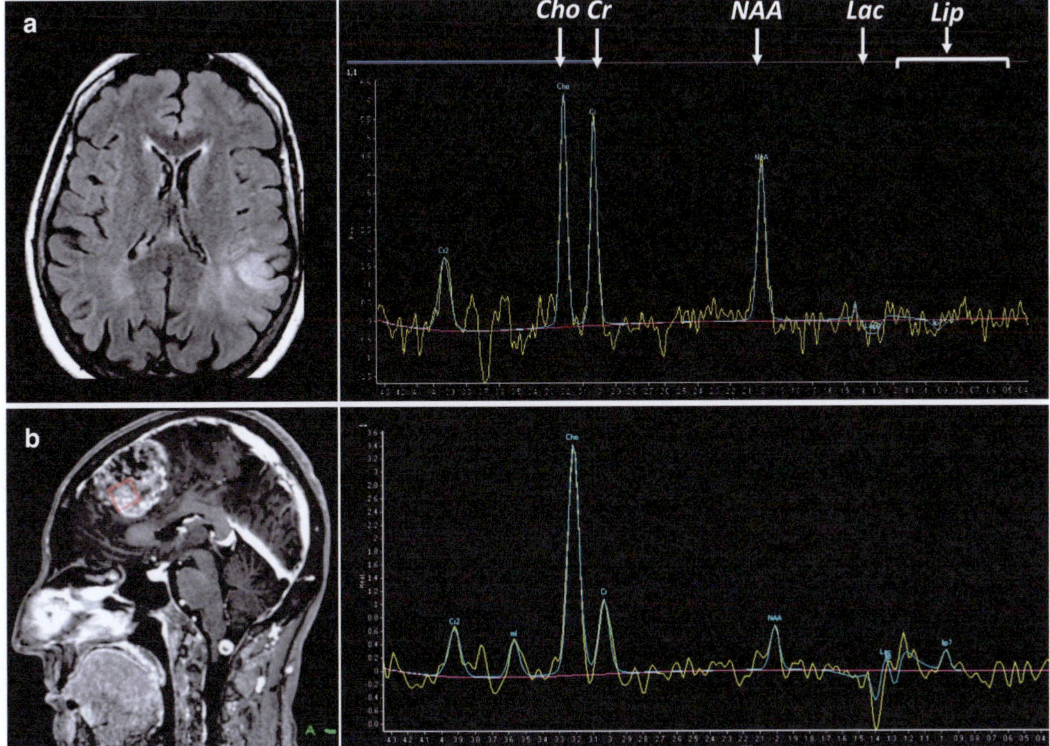

Fig. 1.15 MR spectroscopy. As a general rule in a brain tumor a decrease in NAA peak and an increase in Cho peak is visible, resulting in a progressive increase of Cho/NAA ratio. This increase is usually proportional to the tumor malignancy. In **a** an example of a diffuse infiltrating glioma, in **b** an example of glioblastoma. It is evident in the latter case a dramatic reduction of NAA and also the presence of a small peak of lactate and also of lipids that usually are encountered in presence of tumor necrosis

may not be able to reliably detect functional changes in areas of the brain that have been affected by the tumor, which can complicate surgical planning [23].

1.4.8 How a Brain Tumor Should Be Studied on MRI

A comprehensive study of a brain tumor should encompass the three "conventional" sequences T1WI, T2WI and FLAIR, along with SWI, the diffusion sequence DWI/ADC, a DSC perfusion sequence and in case of particular tumor location, huge calcifications or hemorrhages a DCE perfusion sequence should also be considered. Alternatively ASL acquisition can serve as a substitute of DSC. Additionally, it is advisable to perform single voxel spectroscopy with both short and intermediate echoes. Post-contrast study should be conducted in all cases.

Supplementary sequences could be APT, spectroscopy imaging (or chemical shift imaging), or bSSFP in case of need of very high resolution in some particular conditions.

In any case, before looking at the images, it would be necessary to know at least the age and sex of the patient and before thinking about any diagnosis, keep in mind Tables 1.1 and 1.2 on the frequency of brain tumors considering that the most frequent tumor in adults is also the one that assumes the shapes and the most diverse image characteristics.

1.5 Neuroradiology Features: General Principles

1.5.1 Mass Effect

The presence of mass effect is one of the key features in the neuroradiological diagnosis of a brain tumor.

We can generally divide brain neoplasms according to their mass effect into neoplasm with evident if not dramatic mass effect and in neoplasm with subtle or absent mass effect. The vast majority of brain tumor however causes some degree of mass effect and this may be carefully scrutinized in CT and MR images.

In Fig. 1.16 eight different cases of clear mass effect due to a brain tumor are shown.

Mass effect can be visualized as a deformation of ventricular contour or by a progressive effacement of sulci, when it becomes more clear a shift across midline of the affected side could be appreciable.

However in small neoplasms or in infiltrative gliomas mass effect can be scarcely appreciable as in the cases of Fig. 1.17.

In the cases of Fig. 1.17 the lack of mass effect making the diagnosis of brain tumor is more difficult.

1.5.2 Edema

Together with mass effect the presence of vasogenic edema is suggestive of a brain tumor; however, independently from the size of the tumor the amount of brain edema could be extremely variable. Metastases even small present typically with a conspicuous brain edema (Fig. 1.18), but many aggressive tumors can show extensive vasogenic edema as well.

As shown in Table 1.5 vasogenic edema appears as hyperintense on T2WI and FLAIR sequence, hypointense on T1WI and with an increase in diffusion coefficient. If at least part of the tumor

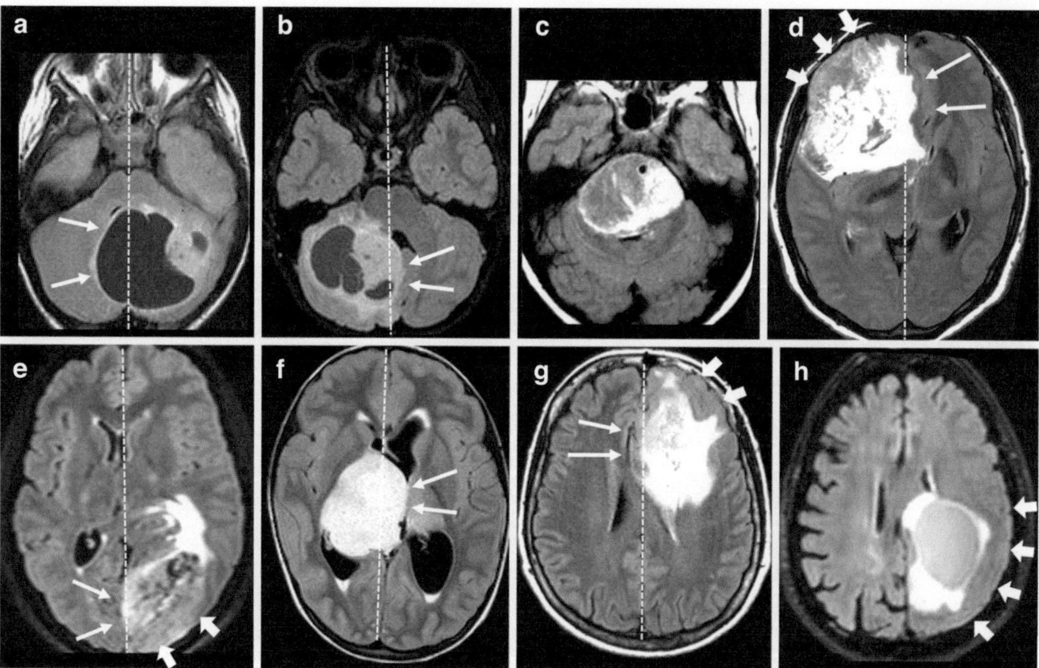

Fig. 1.16 Mass effect. Eight different cases of brain tumors (**a**, **b** pilocytic astrocytoma, **c** diffuse intrinsic pontine glioma, **d** oligodendroglioma, **e**, **g**, **h** glioblastoma, and **f** diffuse thalamic glioma) show different degrees of mass effect (all cases axial FLAIR sequence). In many cases a midline shift of the affected side is appreciable (arrows in **a**, **b**, **d**, **e**, **f**, **g**, dotted line—midline) as well as a mass effect on ventricles (all cases). Effacement of the sulci near the lesion is another typical consequence of mass effect of a brain tumor (small thick arrows **d**, **e**, **g**, **h**)

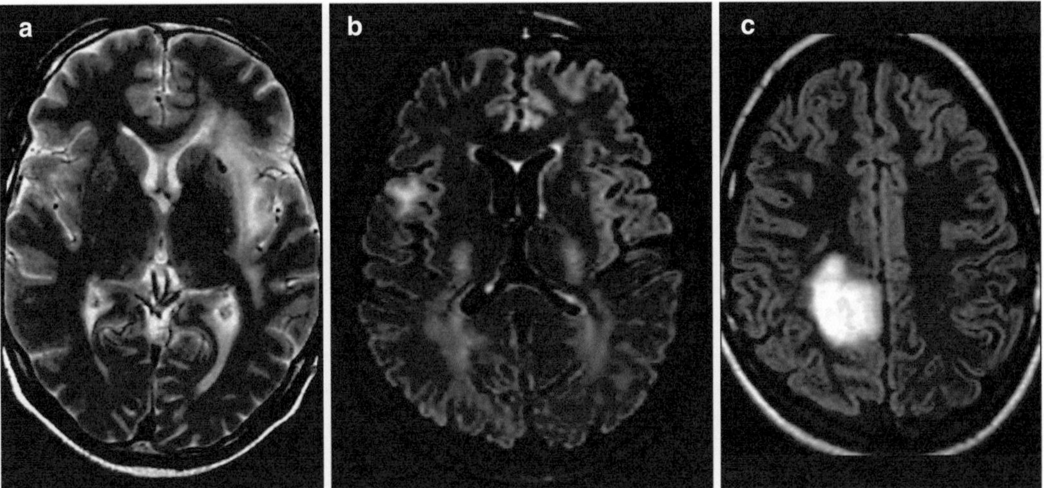

Fig. 1.17 Mass effect. In all these cases mass effect is less evident than in Fig. 1.15. In case **a** the infiltrative glioma does not cause a significative sulci effacement (T2WI). In case **b** the small size of the tumor does not cause any evident mass effect and even in case **c**, where the size of the infiltrative glioma is greater, the mass effect seems to be still trascurable (both cases FLAIR sequences)

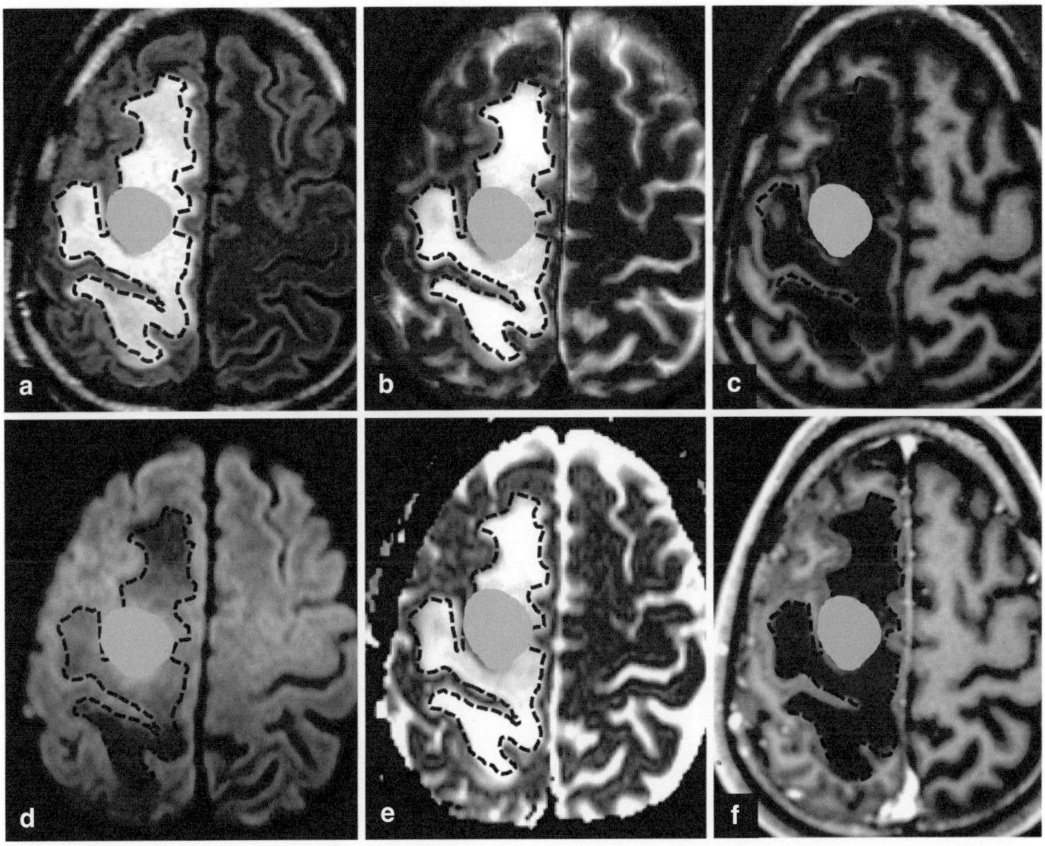

Fig. 1.18 Edema. In brain metastases vasogenic edema is frequently much more larger than the metastases itself. In this case the solid lesion is uniformly covered by a gray layer and the surrounding edema is lined by a dotted line. MRI FLAIR (**a**), T2WI (**b**), T1WI (**c**), DWI (**d**), ADC (**e**), post-contrast T1W1 (**f**)

enhances after contrast a more easy differentiation between tumor and edema can be possible.

Less aggressive tumor such as pilocytic astrocytomas or neuronal tumors, typically exhibit reduced perilesional edema. Nevertheless, it is essential to consider that there are numerous-exceptions to this general rule as demonstrated in Fig. 1.19 particularly concerning medulloblastomas.

Sometimes differentiating edema from tumor itself can be difficult if not impossible. It is especially true in case of low-grade infiltrating tumor which is virtually impossible to delineate a border between tumor, normal parenchyma, and edema (Fig. 1.20).

Table 1.5 Vasogenic edema

T1WI	T2WI	FLAIR	DWI	ADC
Hypo +	*Hyper +*	*Hyper ++*	*Hypo +*	*Hyper +*

1.5.3 Internal Structure

In the differential diagnosis of a tumor and in tumor grading the definition of the internal structure of a tumor is another important step to achieve a correct diagnosis.

First of all we can differentiate *homogeneous* from *inhomogeneous* tumor.

Homogeneous tumor means a tumor with a single solid component that is usually, but not necessarily, enhanced. Examples of potentially homogeneous tumor are primary lymphoma of the CNS (Fig. 1.21), germinoma and diffuse infiltrating glioma in the group of intra-axial tumor. Meningioma can be considered a relatively homogeneous tumor in the group of extra-axial intracranial tumor, even though sometimes it can be extremely heterogeneous.

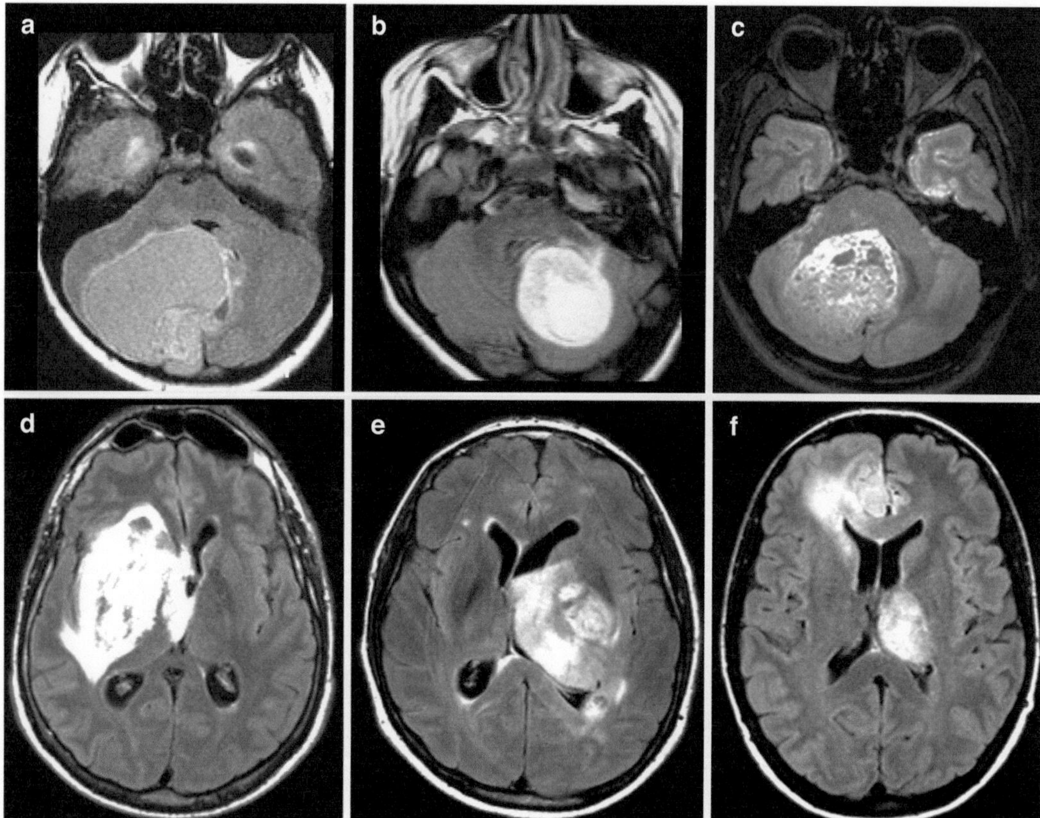

Fig. 1.19 Edema. MRI FLAIR (**a–f**). The three cases of the upper row exhibit few or no edema, case **a** and **b** are pilocytic pstrocytomas, case **c** a medulloblastoma (Shh subtype). The three cases of the lower row exhibit all some degrees of perilesional edema; however, it is difficult if not impossible to discriminate on FLAIR sequence edema from tumor itself. Case **d** oligodendroglioma, case **e** anaplastic astrocytoma, case **f** glioblastoma

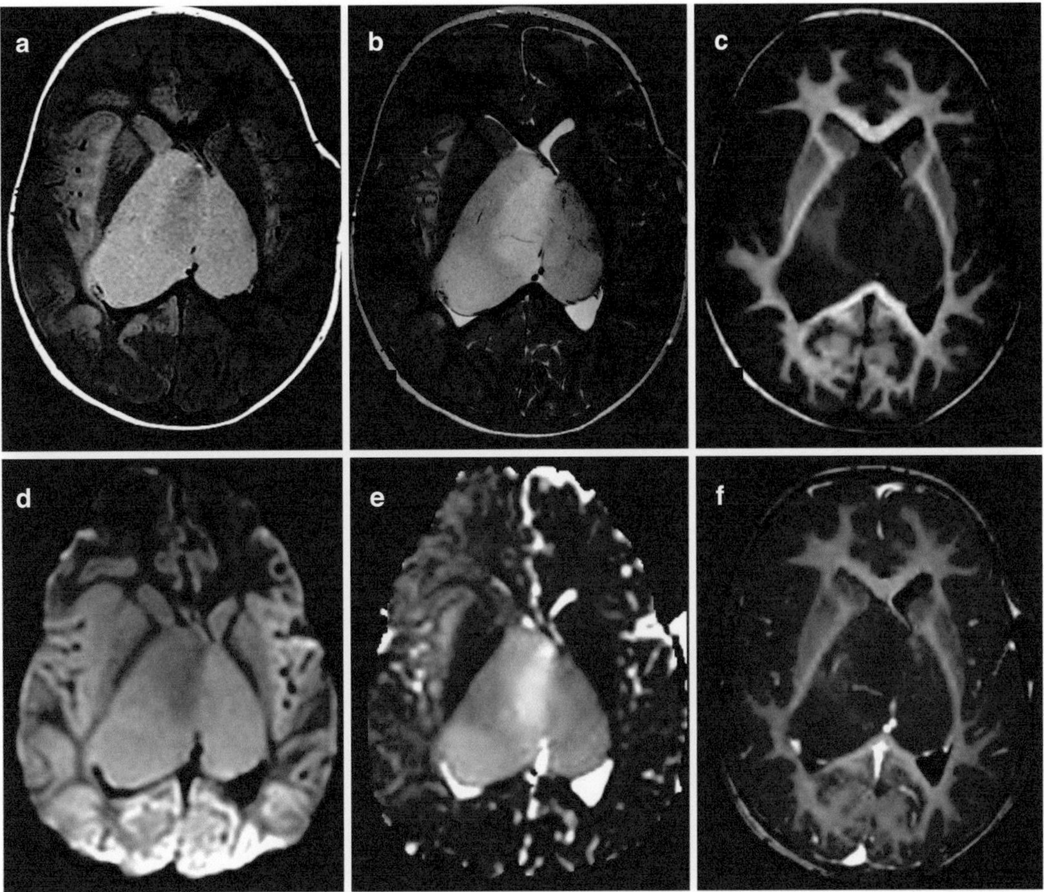

Fig. 1.20 Edema. Midline bithalamic infiltrating glioma. In this case of infiltrating tumor it is not possible to differentiate tumor from edema and normal parenchyma. MRI FLAIR (**a**), T2WI (**b**), T1WI (**c**), DWI (**d**), ADC (**e**), post-contrast T1WI (**f**)

However the majority of the tumor of the CNS are inhomogenous and together with a solid component that can enhance or not after contrast, other components are usually present such as cysts, calcifications, necrosis, hemorrages (Figs. 1.22 and 1.23).

The homogeneity of the internal structure is not necessarily related to the aggressivity of the tumor. For instance the group of homogeneous tumor comprises together with grade II infiltrating gliomas, with a very slow rate of growth, even germinomas that grow very rapidly.

Similarly, within the inhomogeneous group, there are both typically benign tumors like Pilocytic Astrocitoma and more aggressive ones like Glioblastoma.

Through the analysis of different MRI sequences it is possible to achieve a tentative tissue characterization. The tumor behavior on MRI sequences can be summarized as in the follow Table 1.6.

In Figs. 1.24 and 1.25 and in the scheme of Fig. 1.26 are summarized the typical signal intensity patterns of benign and aggressive tumors.

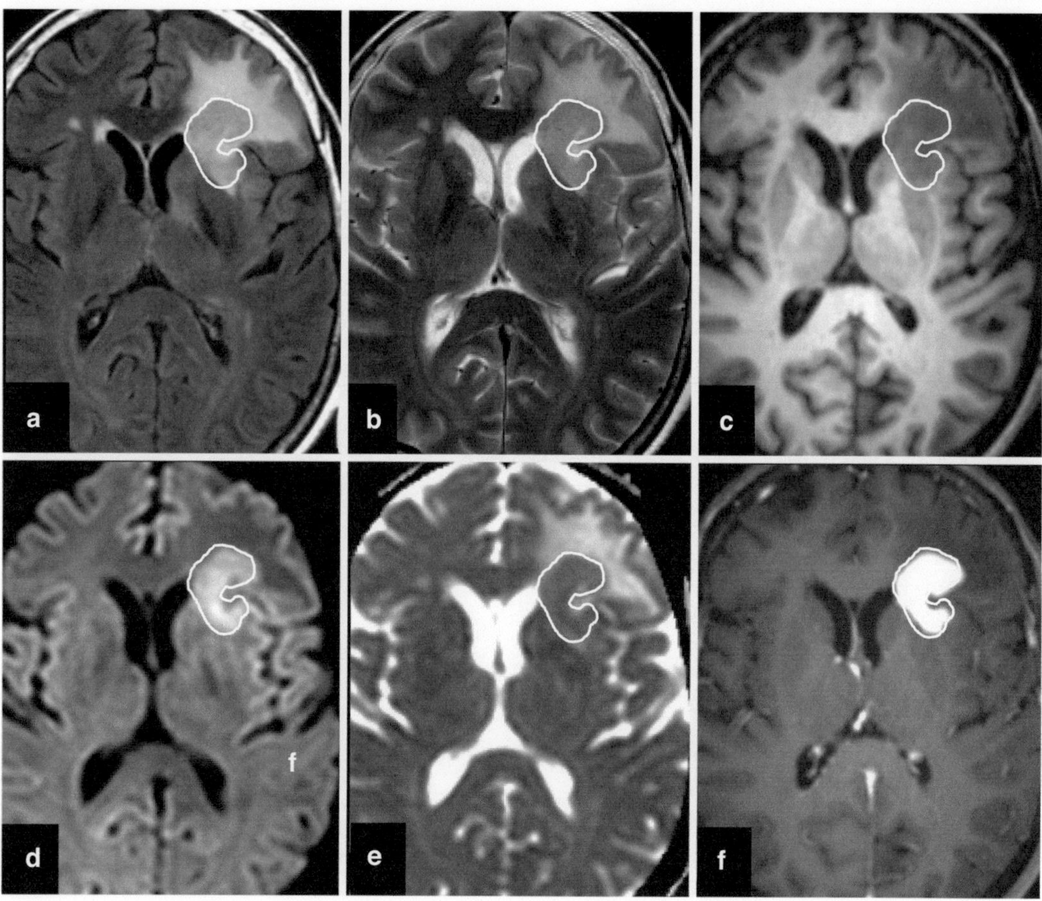

Fig. 1.21 Homogeneous brain tumor, primary CNS lymphoma. The lesion (continuous line) is relatively homogeneous and well differentiable from surrounding vasogenic edema. MRI FLAIR (**a**), T2WI (**b**), T1WI (**c**), DWI (**d**), ADC (**e**), post-contrast T1W1 (**f**)

1.5.4 Location

Brain tumor can grow everywhere within the central nervous system, but any tumor shows, at least in part, some preferential location. For instance pilocytic astrocytoma, even can be theoretically found everywhere, is more typically located in the cerebellar hemispheres or in hypothalamic region. Glioblastoma is almost exclusively supratentorial. Lymphomas are tipically found in proximity to ventricles, and, of course ependymomas are located within or near ventricles as well. In some casse such as for subependymal giant cell astrocytoma or colloid cyst the location itself can be so characteristic that it guides the correct diagnosis.

But apart from the location as a guide for a correct diagnosis location is mostly important for the *prognosis.*

As a general rule for the CNS neoplasm the prognosis is made not only by the aggressiveness of the neoplasm, but in large part by its location. It is a matter of fact that the most benign of tumors in an unresectable area is no longer benign.

In Fig. 1.27 the unresectable areas are schematized. In the posterior fossa a surgical approach

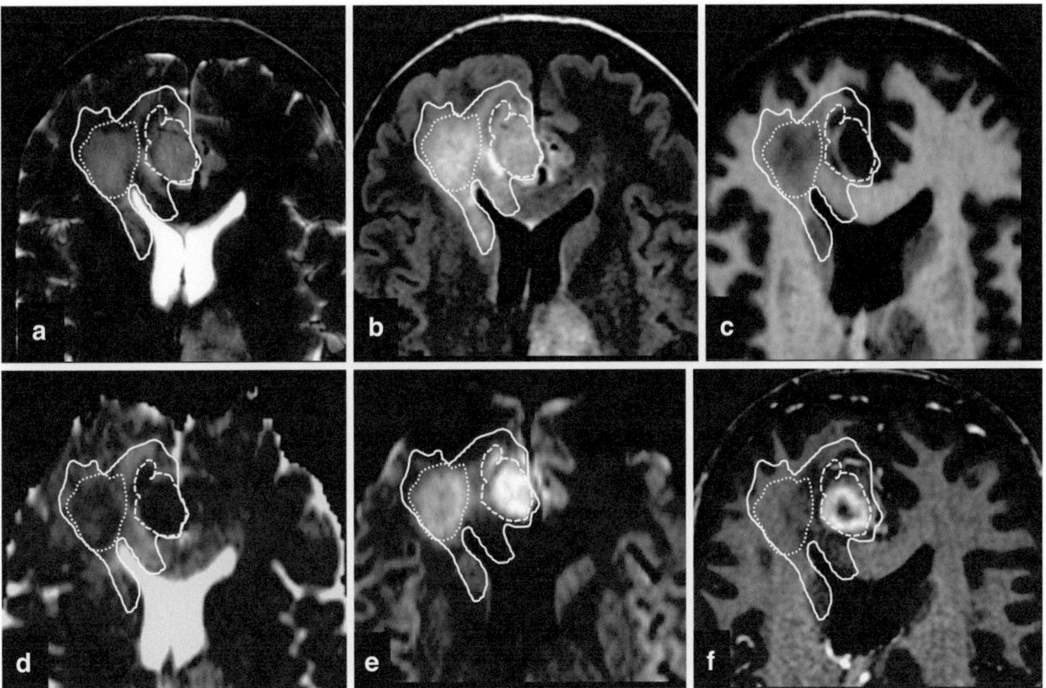

Fig. 1.22 Inhomogeneous brain tumor. Glioblastoma involving right frontal lobe and other structures. T2WI (**a**), FLAIR (**b**), T1WI (**c**), ADC (**d**), DWI (**e**), post-contrast T1WI (**f**). A more aggressive component is delimited by a dotted line, another less aggressive component is identified by a tiny dotted line, the solid line delimited the presumed border of the tumor

to the brainstem is critical in most cases. In the supratentorial compartment a surgical treatment cannot be practicable, or it is critical as well, for the basal ganglia, primary sensorimotor cortex and pyramidal tract, Broca's and Wernicke's area and possibly the arcuate fascicle, the optic radiation and calcarine cortex.

1.5.5 Enhancement

The post-contrast enhancement is another of the most important features in the diagnosis of a brain tumor. In modern diagnostic neuroradiology the injection of contrast media can be used even routinely to obtain data on perfusion and also permeability, but the evidence of post-contrast enhancement still remains one of the pillars for a correct diagnosis (Fig. 1.28).

As a general rule the presence of contrast enhancement is related to a greater aggressiveness of the lesion being expression to a blood–brain barrier (BBB) rupture or malfuncion, but a strong enhancement can be seen also in the mural nodule of the most frequent WHO grade 1 neoplasm, the pilocytic astrocytoma, or in other grade 1 tumors as shown in Fig. 1.5. Conversely it is a well-established fact that certain aggressive tumors, such as WHO grade 3 or even 4 gliomas, may exhibit an increase in cerebral blood flow and permeability without enhancement do not enhance.

1.5.6 General Features and Prognosis

As a general rule brain tumors displaying pronounced mass effect, vasogenic edema, enhancement on MR/CT, along with internally inhomogeneous structure, and located in eloquent areas are inherently associated with a severe prognosis. Conversely brain tumors with

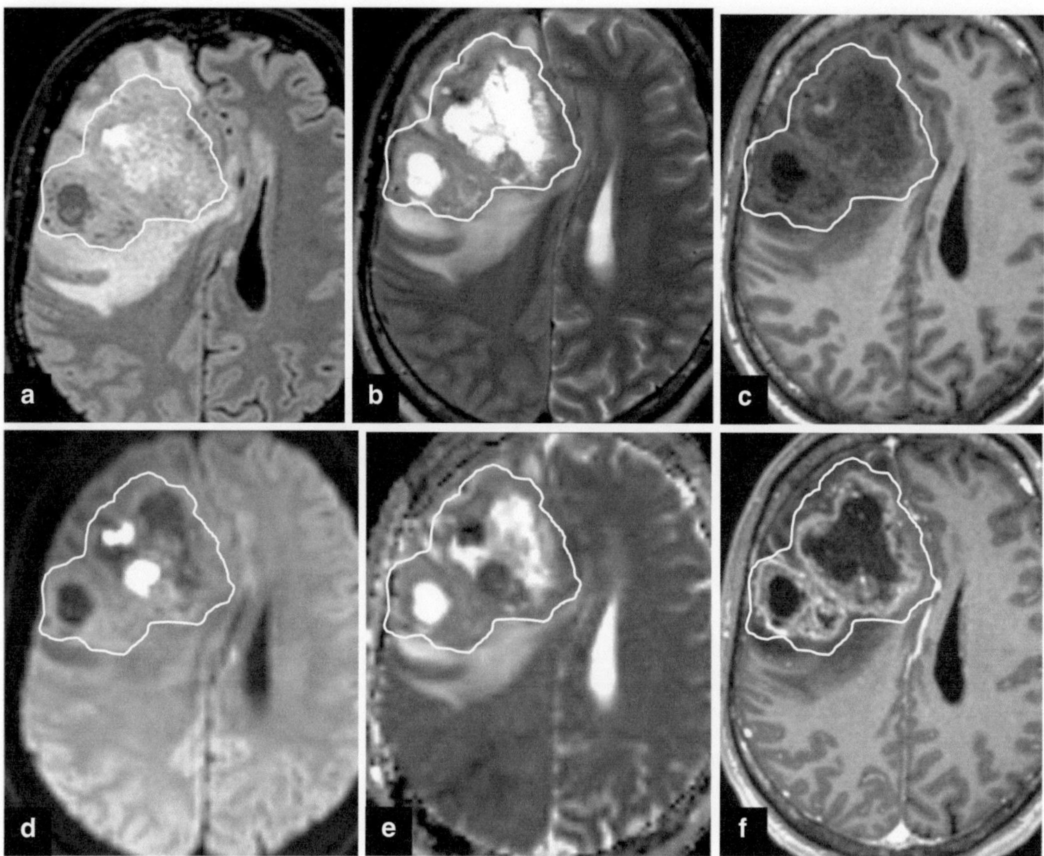

Fig. 1.23 Inhomogeneous brain tumor, glioblastoma. The lesion is extremely inhomogeneous with different components: cysts, necrosis, hemorrhage, irregular enhancement. Vasogenic edema is not completely separable from the lesion (solid line). MRI FLAIR (a), T2WI (b), T1WI (c), DWI (d), ADC (e), post-contrast T1W1 (f)

Table 1.6 A possible MRI characterization of brain tumors

	Benign	Aggressive
CT	Iso/hypo	Hypo/hyper/mix
T1	Iso/hypo	Hypo/mix
T2	Hyper	Hypo/mix
FLAIR	Hyper	Hyper/mix
DWI	Normal/hypo	Hyper/mix
ADC	Hyper	Hypo/mix
Spectroscopy	Slight increase Cho/NAA[a]	Marked increase Cho/NAA + Lac
T1 + Gd	No CE[b]	CE irregular
Perfusion	Normal/slight increase	Moderate/marked imcrease

[a]With the exception of pilocytic astrocytoma
[b]With the exception of grade 1 astrocytic tumor and some rare neuronal tumor

minimal or absent mass effect, edema and enhancement, along with relatively homogeneous internal structure in operable areas, may demonstrate a fovorable prognosis when completely removed. As previously showed many exceptions can be however found to this rule, but nonetheless neuroradiological general features remain an important key to diagnosis (Table 1.7).

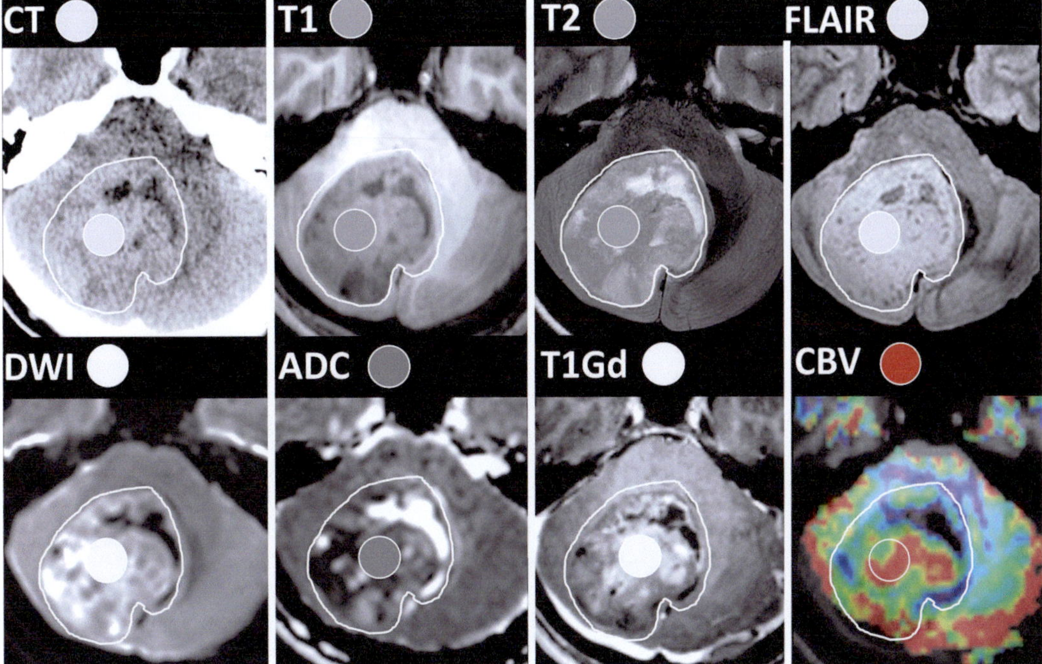

Fig. 1.24 Aggressive tumor pattern. As expression of a high cellularity an aggressive tumor can exhibit an iso-hyperdensity on CT, an iso-hypointensity on T1WI, an iso-hypointensity on T2WI, a mixed signal predominantly hyperintense on FLAIR, a diffusion restriction with an increased signal on DWI and decreased on ADC, an irregular enhancement, and an increase of CBV

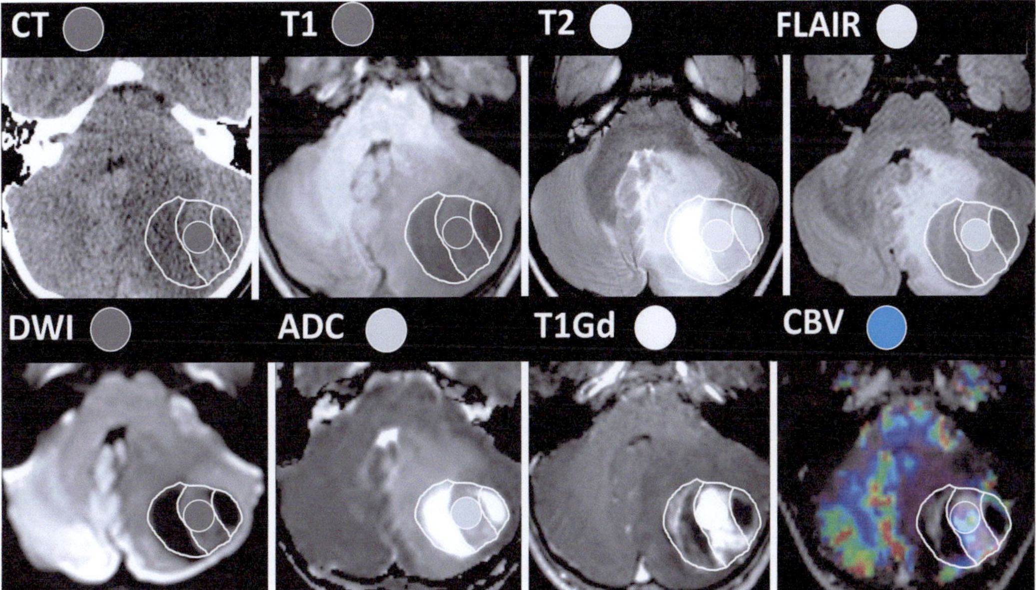

Fig. 1.25 Benign tumor pattern. The MRI typical pattern of a benign tumor such as the mural nodule of a pilocytic astrocytoma is characterized by a hypodensity on CT, a hypointensity on T1WI, a clear hyperintense pattern on T2WI, an intermediate signal on FLAIR, an increase on diffusion with low signal on DWI and high signal on T2WI. In the case of pilocytic astrocytoma enhancement is present with a normal or minimal increase of CBV

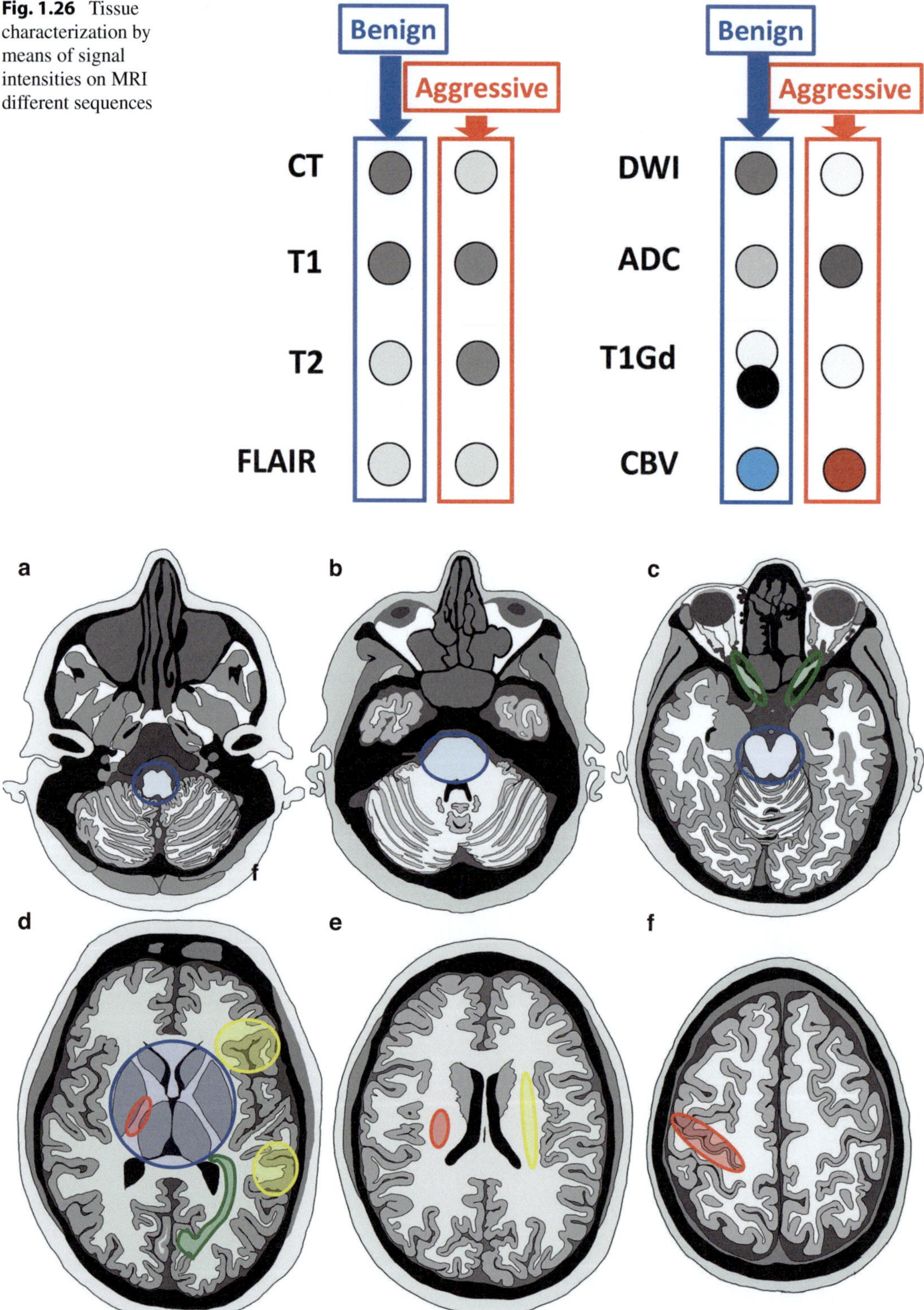

Fig. 1.26 Tissue characterization by means of signal intensities on MRI different sequences

Fig. 1.27 The critical areas for surgery. In blue basal ganglia (d) and brainstem (a-c), in yellow the region of Broca, Wernicke (d) and arcuate fasciculus (f), in green the optic pathways (c). The areas of language are localized in the left hemisphere in 97% of people

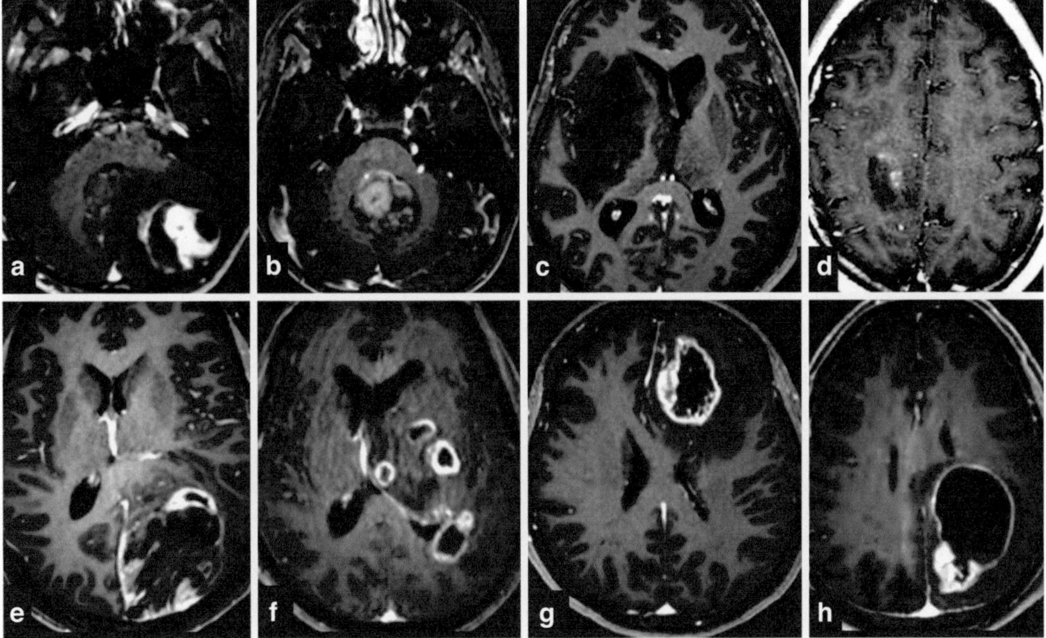

Fig. 1.28 Tumor enhancement. Pylocytic atrocytomas show a marked enhancement of the mural nodule and sometimes of the cyst (**a**), aggressive medulloblastoma shows usually ony a mild enhancement (**b**) WHO grade 3 astrocytomas may exhibit some minimal or scarce enhancement (**c**, **d**), glioblastoma presents an irregular enhancement as one of its more typical feature (**e–h**)

Table 1.7 Neuroradiological general features of brain tumor and prognosis

Mass effect	Marked	Slight/absent
Edema	Marked	Slight/absent
Internal structure	Inhomogeneous	Homogeneous
Location	Inoperable	Operable
Enhancement	Marked/irregular	Slight/absent
PROGNOSIS	(frequently) NEGATIVE	(possibly) POSITIVE

References

1. Ostrom QT, Gittleman H, Truitt G, Boscia A, Kruchko C, Barnholtz-Sloan JS. CBTRUS statistical report: primary brain and other central nervous system tumors diagnosed in the United States in 2011–2015. Neurooncology. 2018;20(S4):1–8.
2. Alentorn A, Hoang-Xuan K, Mikkelsen T. Presenting signs and symptoms in brain tumors. In: Berger MS, Weller M, editors. Handbook of clinical neurology. 3rd series, vol. 134. Amsterdam: Elsevier; 2016. p. 19–26.
3. WHO. Histological typing of tumours of the central nervous system, vol. 21. Geneva: World Health Organization; 1979.
4. WHO. Histological typing of tumours of the central nervous system. Berlin: Springer-Verlag; 1993.
5. WHO. World Health Organization Classification of tumours of the nervous system. Lyon: WHO/IARC; 2000.
6. WHO. World Health Organization histological classification of tumours of the central nervous system. 4th ed. Lyon: International Agency for Research on Cancer; 2007.
7. WHO. World Health Organization classification of tumours of the central nervous system. 4th, updated ed. Lyon: International Agency for Research on Cancer; 2016.
8. Louis DN, Perry A, Reifenberger G, et al. The 2016 World Health Organization classification of tumors of the central nervous system: a summary. Acta Neuropathol. 2016;131(6):803–20.
9. Louis DN, Perry A, Wesseling P, et al. The 2021 WHO classification of tumors of the central nervous system: a summary. Neuro Oncol. 2021;23(8):1231–51.
10. WHO. WHO Classification of Tumours Editorial Board. World Health Organization Classification of Tumours of the Central Nervous System. 5th ed. Lyon: International Agency for Research on Cancer; 2021.

11. Gasparotti R, Pinelli L, Liserre R. New MR sequences in daily practice: susceptibility weighted imaging. A pictorial essay. Insights Imaging. 2011;2:335–47.

12. Cavallaro M, Coglitore A, Tessiore A, et al. Three-dimensional constructive interference in steady state (3D CISS) imaging and clinical applications in brain pathology. Biomedicine. 2022;10:2997.

13. Scheffler K, Lehnardt S. Principles and applications of balanced SSFP techniques. Eur Radiol. 2003;13:2409–18.

14. Drake-Perez M, Boto J, Fitsiori A, Lovblad K, Vargas MI. Clinical applications of diffusion weighted imaging in neuroradiology. Insights Imaging. 2018;9:535–47.

15. Potgieser ARE, Wagemakers M, van Hutzen ALJ, de Jong BM, Hoving EW, Groen RJM. The role of diffusion tensor imaging in brain tumor surgery: a review of the literature. Clin Neurol Neurosurg. 2014;124:51–8.

16. Xiao X, Kong L, Pan C, et al. The role of diffusion tensor imaging and tractography in the surgical management of brainstem gliomas. Neurosurg Focus. 2021;50:E10.

17. Kelker K, Boxweman J, Kalnin A, Shiroishi M, Wintermak M. ASFNR recommendations for clinical performance of MR dynamic susceptibility contrast perfusion imaging of the brain. AJNR Am J Neuroradiol. 2015;36:E41–51.

18. Zhou J, Lal B, Wilson DA, Laterra J, van Zijl PCM. Amide proton transfer (APT) contrast for imaging of brain tumors. Magn Reson Med. 2003;50:1120–6.

19. Friismose AI, Markovic L, Nghuyen N, Gerke O, Schulz MK, Mussmann BR. Amide proton transfer-weighted MRI in the clinical setting—correlation with dynamic susceptibility contrast perfusion in the post-treatment imaging of adult glioma patients at 3T. Radiography. 2022;28:95–101.

20. Zhu H, Barker PB. MR spectroscopy and spectroscopic imaging of the brain. Methods Mol Biol. 2011;711:203–26.

21. Castillo M, Smith JK, Kwock L. Correlation of Myo-inositol labels and grading of cerebral astrocytomas. AJNR Am J Neuroradiol. 2000;21:1645–9.

22. Hollingworth W, Medina LS, Lenkinski RE, et al. A systematic literature review of magnetic resonance spectroscopy for the characterization of brain tumor. AJNR Am J Neuroradiol. 2006;27:1404–11.

23. Silva MA, See AP, Essayed WI, Golby AJ, Tie Y. Challenges and techniques for presurgical brain mapping with functional MRI. Neuroimage Clin. 2018;17:795–803.

Gliomas, Glioneuronal Tumors, and Neuronal Tumors: Adult-Type Diffuse Glioma

2.1 Adult-Type Diffuse Gliomas

2.1.1 Astrocytoma, IDH-Mutant

WHO definition. A diffusely infiltrating IDH1- or IDH2-mutant glioma with frequent *ATRX* and/or *TP53* mutation and absence of 1p/19q codeletion. CNS WHO grade 2, 3, or 4.

This is an astrocytoma with a moderate pleomorphic cell with a high degree of cellular differentiation and slow growth; however, it has the potential to progress in grade 3 and grade 4 astrocytoma.

Epidemiology. Atrocytoma IDH-mutant grade 2 affects the younger population in comparison with glioblastoma (GBM) and astrocytoma grade 3 and 4 with a median age between 30 and 40 years. The incidence rate of grade 2 is 0.75 cases for 100,000 population for year, doubling the incidence rate of astrocytoma grade 3, but consistently lower than GBM.

Location. It can occur everywhere within the CNS; however, this tumor is more frequently found supratentorially and in the frontal lobes.

Clinical features. Can be diagnosed incidentally due to the slow growth and paucity of symptoms, when symptoms and signs occur they are mainly related to epileptic seizure or to some subtle sensory-motor deficits with insidious onset sometimes, considering the main age of patients, confounded with the onset of a demyelinating disease.

Prognosis. For grade 2 a median survival of more than 10 years was reported with a progressive shortening for grade 3 and 4.

2.1.1.1 Astrocytoma IDH-Mutant, Grade 2 *(Diffuse Astrocytoma WHO 2016)*

WHO definition. A diffusely infiltrative astrocytic glioma with an IDH1 or IDH2 mutation that is well differentiated and lacks histological features of anaplasia.

Mitotic activity is not detected or is very low.

Microvascular proliferation, necrosis, and homozygous deletions of CDKN2A or CDKN2B are absent.

Imaging. The typical appearance of astrocytoma IDH-mutant grade 2 is an infiltrative lesion with no clearly defined margins with a slight to more evident hyperintensity aspect on T2WI, a slight to more clear hypointensity on T1WI, and a variable aspect on FLAIR image from diffuse hyperintensity such as for T2WI to a more heterogeneous aspect with diffuse areas of iso- to hypointensity.

T2-FLAIR mismatch sign. The different signal behaviors between T2 and FLAIR in low-grade astrocytoma were observed for the first time in 2017 by Patel et al. [1]. This sign was described as follows: a complete or near-complete homogenous high signal on T2WI and central hypointense signal and peripheral high intensity rim on FLAIR images. Additional features better char-

Table 2.1 T2-FLAIR mismatch sign in low-grade IDH-mutant noncodeleted astrocytomas

Original signs
(a) Complete or near-complete homogeneous high signal on T2WI
(b) Central hypointense signal and peripheral high intensity rim on FLAIR
Additional signs
(a) No enhancement
(b) Nonperipheral edema
(c) No cystic/necrotic regions
(d) FLAIR hypointense can be inhomogeneous within the tumor

acterizing this sign were successively reported: no contrast enhancement or evident surrounding edema should be present, the FLAIR hypointense region should not represent cystic/necrotic regions, FLAIR hypointense aspect can be inhomogeneous within the tumor (Table 2.1) [2].

Up to date two different metanalysis studies [3, 4] have already addressed the sensitivity and the specificity of this sign. Both studies showed a very high specificity (95–100%) but a low sensitivity (40–45%).

In other words, the presence of the MRI features reported in Table 2.1 are extremely confident to make a diagnosis of a low-grade IDH-mutant noncodeleted astrocytoma, but some debate is present on the reproducibility of this sign [2] and it should be evaluated with caution. For instance, the relative "hypointensity" on FLAIR with respect to T2WI could simply depend on the window used to evaluate the images and it is quite difficult to standardize. Furthermore, these data are generically reported encompassing both grade 2 and 3 among low-grade gliomas. Consequently this sign should only serve to distinguish these astrocytomas only from GBM, not between grade 2 and grade 3.

From a pathological point of view accordingly to Deguchi et al. [5], T2-FLAIR mismatch sign may reflect microcyst formation in IDH-mutant astrocytomas and be common in IDH-mutant protoplasmic astrocytoma. According to the WHO 2021 the macroscopic appearance of a low-grade IDH-mutant astrocytoma is the fol-

lowing "…they enlarge and distort invaded anatomical structures and may show large or small cysts. Extensive microcystic formation occasionally produces a gelatinous appearance…." Hence the typical microcystic appearance of IDH-mutant noncodeleted astrocytoma and consequently the increased amount of water should be the histological basis of the T2-FLAIR mismatch. This could explain the other typical MR features of this type of gliomas with a relative hypointensity on T1WI and an increase in ADC.

Figure 2.1 shows astrocytoma IDH-mutant grade 2 with a different signal intensity on T2 and FLAIR. It appears to meet all the criteria for the T2-FLAIR mismatch sign, even thiugh the hyperintense rim on FLAIR is not particularly pronounced. What is clear is the increase of water with T1WI hypointensity and ADC increase. The FLAIR is quite inhomogeneous probably due to the different sizes and concentrations of microcysts.

Another case of possible T2-mismatch is reported in Fig. 2.2. In this case a central area of FLAIR hypointensity corresponding to T1WI hypointensity and ADC increase is well evident; however, the peripheral part of the tumor shows a normalization of ADC and the CBV seems similar at least to normal cortex. In this case proton spectroscopy is normal.

Other astrocytomas IDH-mutant grade 2 does not show the T2-FLAIR mismatch probably due to less content in microcysts. The case in Fig. 2.3 exhibits many features quite typical for the T2-FLAIR mismatch cases such as a diffuse homogeneous T2 hyperintensity, a diffuse homogeneous T1 hypointensity, and a homogeneous increase in ADC, all features quite typical for a water increase and a presumably microcystic content; however, the signal intensity on FLAIR still remains a little bit hyperintense with respect to brain parenchyma, even not so hyperintense like on T2WI. This case highlights the potential ambiguity in defining the T2-FLAIR mismatch sign. Nevertheless, histologically this case result to be very similar to the previous one of Figs. 2.1 and 2.2.

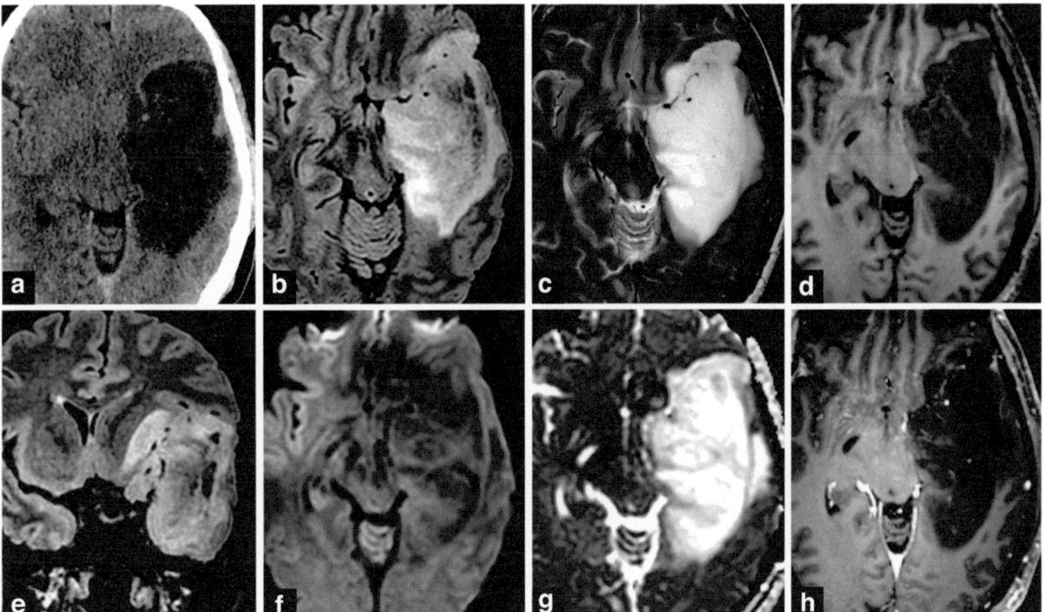

Fig. 2.1 Astrocytoma IDH-mutant, grade 2. Huge left fronto-temporo-insular tumor with T2-FLAIR mismatch. CT (**a**). MRI FLAIR (**b, e**), T2WI (**c**), T1WI (**d**), DWI (**f**) ADC (**g**), post-contrast T1WI (**h**). The signal intensity of the lesion is inhomogeneous on FLAIR. No contrast enhancement is evident

The case in Fig. 2.4 presents some aspects of the typical T2-FLAIR mismatch sign, but a small area of enhancement was visible after contrast. In case in Fig. 2.5 the tumor shows a moderate to slight hyperintensity on both T2 and FLAIR and a slight increase of ADC, CBV is reduced but there is an increase in Cho/NAA ratio. This case was operated and does not show any recurrence in the 4 years follow-up MR study.

Contrast enhancement. In the great majority of astrocytomas IDH-mutant grade 2 the lesion does not enhance after contrast administration. This sign has been considered an important caveat to differentiate the grade 2 gliomas from more aggressive gliomas. However it is now well known that some astrocytoma grade 2 can show post-contrast enhancement (Figs. 2.4 and 2.7) and on the contrary more aggressive gliomas or even GBMs cannot enhance contrast administration.

Diffusion. Diffusion is usually increased and more strikingly in case with T2-FLAIR mismatch. Areas of diffusion restriction are normally not detected in grade 2 astrocytoma and the pres-

ence of diffusion restriction is one of the major signs to differentiate a grade 2 from a higher grade.

Spectroscopy. Proton spectroscopy exhibits an increase of Cho/NAA but usually not so striking such as in grade 4 or in GBM. Different authors have claimed that some cut-off value of Cho/NAA ratio can be used to differentiate low-grade from high-grade gliomas, this can be true on a large scale but in a single case it is more important to consider all the different features of an MRI study than the single technique.

With specific acquisition technique and dedicated postprocessing [6, 7] it is however possible to determine the IDH status of patients with brain gliomas through the detection of the oncometabolite 2-hydroxyglutarate (2HG) (see Fig. 2.29).

Perfusion. CBV can be reduced or normal, rarely it increases and if so a higher grade should be suspected.

Calcification is rare and definitely more characteristic of oligodendrogliomas, but they are not impossible to find also in an astrocytoma (Fig. 2.6).

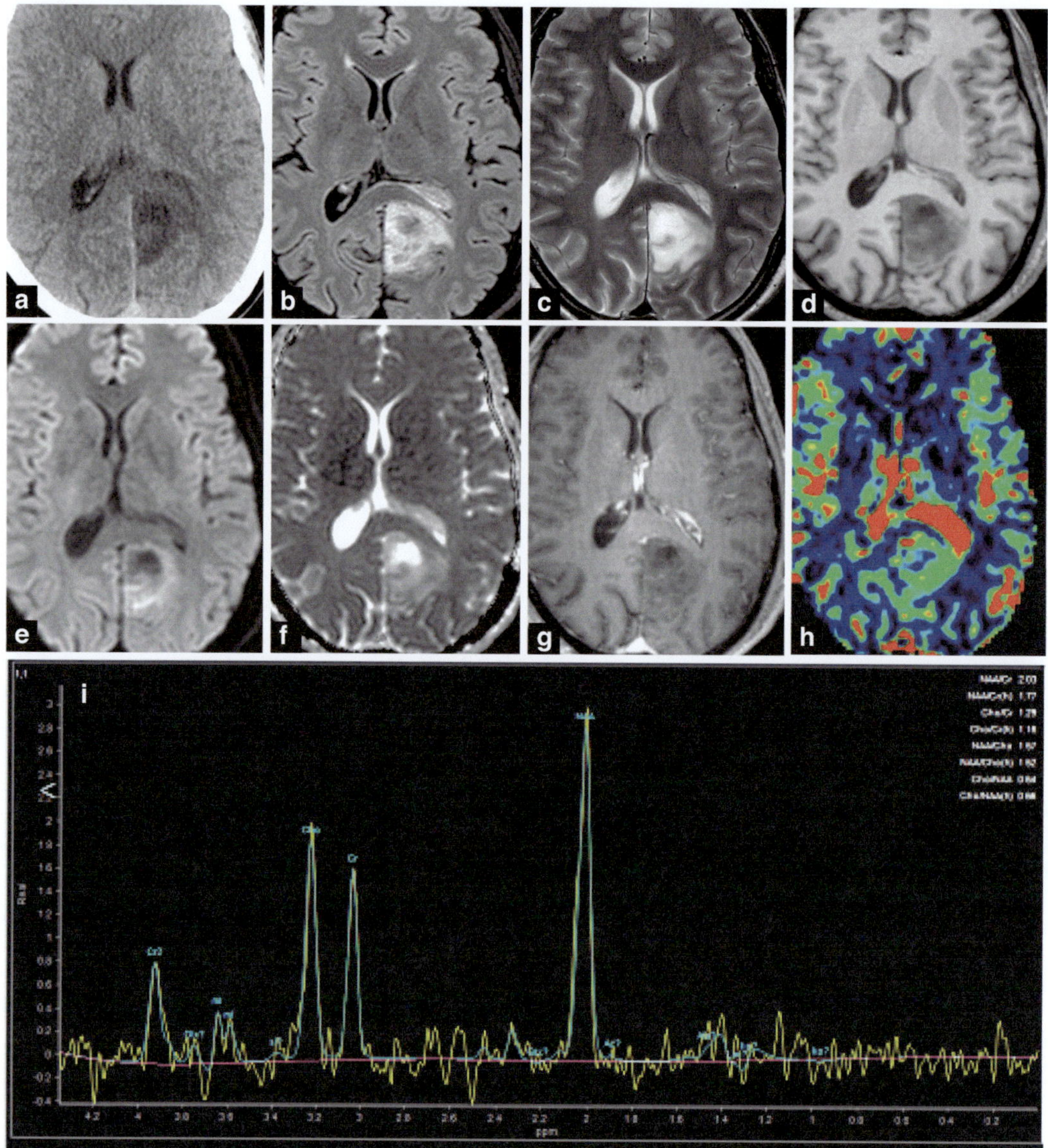

Fig. 2.2 Astrocytoma IDH-mutant, grade 2. Left parieto-occipital mesial tumor with T2-FLAIR difference in signal intensity. CT (**a**). MRI FLAIR (**b**), T2WI (**c**), T1WI (**d**), DWI (**e**) ADC (**f**), post-contrast T1WI (**g**), CBV (**h**), MR spectroscopy (**i**). The signal intensity of the lesion is inhomogeneous on FLAIR. Some inhomogeneities are visible on T2WI and DWI-ADC as well. No contrast enhancement is visible. The spectroscopy of the tumor does not differ from the normal parenchyma

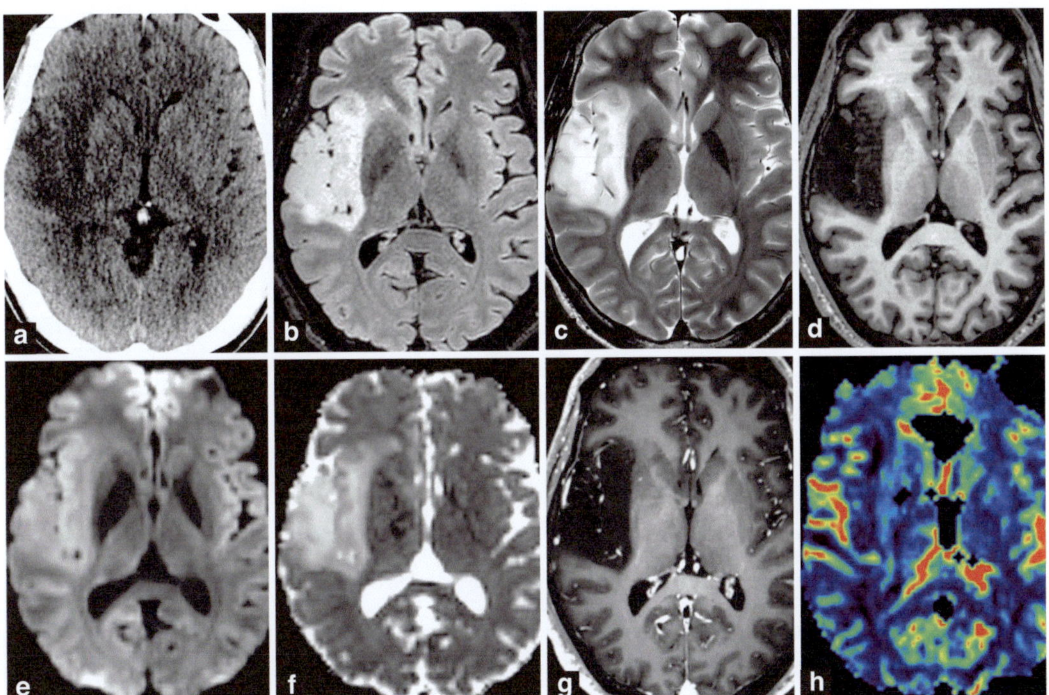

Fig. 2.3 Astrocytoma IDH-mutant, grade 2. CT (**a**). MRI T1WI (**b**), FLAIR (**c**), T2WI (**d**), DWI (**e**), ADC (**f**), post-contrast T1WI (**g**), CBV (**h**). A right temporo-insular lesion is visible with a clear hyperintensity on T2WI and hypointensity on T1WI. FLAIR still exhibits a slight hyperintense signal and CBV is normal. No contrast enhancement is visible

Gemistocytic differentiation is the second most common histological feature of an astrocytoma. According to WHO 2022 *"..it can be found focally, regionally or nearly uniformly in all grade of IDH-mutant astrocytoma, but this pattern is not specific to IDH-mutant gliomas and can be found also in IDH-wildtype gliomas…they are characterized by plump, glassy, eosinophilic cell bodies and stout, randomly oriented processes that form a coarse fibrillary network."*

This histological variant does not show any definite association with a determinate clinical behavior. On neuroimaging many different patterns are described but no one is specific. The case in Fig. 2.6 seems a typical astrocytoma IDH-mutant grade 2 and the only oddity is the presence of a calcification that however is not typical for the gemistocytic variant.

The case in Fig. 2.7 is more peculiar. It is a huge lesion with a slight hyperintense signal on both T2 and FLAIR and diffuse hypointense sig-

nal on T1WI. ADC is almost normal and CBV is quite similar to normal gray matter. After contrast administration an irregular and diffuse enhancement is visible. In Table 2.2 are summarized the imaging features of the Astrocytoma IDH-mutant grade 2.

2.1.1.2 Astrocytoma IDH-Mutant, Grade 3 *(Anaplastic Astrocytoma WHO 2016)*

WHO definition. A diffusely infiltrative astrocytic glioma with an IDH1 or IDH2 mutation that exhibits focal or dispersed anaplasia and displays significant mitotic activity.

Microvascular poliferation, necrosis, and homozygous deletions of CDKN2A or CDKN2B are absent.

Imaging. As a general rule astrocytoma IDH-mutant, grade 3 shows less heterogeneous aspects than GBM but more heterogeneous features than the typical astrocytoma IDH-mutant grade 2.

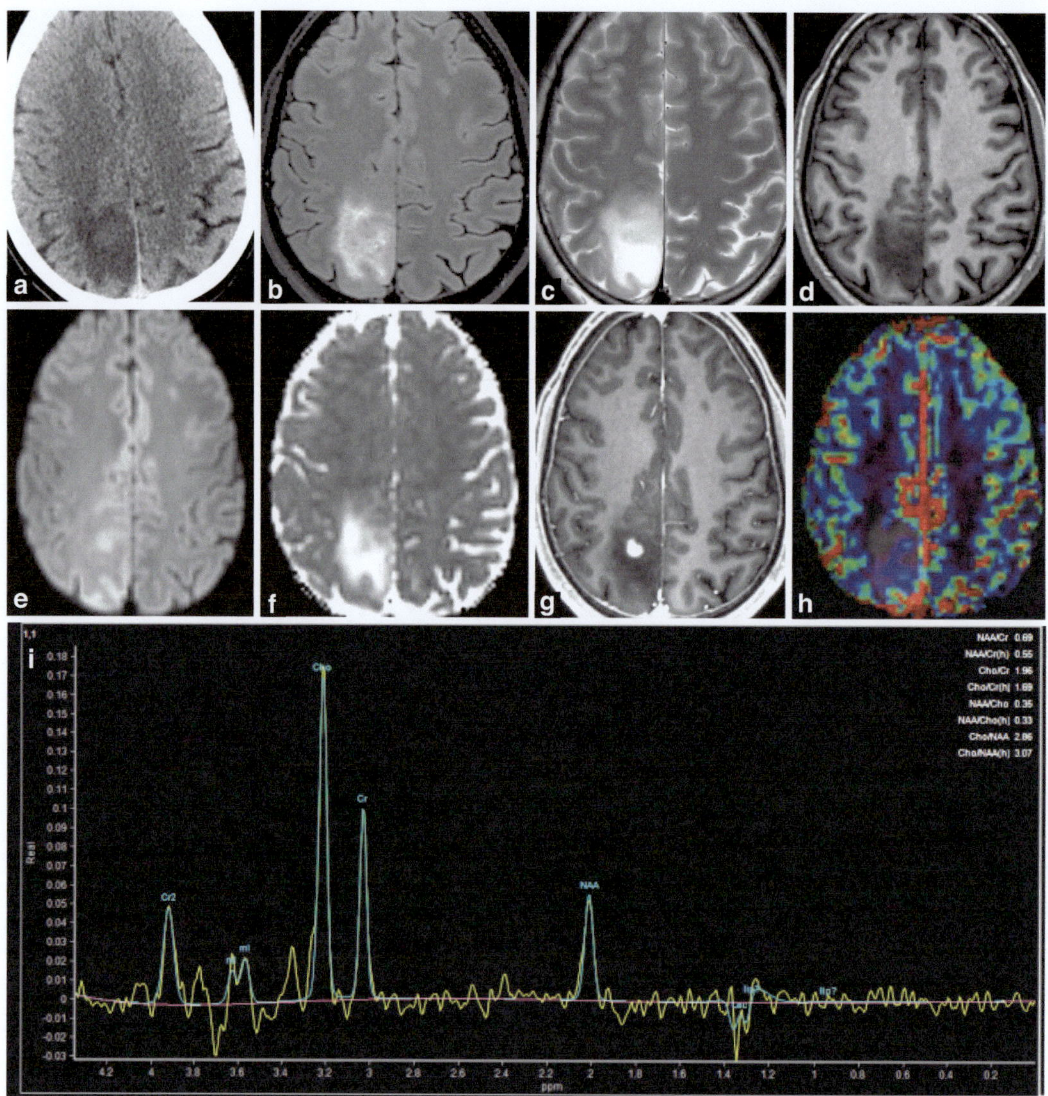

Fig. 2.4 Astrocytoma IDH-mutant, grade 2. CT (**a**). MRI FLAIR (**b**), T2WI (**c**), T1WI (**d**), DWI (**e**), ADC (**f**), post-contrast T1WI (**g**), CBV (**h**). A right parietal lesion is visible as a clear hyperintensity on T2WI and hypointensity on T1WI. FLAIR still exhibits a slight hyperintense signal and CBV is reduced. After contrast administration a small area of enhancement is visible (**g**). (**b**). MR spectroscopy (**i**) shows a clear increase of Cho/NAA ratio and a small doublet peak of lactate

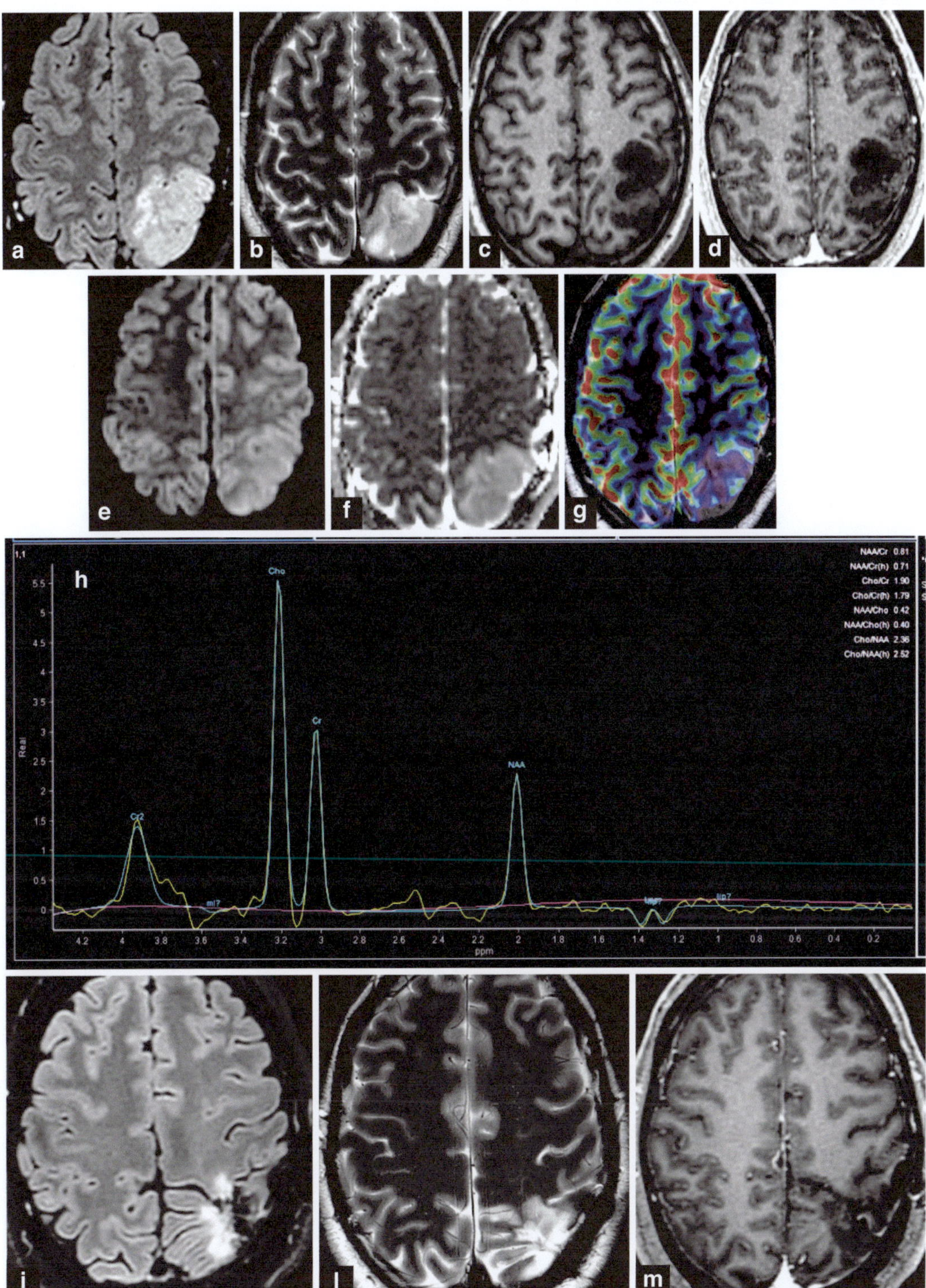

Fig. 2.5 Astrocytoma IDH-mutant, grade 2. MRI FLAIR (**a**), T2WI (**b**), T1WI (**c**), post-contrast T1-WI (**d**), DWI (**e**), ADC (**f**), CBV (**g**), MR spectroscopy (**h**). A left parietal lesion is visible as a slight and inhomogeneous hyperintensity on both T2WI and FLAIR, a slight increase of ADC and a decrease of CBV are evident as well. (**b**). Spectroscopy documented an increase of cho/NAA ratio. Post-surgical follow-up at 4 years. MRI FLAIR (**i**), T2WI (**l**), post-contrast T1WI (**m**). MR study does not show any recurrence

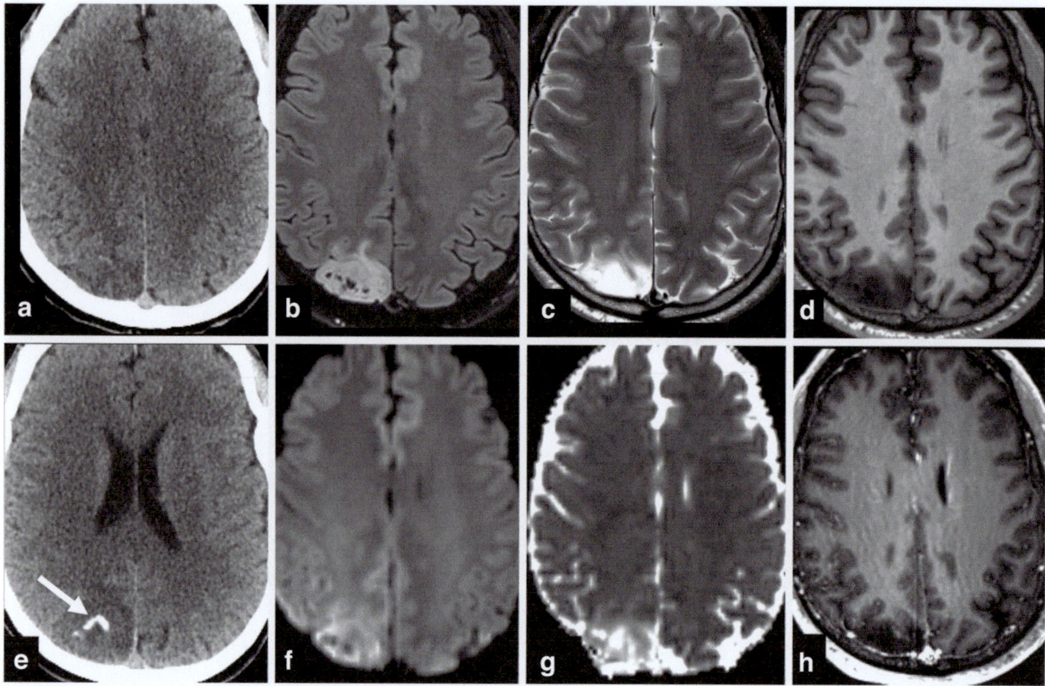

Fig. 2.6 Gemistocytic astrocytoma IDH-mutant, grade 2. CT (**a**, **e**); MRI FLAIR (**b**), T2WI (**c**), T1WI (**d**), DWI (**f**), ADC (**g**), post-contrast T1WI (**h**). A right parietal lesion is visible with a marked hyperintensity on T2WI and hypointensity on T1WI. Signal intensity on FLAIR is only slightly increased and some small cysts seem to be detectable in the subcortical area. ADC is increased and a calcification is clearly visible on CT (arrow **e**)

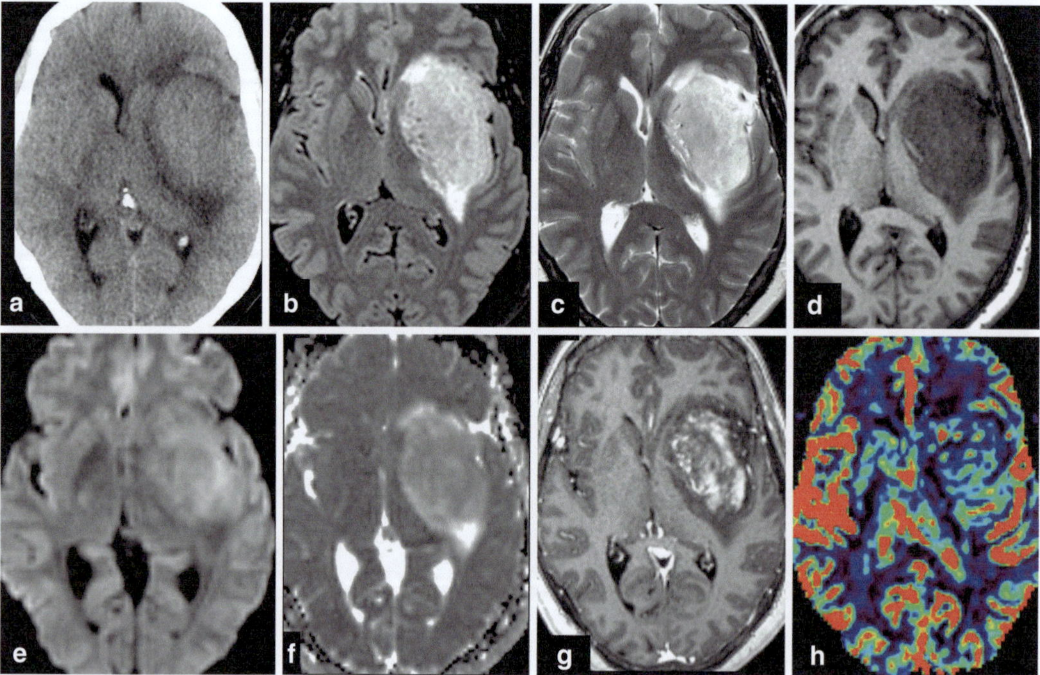

Fig. 2.7 Gemistocytic astrocytoma IDH-mutant, grade 2. CT (**a**); MRI FLAIR (**b**), T2WI (**c**), T1WI (**d**), DWI (**e**), ADC (**f**), post-contrast T1WI (**g**), CBV (**h**). A large left insular lesion is visible with a slight hyperintensity on T2WI and FLAIR and diffusely hypointense on T1WI. CBV is similar to normal gray matter and after contrast an irregular and diffuse enhancement is visible

Contrast enhancement can be present, but it is not a rule and cannot be used as a sign to differentiate grade 3 from grade 2. The cases in Figs. 2.8, 2.9, and 2.10 do not enhance, whereas the cases in Figs. 2.11 and 2.12 do enhance.

T2-FLAIR mismatch sign was reported in astrocytoma IDH-mutant series of both grade 2 and grade 3 [8]; however, it should be expected a less homogeneous high signal on T2WI.

In Figs. 2.8, 2.9, and 2.10 are reported three cases in which on FLAIR images the tumor presents central area of slight hypointense signal, and in cases of Figs 2.8 and 2.9 some real multiple cysts. All these tumors are heterogeneous on both

Table 2.2 Astrocytoma IDH-mutant, grade 2 imaging features

Mass effect		Edema	Inhomogeneity		Cysts	Necrosis		Hemorrhage	Calcifications
+/+++		0 / ++	+		Rare	0		0	Rare

CT	T1	T2	FLAIR	DWI	ADC	T1 Gd	CBV	Spec
⬤	⬤	◯	◯ ◯	⬤	◯ ◯	Rare	🔵	↑ Cho/NAA ↑ 2HG

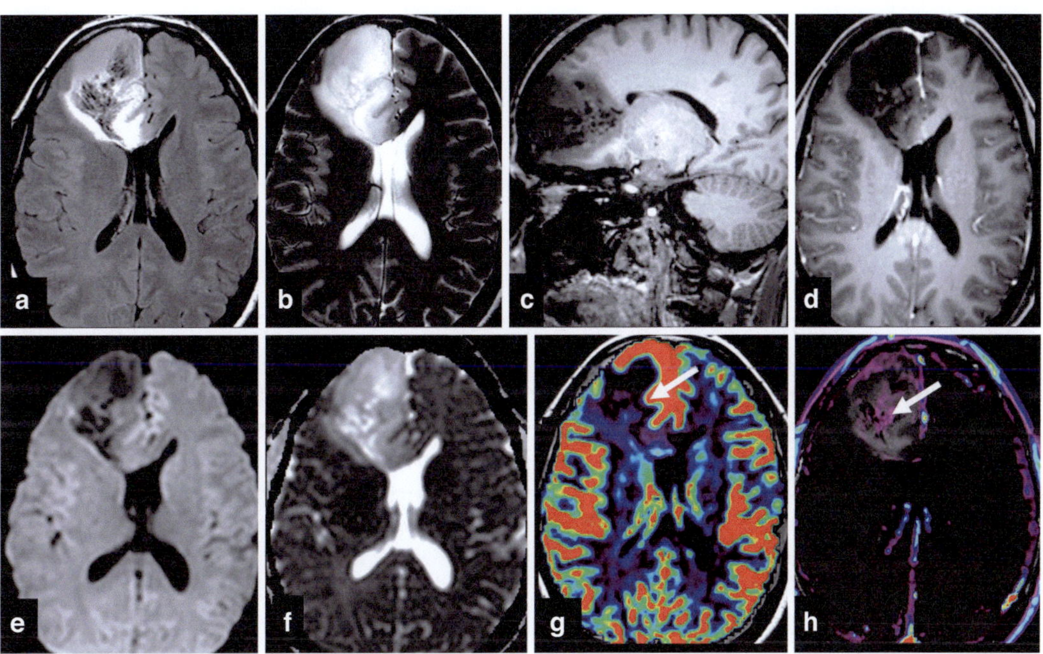

Fig. 2.8 Astrocytoma IDH-mutant, grade 3. MRI FLAIR (**a**), T2WI (**b**), T1WI (**c**), post-contrast T1WI (**d**), DWI (**e**), ADC (**f**), CBV (**g**), K-trans (**h**). A large inhomogeneous right frontal tumor is visible with a central area of FLAIR hypointensity with multiple microcysts. No enhancement is clearly visible after contrast administration. ADC signal intensity is inhomogeneous as well as T2WI. Small area of CBV and k-trans increase are present (arrows **g** and **h**). Six years follow-up after surgery and radio-chenotherapy. MRI FLAIR (**i**), T2WI (**j**), T1WI (**k**), DWI (**l**), ADC (**m**), post-contrast T1WI (**n**). No tumor recurrence is visible on MR images

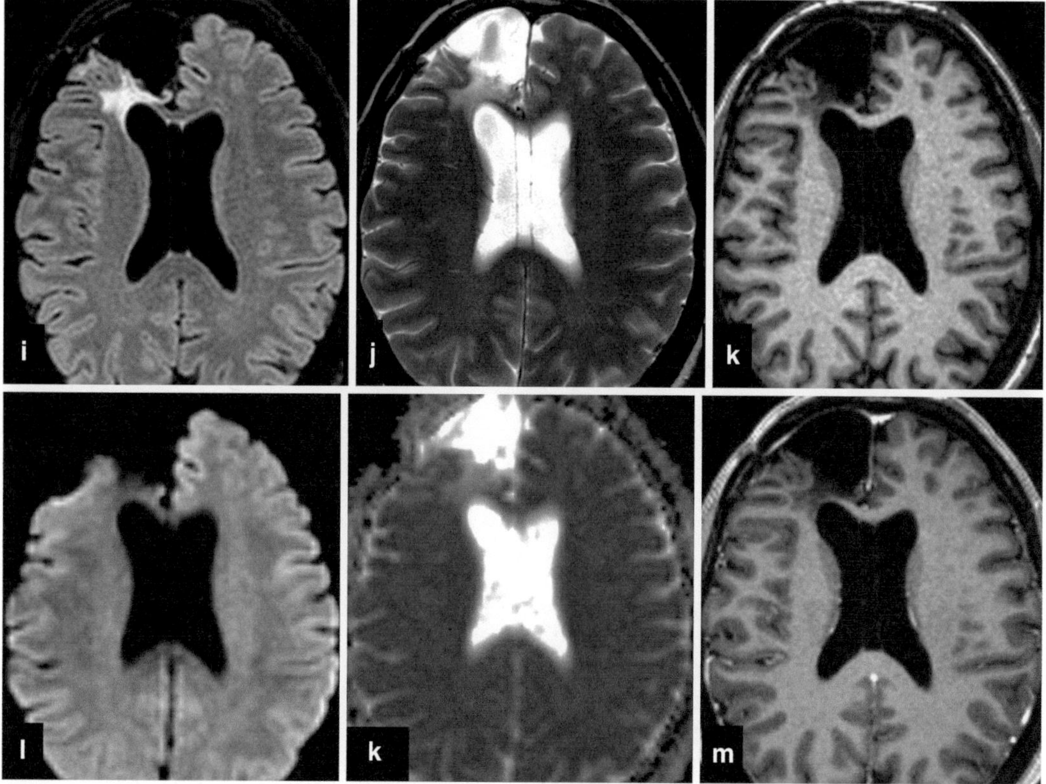

Fig. 2.8 (continued)

ADC and T2WI, but demonstrated a different behavior after treatment with a favorable course in case in Fig. 2.8 and unfavorable in case of Fig. 2.10.

Diffusion. DWI-ADC images should be carefully examined in order to evaluate areas of restricted diffusion that is different from astrocytoma IDH-mutant grade 2 should be expected in grade 3. This is one of the most reliable signs to differentiate the most aggressive behavior of grade 3 from grade 2 in which diffusiom should be normal or increased (see Fig. 2.10).

Spectroscopy shows a clear increase of Cho/NAA but it is impossible only in the basis of this data to differentiate grade 3 from grade 2 or grade 4.

Perfusion and permeability could be helpful to differentiate grade 3 from grade 2 being particularly sensitive to a more aggresiveness of the tumor due to the increase in vascularity.

The cases in Figs. 2.11 and 2.12 show more criteria suggestive to a clear increase of the tumor malignancy, in all case lesions are inhomogeneous, contrast enhancement is present, diffusion is somewhat restricted, the Cho/NAA is clearly increases as well as CBV and permeability.

The case in Fig. 2.12 is highly nonspecific: a single lesion with a ring enhancement and diffusion restriction may have many differential diagnosis issues. Imaging geatures of Astrocytoma IDH-mutant are summarized in Table 2.3.

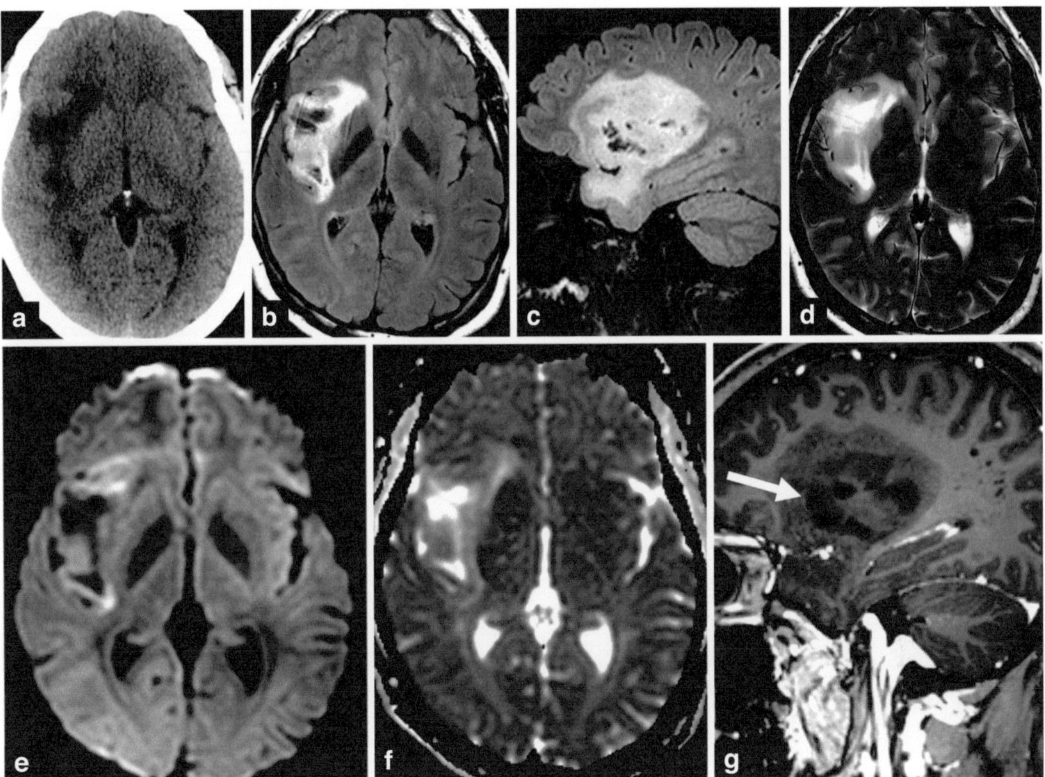

Fig. 2.9 Astrocytoma IDH-mutant, grade 3. CT (**a**); MRI FLAIR (**b, c**), T2WI (**d**), T1WI (**c**), DWI (**e**), ADC (**f**); post-contrast T1WI (**g**). Similarly to the case of Fig. 2.8 also in this case a central tumoral area of FLAIR hypointensity with multiple microcysts is visible (arrow **g**) with no enhancement after contrast administration. The signal intensity on both T2WI and DWI/ADC sequences is clearly inhomogeneous

2.1.1.3 Astrocytoma IDH-Mutant, Grade 4 *(Glioblastoma IDH-Mutant WHO 2016)*

WHO definition. A diffusely infiltrative astrocytic glioma with an IDH1 or IDH2 mutation that exhibits microvascular poliferation, necrosis, and homozygous deletions of CDKN2A or CDKN2B or any combination of these features.

Imaging. It is not possible to differentiate by means of conventional qualitative MRI evaluation a GBM IDH-wildtype from an astrocytoma IDH-mutant group 4. In group analysis a prevalence of fronto-insular location is reported for IDH-mutant types, but the analysis of single cases does not allow to make any reliable differences among the two types (Figs. 2.13 and 2.14).

All the typical signs of tumor aggressiveness can usually encounter with an heterogeneous pattern on both FLAIR and T2WI, presence of cystic necrotic areas, and solid component with diffusion restriction, marked increase of Cho/NAA, and increase of CBV and permeability. The post-contrast enhancement is frequently present with an inhomogeneous pattern as well (Figs. 2.13 and 2.14).

Prognosis. The median survival time of astrocytoma IDH-mutant grade 4 is greater than in GBM IDH-wildtype and can reach even 4–6 years. Imaging feature of Astrocytoma IDH-mutant grade 4 are reported in Table 2.4.

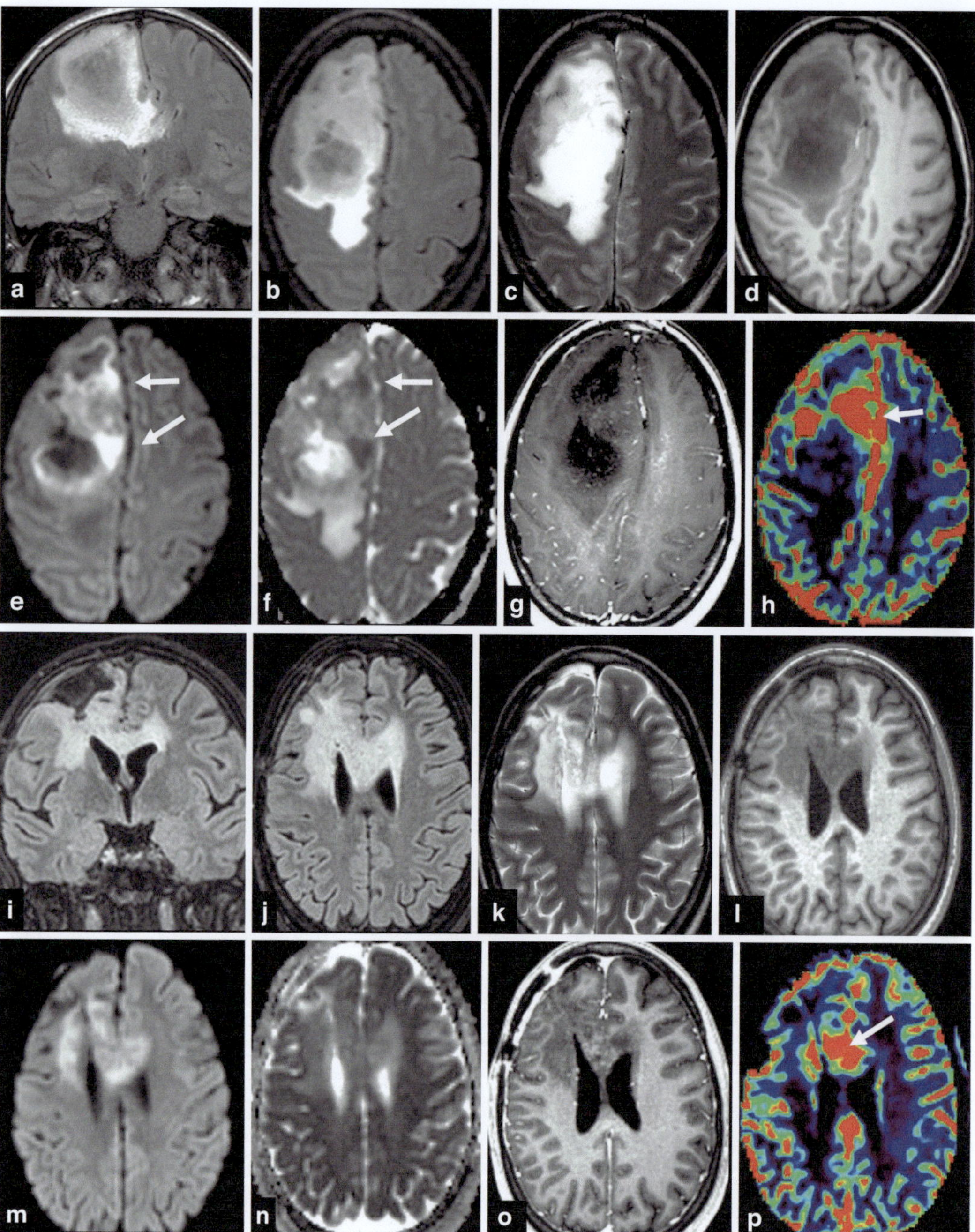

Fig. 2.10 Astrocytoma IDH-mutant, grade 3. MRI FLAIR (**a**, **b**), T2WI (**c**), T1WI (**d**), DWI (**e**), ADC (**f**), post-contrast T1WI (**g**), CBV (**h**). On coronal FLAIR section (**a**) this huge right frontal tumor can resemble an astrocytoma IDH-mutant grade 2 with the typical T2-FLAIR mismatch sign. On the axial section it appears very clear how this tumor is inhomogeneous, showing multiple areas of diffusion restriction (arrows **e**, **f**) and CBV increase (arrow **h**). There is no apparent enhancement after contrast administration. MRI follow up study after 8 months from surgery and radio-chemotherapy. MRI FLAIR (**i**, **j**), T2WI (**k**), T1WI (**l**), DWI (**m**), ADC (**n**), post-contrast T1WI (**o**), CBV (**p**). Differently from case 2.8 this case with a similar histological diagnosis had an unfavorable course and after only 8 months from surgery and subsequent radio-chemotherapy exhibits a diffuse growth through the genu of the corpus callosum and surrounding deep white matter with a corresponding increase in CBV (arrow **h**) and restriction in diffusion (**e**, **f**)

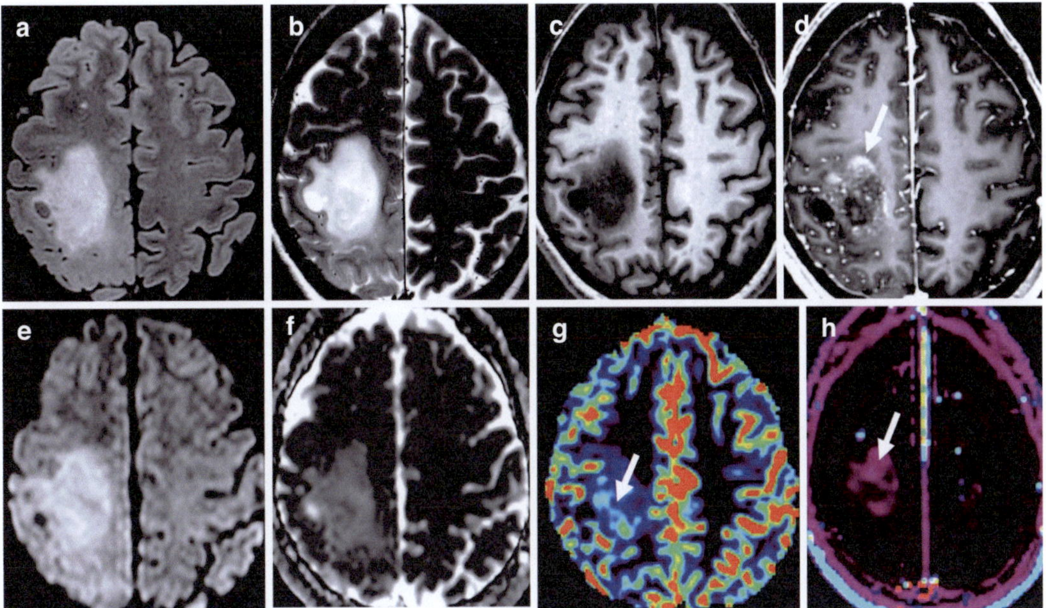

Fig. 2.11 Astrocytoma IDH-mutant, grade 3. MRI FLAIR (**a**), T2WI (**b**), T1WI (**c**), post-contrast T1WI (**d**), DWI (**e**), ADC (**f**), CBV (**g**), k-trans (**h**). A right rolandic tumor with a heterogeneous pattern and irregular enhancement. CBV and k-trans are increased, diffusion is slightly restricted

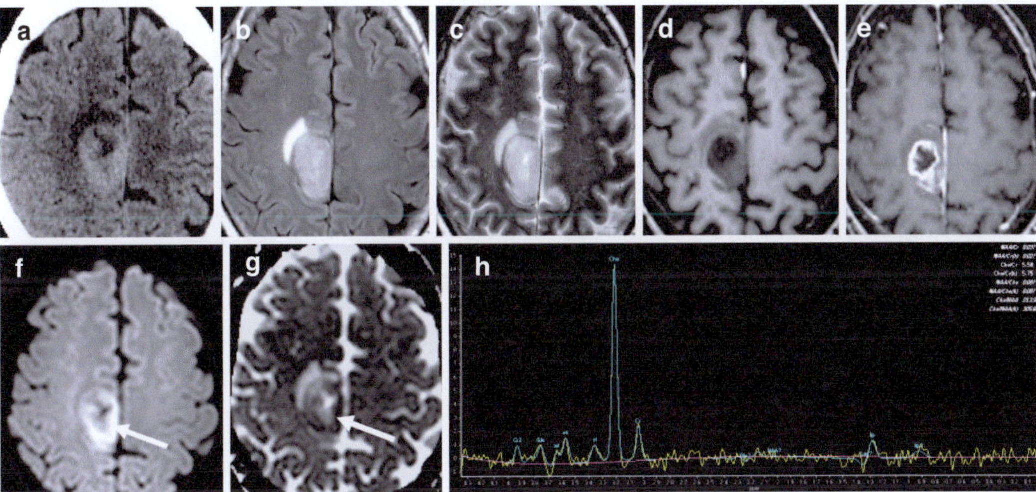

Fig. 2.12 Astrocytoma IDH-mutant, grade 3. CT (**a**). MRI FLAIR (**b**), T2WI (**c**), T1WI (**d**), post-contrast T1WI (**e**), DWI (**f**) ADC (**g**), spectroscopy (**h**). This focal lesion shows an irregular and peripheral enhancement with a clear diffusion restriction with a possible necrotic core. In the proton spectra NAA is virtually undetectable

Table 2.3 Astrocytoma IDH-mutant, grade 3 imaging features

Mass effect		Edema	Inhomogeneity		Cysts	Necrosis		Hemorrhage		Calcifications
+/+++		+/+++	++		+	++		+		0/+

CT	T1	T2	FLAIR	DWI	ADC	T1 Gd	CBV	Spec
◯	●	◯	◯ ◯	◯	◯	0/++	◯	↑↑Cho/NAA ↑ 2HG

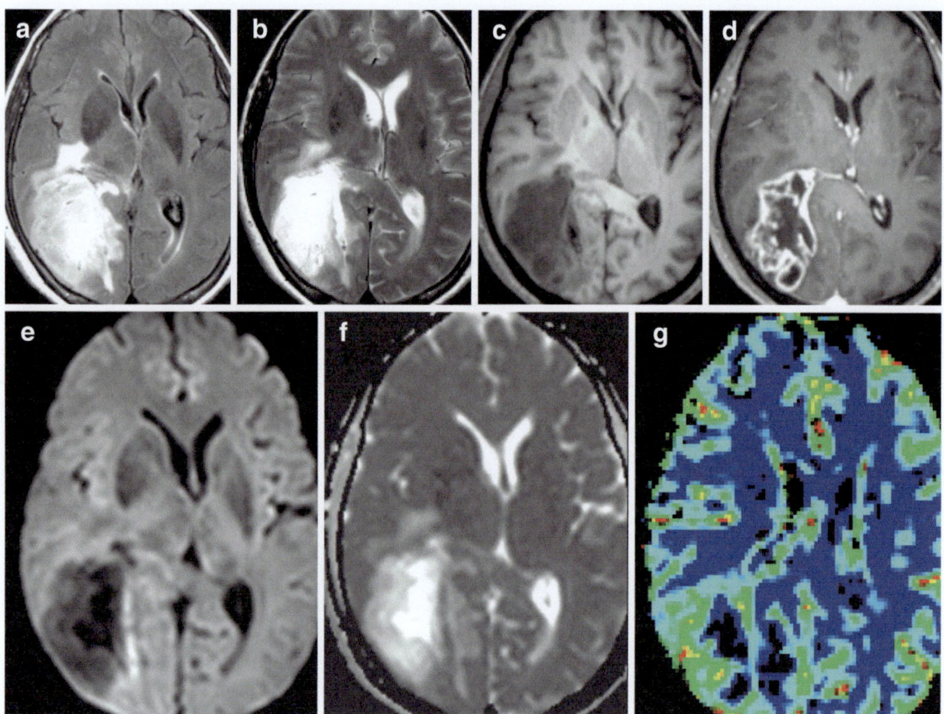

Fig. 2.13 Astrocytoma IDH-mutant, grade 4. MRI FLAIR (**a**), T2WI (**b**), T1WI (**c**), post-contrast T1WI (**d**), DWI (**e**), ADC (**f**) CBV (**g**). Heterogeneous right occipital lesion with mass effect, perilesional edema, and irregular enhancement. DWI/ADC restriction is only partly visible, no differences with GBM IDH-wildtype are clearly detectable

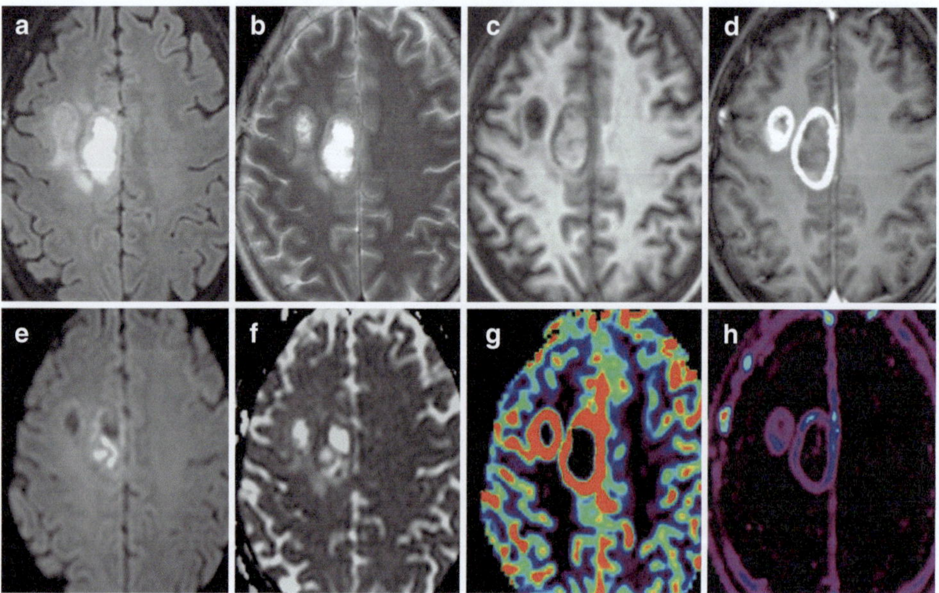

Fig. 2.14 Astrocytoma IDH-mutant, grade 4. MRI FLAIR (**a**) T2WI (**b**) T1WI (**c**), post-contrast T1WI (**d**), DWI (**e**), ADC (**f**), CBV (**g**), K-trans (**h**). Heterogeneous pre-rolandic lesion with mass effect, perilesional edema, necrosis, ADC/DWI restriction, and irregular enhancement with marked increase in both CBV and permeability. All the typical features of an aggressive glioma are shown with no differences with the GBM IDH-wildtype

Table 2.4 Astrocytoma IDH-mutant, grade 4 imaging features

Mass effect	Edema	Inhomogeneity	Cysts	Necrosis	Hemorrhage	Calcifications
+/+++	+/+++	+++	++	+++	0/++	0/+

CT	T1	T2	FLAIR	DWI	ADC	T1 Gd	CBV	Spec
○	●	●	○	○	●	+++	●	↑↑↑Cho/NAA ↑ 2HG?

2.1.2 Oligodendroglioma, IDH-Mutant and 1p/19q-Codeleted

WHO definition. Oligodendroglioma, IDH-mutant and 1p/19q-codeleted, is a diffusely infiltrating glioma composed with IDH1 or IDH2 mutation and codeletion of chromosome arms 1p and 19q.

Presence IDH mutation and 1p/19q codeletion are necessary to make the diagnosis; however, loss of nuclear ATRX is sufficient to diagnose an IDH-mutant astrocytoma, being the loss of nuclear ATRX absent in oligodendroglioma.

It is a WHO grade 2 or 3 tumor.

Epidemiology. Olidogendroglioma grade 2 occurs at a median age approximately equal to astrocytoma IDH-mutant grade 2 (between 35 and 40 years) with an incidence rate of 0.28 cases for 100.000 population for a year, it is rare in children and shows a little prevalence in men (ratio M/F 1.3) and in USA it is more common in White than in Black (ratio 2.3:1).

The median age of patients affected by oligodendroglioma grade 3 is around 50 years (45–55 years) with an incidence rate of 0. 11 cases for 100,000 population for a year. As for grade 2 there is a little prevalence in male vs. female.

Location. According to CBTRUS database [9] 59% are located in frontal lobes, 14% in temporal lobes, 10% in parietal lobes, and 1% in occipital lobes. According to the POLA network regarding 470 defined oligodendroglioma grade 3 [10], 62% are located in frontal lobes, 16% in temporal lobes, 15% in parietal lobes, and 6% in occipitale lobes. Other locations are very rare even though primary leptomeningeal origin has also been reported.

Clinical features. Among the more typical signs of brain tumors, seizures are the most frequent followed by headache and signs of increased intracranial pressure.

Prognosis. Overall prognosis is quite similar to Astrocytoma IDH-mutant grade 2 with a median survival time around 10 years (Fig. 2.15), some data on patients with oligodendroglioma grade 3 IDH-mutant and 1p/19q codeleted in prospective clinical trial with new chemotherapy treatment showed a median survival of approximately 14 years (Fig. 2.20).

2.1.2.1 Oligodendroglioma, IDH-Mutant and 1p/19q-Codeleted, Grade 2

WHO definition. Olidendrogliomas comprise a continuum spectrum from the histological point of view and the criteria for distinction between grades are not well defined. Low cellularity, scarce cytological atypia, low mitotic activity, and absence od pathological microvascular proliferation are the typical hystological markers of grade 2.

Imaging. Oligodendroglioma is typically a cortico-subcortical tumor generally quite well demarcated, slightly more inhomogeneous than astrocytoma and with frequent, but not diagnostic calcifications clearly visible on CT images or on T2*WI or SWI MR images (Fig. 2.15).

On T1WI Oligodendroglioma grade 2 is inhomogeneously hypointense, but differently from astrocytoma IDH-mutant grade 2 or 3, it does not show the T2-FLAIR mismatch sign and the signal intensity on both sequences is quite similar and predominantly hyperintense.

Contrast. Oligodendroglioma grade 2 usually does not enhance after contrast media administration (Figs. 2.15, 2.16, and 2.17).

Diffusion and spectroscopy. On DWI/ADC images this tumor shows usually a slight increase

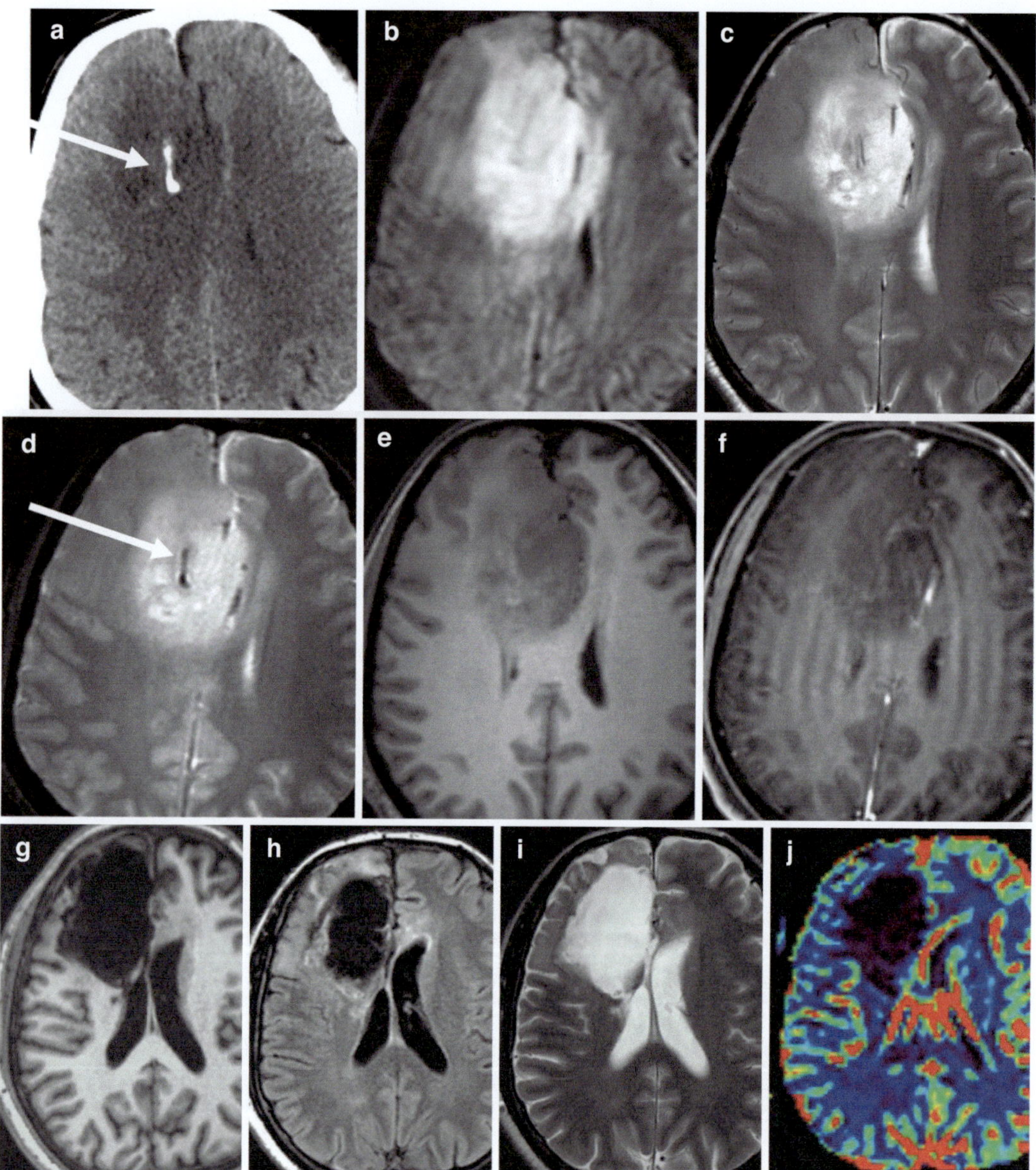

Fig. 2.15 Oligodendroglioma, IDH-mutant, 1p/19q codeleted, grade 2. CT (**a**). MRI FLAIR (**b**), T2WI (**c**) T2* (**d**), T1WI (**e**) post-contrast T1WI (**f**). Large right frontal infiltrative tumor showing hyperintense but heterogeneous signal on T2WI/FLAIR and a relatively large cal-cification (arrow **A** and **D**). Tumor enhancement after gadolinium is not clearly visible. MRI follow-up study 2 years after surgery and radio-chemotherapy. MRI T1WI (**g**), FLAIR (**h**), T2WI (**i**), CBV (**j**). The follow-up study does not show any residual tumor or recurrence

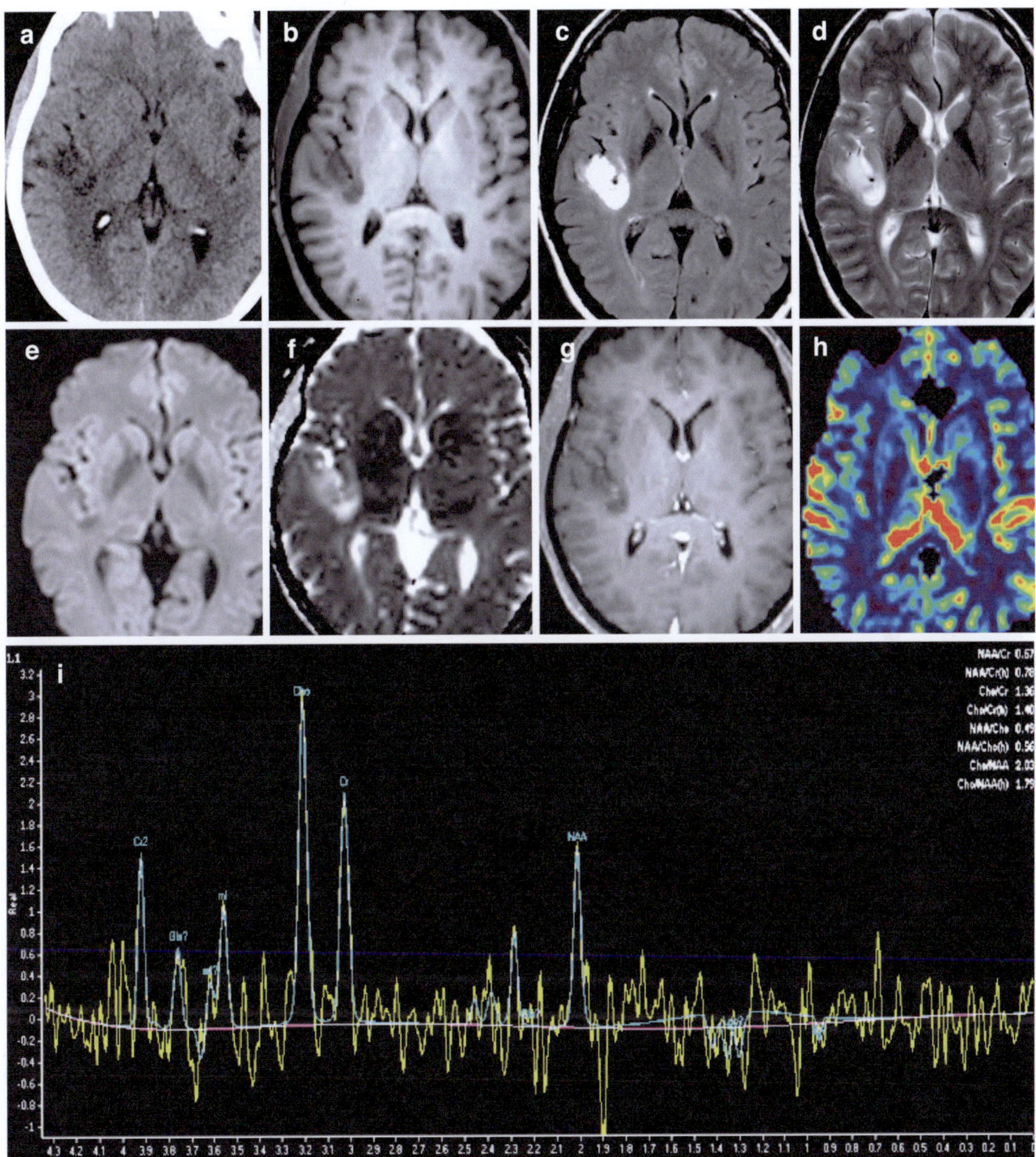

Fig. 2.16 Oligodendroglioma, IDH-mutant, 1p/19q codeleted, grade 2. CT (**a**), MRI T1WI (**b**), FLAIR (**c**), T2WI (**d**), DWI (**e**) ADC (**f**), post-contrast T1WI (**g**), CBV (**h**), single voxel spectroscopy (**i**). Right temporo-insular tumor with no calcification and enhancement. There is no T2-FLAIR mismatch sign but the differential diagnosis with astrocytoma IDH-mutant is quite impossible. Single voxel spectroscopy (**i**) shows a moderate increase of Cho/NAA ratio

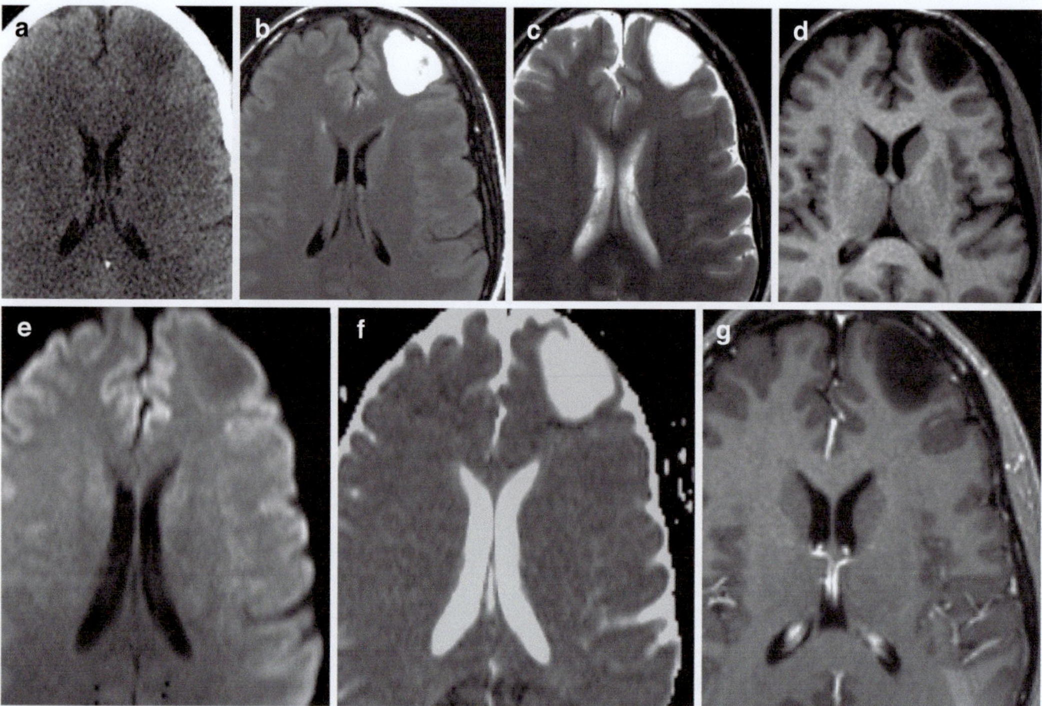

Fig. 2.17 Oligodendroglioma IDH-mutant, 1p/19q codeleted, grade 2. CT (**a**). MRI FLAIR (**b**), T2WI (**c**), T1WI (**d**), DWI (**e**), ADC (**f**), post-contrast T1WI (**g**). Left cortico-subortical frontal tumor with no calcifications and enhancement. Signal intensity in this case is homogeneous, the T2-FLAIR mismatch sign is absent

Table 2.5 Oligodendroglioma, IDH-mutant, and 1p/19q-codeleted, grade 2 imaging features

Mass effect	Edema	Inhomogeneity	Cysts	Necrosis	Hemorrhage	Calcifications
+/++	+/++	++	0/+	0	0	0/+++

CT	T1	T2	FLAIR	DWI	ADC	T1 Gd	CBV	Spec
◐	◐	○	◔	◔	◔	0/+	🔵	↑ Cho/NAA ↑ 2HG

of diffusion (Figs. 2.16 and 2.17), whereas on spectroscopy shows an increase of Cho/NAA ratio usually compatible with a slow growing tumor (Fig. 2.16).

As for astrocytomas IDH-mutant it is possible with specific spectroscopic sequences to determine the IDH status of patients through the detection of the oncometabolite 2-hydroxyglutarate (2HG) (see Fig. 2.29).

Perfusion, permeability. Large calcifications can interfere with dynamic susceptibility contrast (DSC) perfusion sequence, and in this case dynamic contrast enhancement (DCE) technique should be preferred. CBV is normal or decreases, and permeability is normal.

Differential diagnosis with astrocytoma IDH-mutant non-codeleted. The presence of the T2-FLAIR mismatch sign can be suggestive of the presence of an astrocytoma, but as previously reported this sign is not always present in astrocytic noncodeleted tumors and in case of absence of T2-FLAIR mismatch sign and absence of calcification too, the differential diagnosis between these two tumors could be quite impossible. Imaging features of Oligodendroglioma, IDH-mutant, and 1p719q-codeletd, grade 2 are summarized in Table 2.5.

2.1.2.2 Oligodendroglioma, IDH-Mutant, and 1p/19q-Codeleted, Grade 3

WHO definition. High cellularity, marked cytological atypia, high mitotic activity, and presence of pathological microvascular proliferation are the typical histological markers of grade 3.

Imaging. Oligodendroglioma, IDH-mutant and 1p/19q-codeleted, grade 3 is typically a cortico-subcortical heterogeneous neoplasm showing other than calcifications also cysts, necrosis, and hemorrhagic components. MRI appearance can partly mimic more aggressive astrocytomas, even though the presence of calcifications is a typical hallmark of oligodendrogliomas (Fig. 2.18) as well as the frontal cortico-subcortical location.

The signal intensity on T1WI, T2WI, and FLAIR images is typically heterogeneous (Figs. 2.18, 2.19, and 2.20).

Contrast enhancement is commonly present even if it is not the rule.

Diffusion and spectroscopy. Areas of diffusion restriction are usually evident (Figs. 2.18 and 2.20) and the ratio Cho/NAA is usually markedly increased (Fig. 2.20).

Perfusion and permeability. CBV is usually increased even not as in GBM (Fig. 2.19). Imaging features of Oligodendroglioma IDH-mutant and 1p/19q-codeleted, grade 3 are summarized in Table 2.6.

2.1.3 Glioblastoma, IDH-Wildtype

WHO definition. Glioblastoma (GBM), IDH-wildtype is a diffuse astrocytic glioma that is IDH-wildtype and H3-wildtype and has one or more of the following histological or genetic features: microvascular proliferation, necrosis, *TERT* promoter mutation, *EGFR* gene amplification, +7/−10 chromosome copy-number changes.

It is a CNS WHO grade 4 tumor.

Epidemiology. GBM is the <u>most frequent intra-axial brain tumor of adults</u> with an inci-

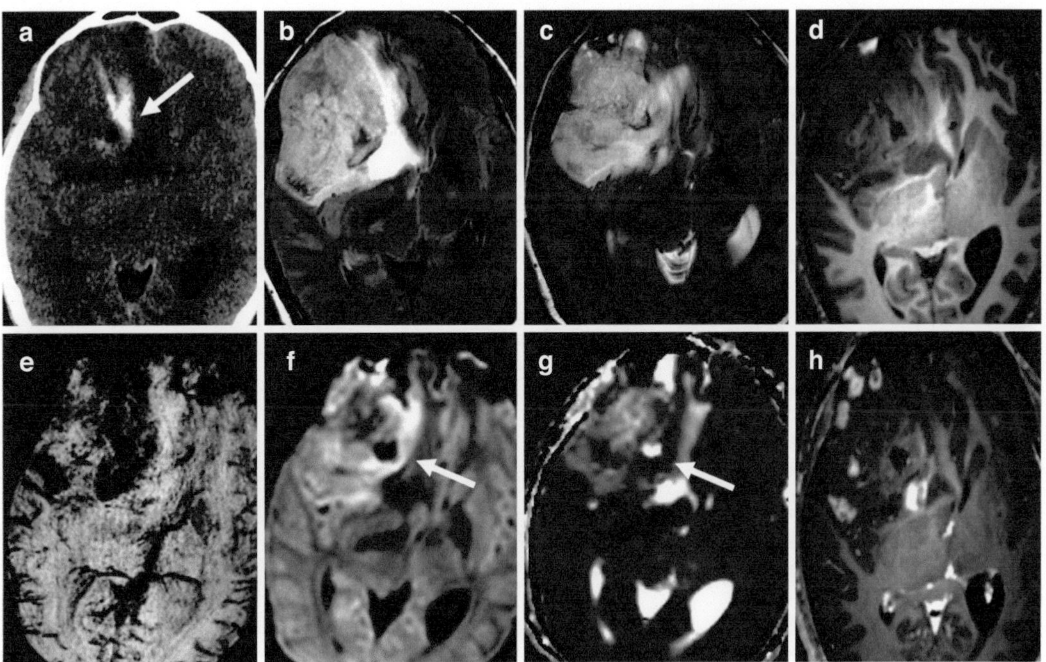

Fig. 2.18 Oligodendroglioma, IDH-mutant, 1p/19q codeleted, grade 3. CT (**a**). MRI FLAIR (**b**), T2WI (**c**), T1WI (**d**), SWI (**e**), DWI (**f**), ADC (**g**), post-contrast T1WI (**h**). Large right cortico-subcortical frontal tumor with calcification (**a** and **e**), enhancement, areas of diffusion restriction (arrow **f** and **g**), and huge mass effect

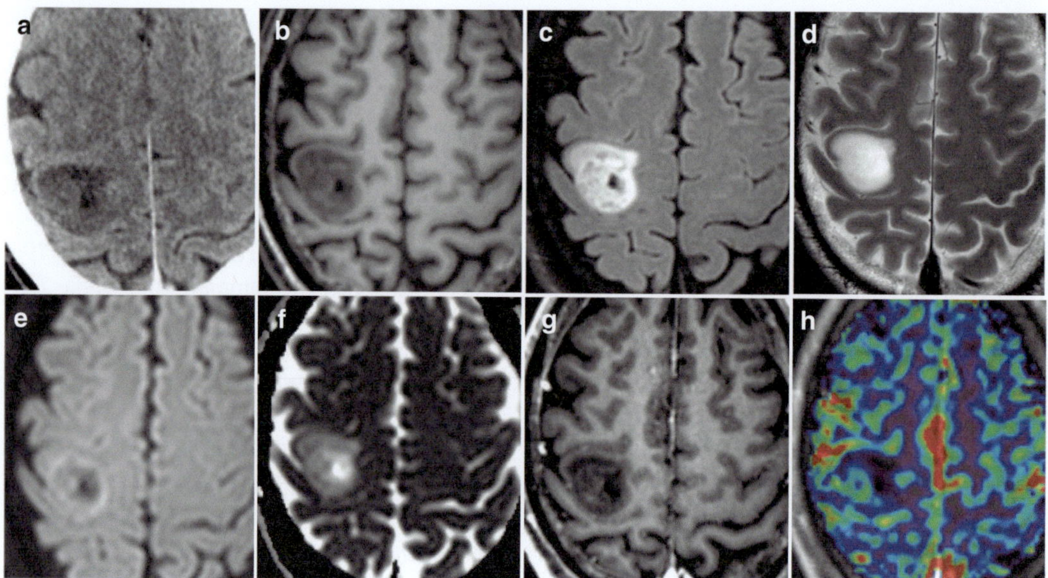

Fig. 2.19 Oligodendroglioma, IDH-mutant, 1p/19q codeleted, grade 3. CT (**a**). MRI T1WI (**b**), FLAIR (**c**), T2WI (**d**), DWI (**e**), ADC (**f**), post-contrast T1WI (**g**), CBV (**h**). Right cortico-subcortical pre-rolandic lesion without calcification and heterogeneous pattern. A doubtful enhancement is present in correspondence with the small area of increased CBV

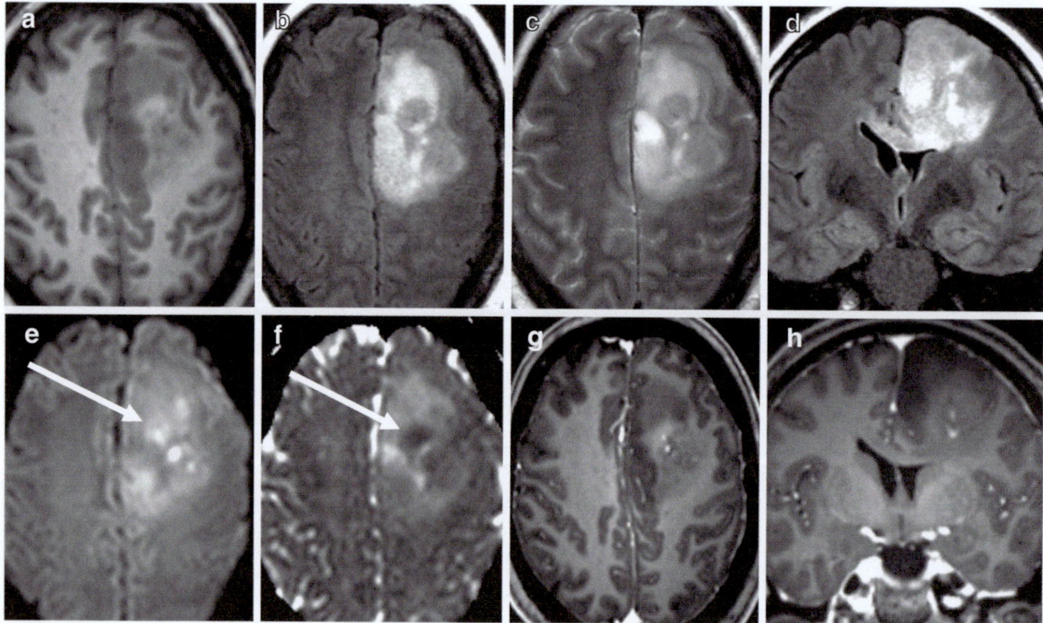

Fig. 2.20 Oligodendroglioma, IDH-mutant, 1p/19q codeleted, grade 3. MRI T1WI (**a**), FLAIR (**b, d**), T2WI (**c**), DWI (**e**), ADC (**f**), post-contrast T1WI (**g, h**), single voxel spectroscopy (**i**) Large and heterogeneous left cortico-subcortical frontomesial tumor with mass effect. Areas of diffusion restriction are evident in **E** and **F** (arrow). Subtle areas of contrast enhancement are present. Spectroscopy (**I**) shows a marked increase of Cho/NAA ratio. Four years follow-up study. MRI T1WI (**j**), T2WI (**k**), FLAIR (**l**), post-contrast T1WI (**m**). At the 4 years follow-up study after surgery and combined therapy no signs of residual tumor or recurrence are visible

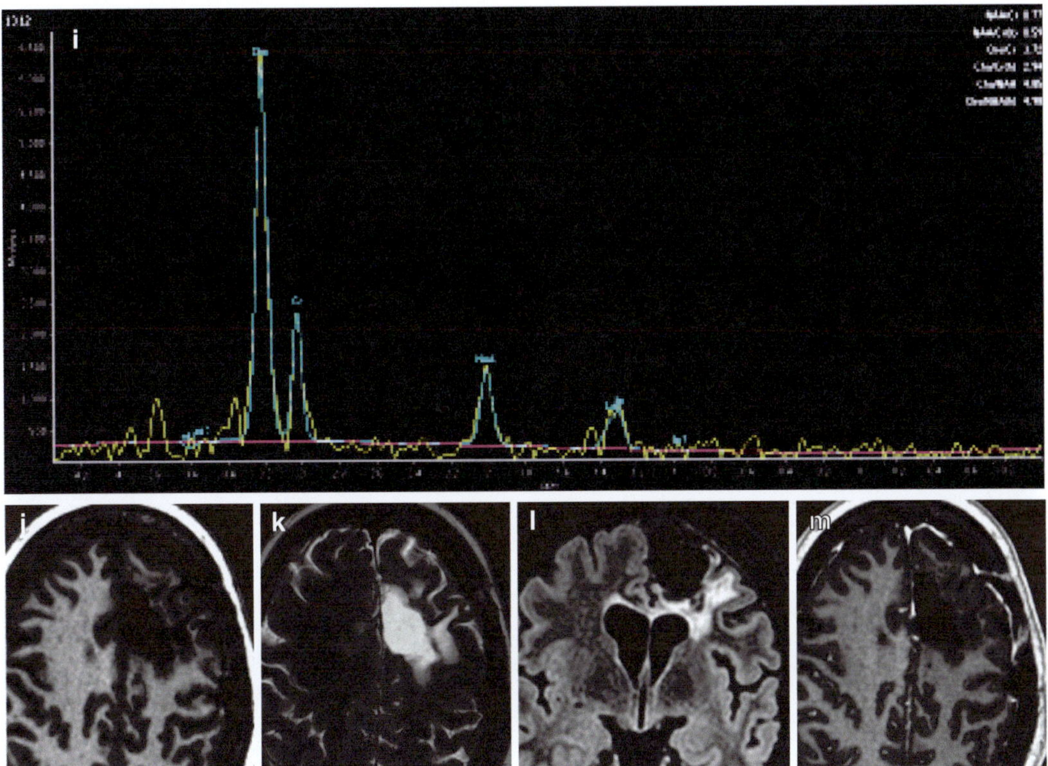

Fig. 2.20 (continued)

Table 2.6 Oligodendroglioma, IDH-mutant and 1p/19q-codeleted, grade 3 imaging features

Mass effect	Edema	Inhomogeneity	Cysts	Necrosis	Hemorrhage	Calcifications
+/+++	+/++	+++	0/++	0/++	0/++	0/+++

CT	T1	T2	FLAIR	DWI	ADC	T1 Gd	CBV	Spec
◖	◖	○	◌	○	◉	+/++	◉	↑↑Cho/NAA ↑ 2HG

dence rate of 3.5 cases for 100,000 subjects. GBM can be found at any age but the median age of patients with this kind of tumor is around 65 years. There is an overall slight prevalence in men (1.6/1.0), but females show an earlier presentation.

Localization. Even potentially present everywhere, GBM shows a predilection for subcortical white matter and deeper gray matter of cerebral hemispheres with a slight prevalence of temporal lobe (1/3 of cases).

In the WHO 2016 classification GBM was genetically subdivided into two main categories: GBM without the mutation of IDH genes or GBM wildtype, and GBM that carries the mutation in either the IDH1 and IDH2 genes, the GBM "IDH-mutant." In the WHO 2021 classification astrocytic gliomas carrying the IDH mutation are all classified in the same group and what was previously defined as GBM IDH-mutant is now classified as astrocytoma IDH-mutant, grade 4.

GBM IDH-wildtype represents the vast majority of astrocytic gliomas grade 4 (approximately 90%).

GBM IDH-wildtype and astrocytoma IDH-mutant, grade 4 exhibit some clinical and prognostic differences summarized in Table 2.7 (from WHO 2016 classification).

Clinical presentation. Symptoms depend on the tumor's location and can range from epileptic seizures, to focal neurological deficits (such as hemiparesis or aphasia) as weel as behavioral and cognitive symptoms. Generally, given that GBM a rapid developing tumor, the time between the onset of the first symptom and diagnosis is usually brief, tipically around 3 months.

Prognosis. According to WHO 2021 the survival rate at 5 years is still very low (around 6–7% in the USA between 2012 and 2016) and most GBM patients die 15–18 months after 15–18 from therapy.

Imaging. Glioblastomas IDH-wildtype shows all the typical features described for an aggressive tumor and usually exhibit a clear mass effect, perilesional edema, and a deeply inhomogeneous structure with irregular enhacement. All these features are shown in Figs. 2.21, 2.22, 2.23, and 2.24.

The signal intensity on conventional sequence is extremely variable, but predominantly heterogeneous and even in the presence of a relatively homogeneous lesion such as in the case of Fig. 2.25 the signal intensity on T2-FLAIR sequences is only very slightly hyperintense.

Table 2.7 Main differences between GBM wildtype and mutant (from WHO 2016/2021)

Astrocytic glioma	GBM IDH-wildtype	Astrocytoma IDH-mutant, grade 4
Percentage of total grade 4	90%	10%
Median age at diagnosis	~ 60 years	~ 45 years
Male, female ratio	1.6/1	1/1
Mean length of clinical history	4 months	15 months
Median overall survival	9–15 months	24–31 months
Location	Supratentorial	Frontal
Necrosis	Extensive	Limited

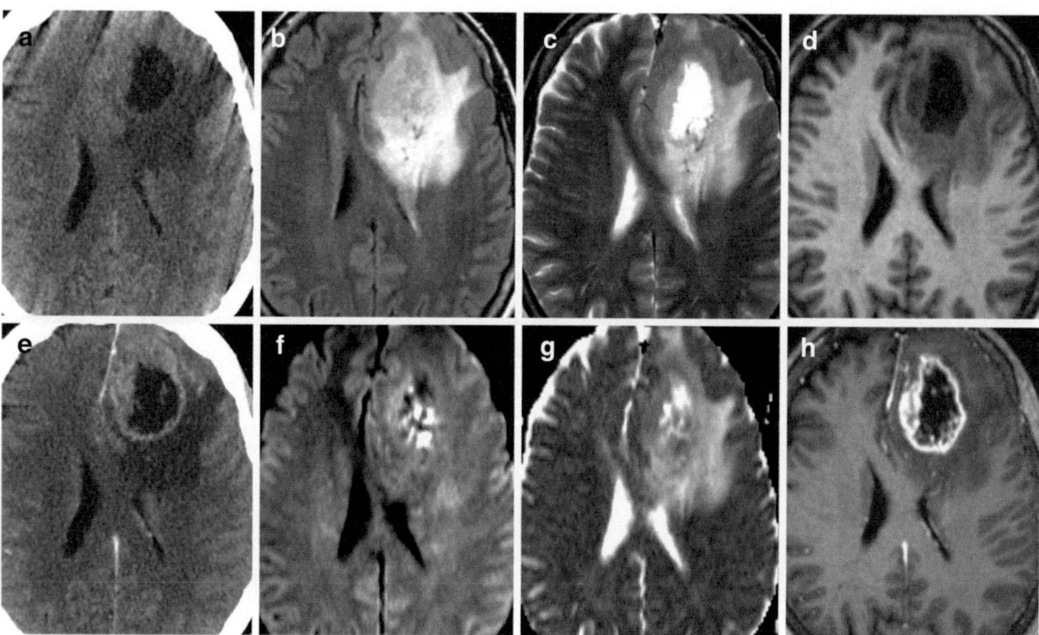

Fig. 2.21 GBM IDH-wildtype. CT pre (**a**) and post (**e**) contrast. MRI FLAIR (**b**), T2WI (**c**), T1WI (**d**), DWI (**f**), ADC (**g**), post-contrast T1WI (**h**). Heterogeneous frontal lesion with mass effect, perilesional edema, necrosis, ADC/DWI restriction, and irregular enhancement

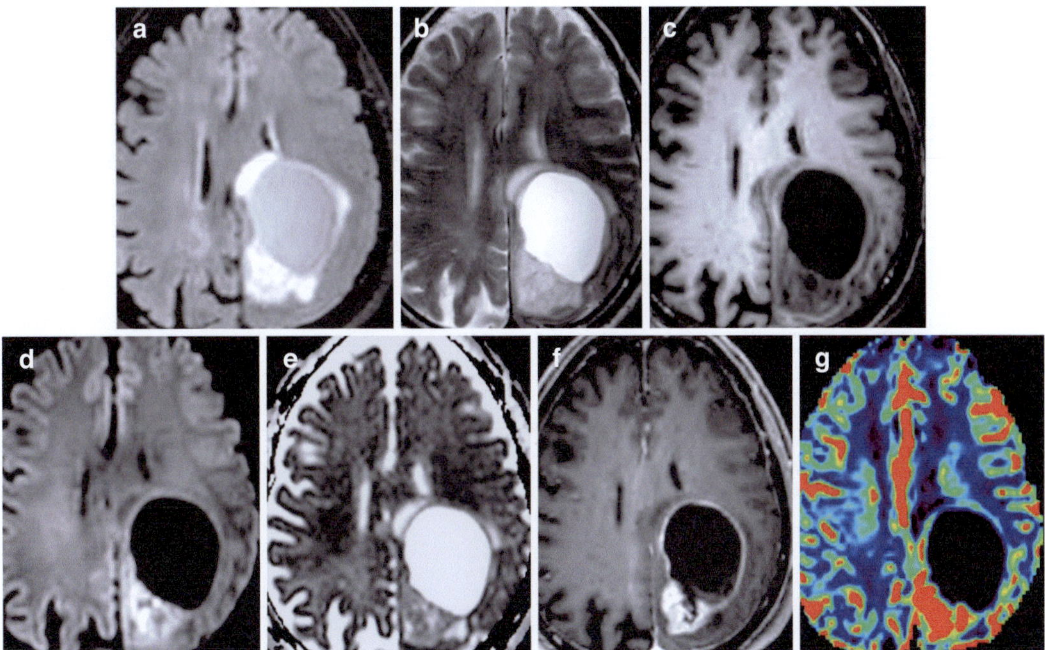

Fig. 2.22 GBM IDH-wildtype. MRI FLAIRI (**a**), T2WI (**b**), T1WI (**c**), DWI (**d**) ADC (**e**), post-contrast T1WI (**f**), CBV (**g**). Heterogeneous parietal lesion with mass effect, perilesional edema, necrosis, ADC/DWI restriction, increased cerebral blood volume and irregular enhancement

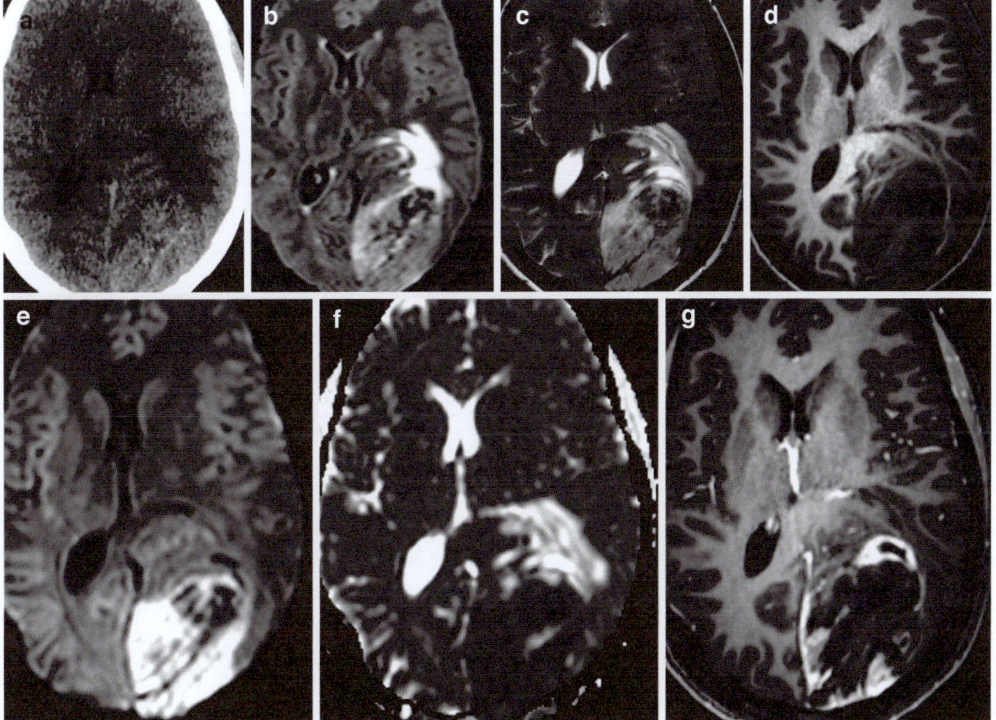

Fig. 2.23 GBM IDH-wildtype. CT (**a**). MRI FLAIR (**b**), T2WI (**c**), T1WI (**d**), DWI (**e**), ADC (**f**), post-contrast T1WI (**g**). Heterogeneous occipital lesion with mass effect, perilesional edema, ADC/DWI restriction, and irregular enhancement

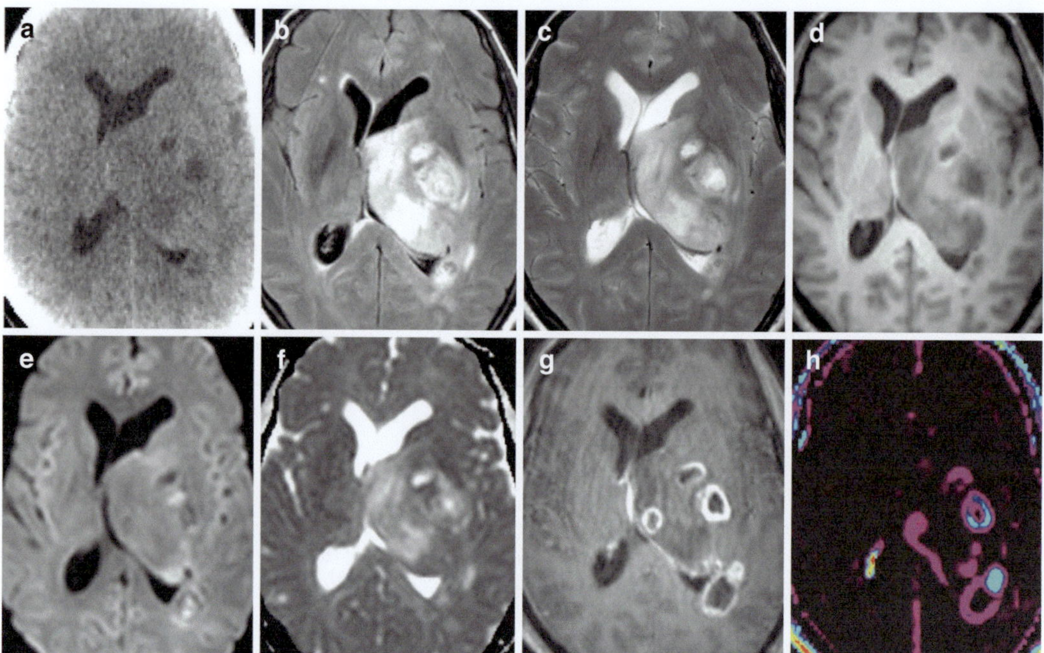

Fig. 2.24 GBM IDH-wildtype. CT (**a**). MRI FLAIR (**b**), T2WI (**c**), T1WI (**d**), DWI (**e**), ADC (**f**), post-contrast T1WI (**g**), K-trans (**h**). Heterogeneous infiltrating left tha- lamic lesion with areas of diffusion restriction, enhance- ment, and high permeability (increase of K-trans)

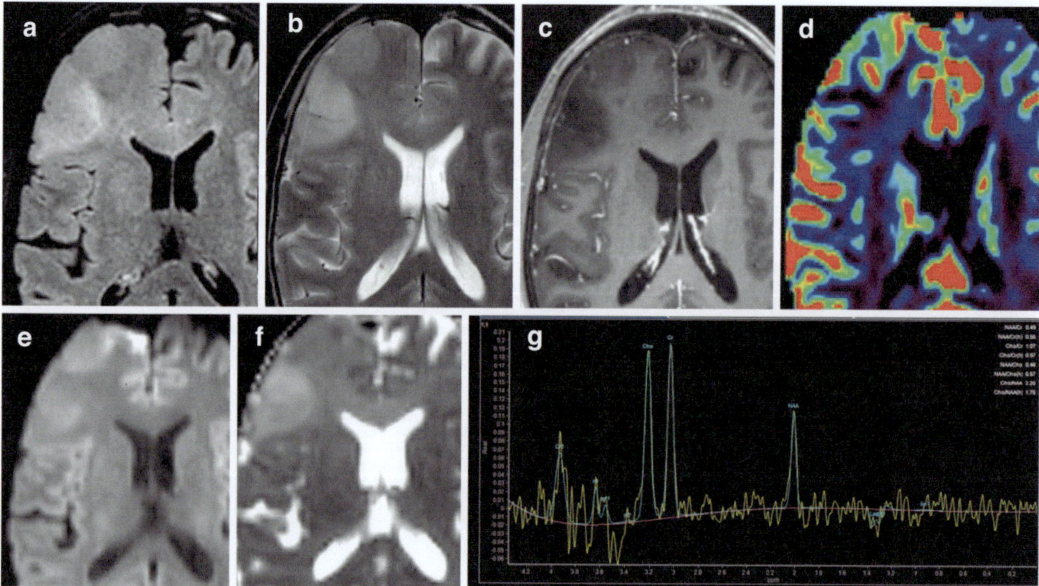

Fig. 2.25 GBM IDH-wildtype. MRI FLAIR (**a**), T2WI (**b**), post-contrast T1WI (**c**), CBV (**d**), DWI (**e**), ADC (**f**), spectroscopy (**g**). Left frontal neoplasm with an infiltra- tive behavior and apparently no enhancement and only a mild increase of Cho/NAA ratio. The first histological diagnosis was an astrocytoma grade 2. On CBV image some superficial areas of CBV increase are however visi- ble and on ADC map an involvement of the genu of the corpus callosum seems to be present. On T2WI and FLAIR images the hyperintensity is extremely mild. MRI follow-up study at 4 months after surgery and combined therapy. MRI FLAIR (**i**), DWI (**j**), ADC (**k**), post-contrast T1WI (**l**). MRI follow-up 5 months MRI FLAIR (**m**), DWI (**n**), ADC (**o**), post-contrast T1WI (**p**). Follow-up studies show a rapid increase and infiltration of the neo- plasm through the genus of the corpus callosum, the ipsi- lateral basal ganglia, and temporo-insular region

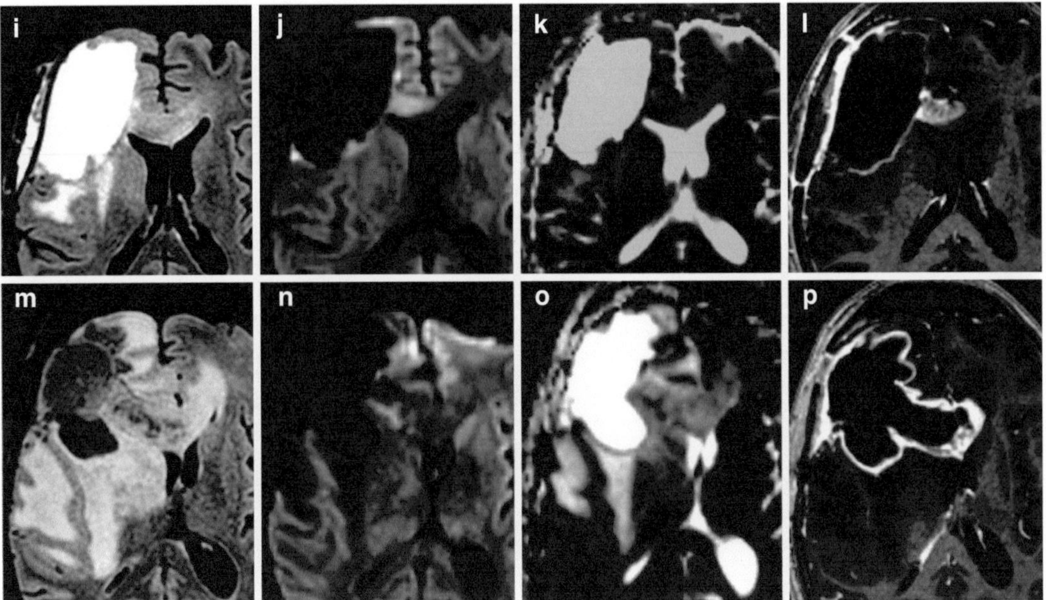

Fig. 2.25 (continued)

This aspect is of great importance, considering also the relatively mild increase of Cho/NAA, this neoplasm can be misdiagnosed as a more benign glioma, but the signal intensity on T2WI definitely does not fit with a benign lesion.

Contrast enhancement. The enhancement of GBMs after contrast administration is quite always present and irregular, but in some case can be initially absent (Fig. 2.25) or apparently so (Fig. 2.26).

Diffusion. High cellularity of the aggressive tumors is usually associated with a diffusion restriction and diffusion sequences still remain one of the most reliable imaging techniques to detect a possible malignancy and the overall aggressiveness of the tumor. An illustrative example is shown in Fig. 2.27, where, in the case of a multifocal glioma, diffusion images can identified regions of increased malignancy. It is worth noting that the increased cellularity of a neoplasm not only result in diffusion restriction, but also leads to a relative hyperdensity on CT. On T2WI the signal intensity can be confused with that of the normal cortex (Fig. 2.27).

Spectroscopy. As a general rule the Cho/NAA ratio progressively increases as tumor malignancy increases. Other indicators of tumor invasiveness may include the presence of lactate, primarly attributable to necrosis or to a lipid peak, which also signifies necrosis and tissue destruction (Fig. 2.28).

As previously mentioned with specific acquisition techniques and dedicated postprocessing [6, 7] it is possible to determine the IDH status of patients with brain gliomas through the detection of the oncometabolite 2-hydroxyglutarate (2HG) (Fig. 2.29).

Perfusion and permeability. Microvascular proliferation is one of the hallmarks of glioblastomas. Sometimes microvessel proliferation is so prominent that the vessels acquired a glomeruloid shape (WHO 2021). Perfusion and permeability imaging are consequently of great importance in the evaluation of these neoplasms and CBF, but in particular CBV (Fig. 2.26) and permeability (K-trans) (Fig. 2.24) are greatly increased. On the contrary a reduction of perfusion could be an important feature to make the diagnosis of an aggressive glioma less probable.

Multifocal/multicentric glioblastomas. The presence of a multifocal glioblastoma is reported up to 35% in the various series. Multifocal glio-

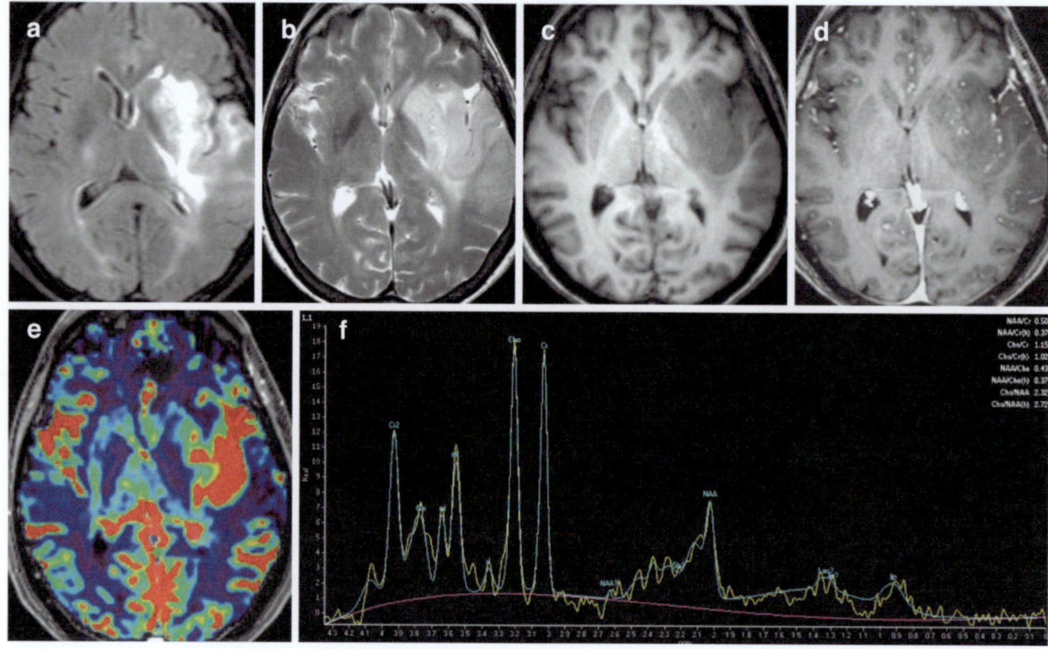

Fig. 2.26 GBM IDH-wildtype. MRI FLAIR (**a**), T2WI (**b**) T1WI (**c**), post-contrast T1WI (**d**) CBV (**e**), spectroscopy (**f**). A large left temporo-insular infiltrative tumor shows apparently no enhancement after contrast administration, but a clear increase in perfusion (CBV) and an evident increase of Cho/NAA ratio. As for the case of Fig. 2.25 the signal intensity on T2WI is only mildly increased

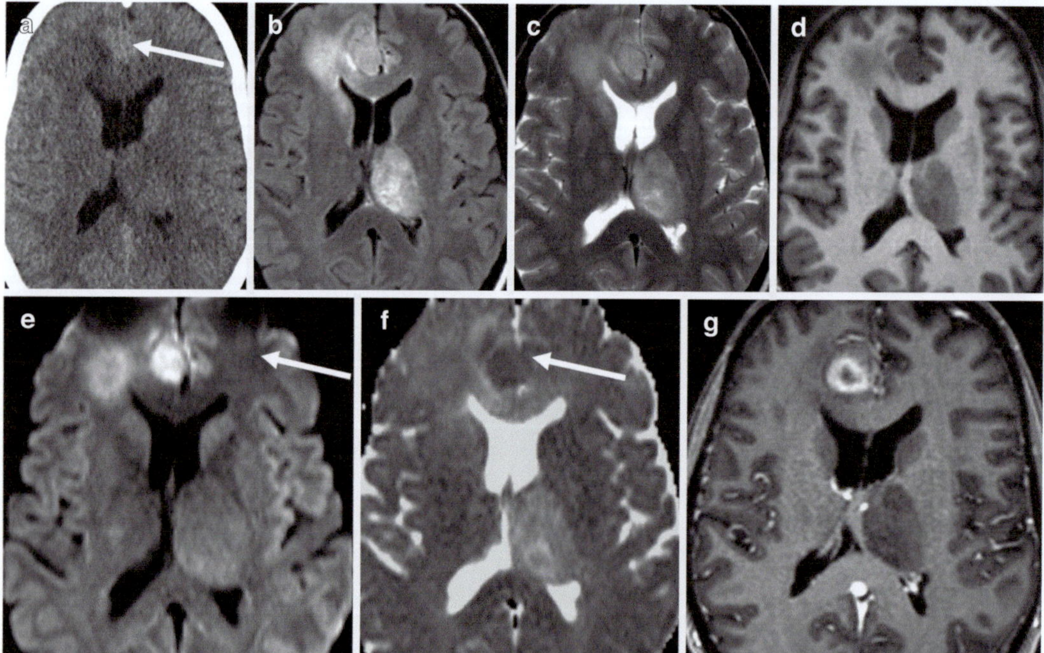

Fig. 2.27 Multifocal/multicentric GBM IDH-wildtype. CT (**a**) MRI FLAIR (**b**) T2WI (**c**) T1WI (**d**), DWI (**e**), ADC (**f**), post-contrast T1WI (**g**). The right frontal lesion is heterogeneous with areas of DWI/ADC restriction (arrows **e** and **f**), CT slight hyperdensity (arrow **a**), and post-contrast enhancement (**g**). The thalamic lesion is relatively more homogeneous with no enhancement after contrast

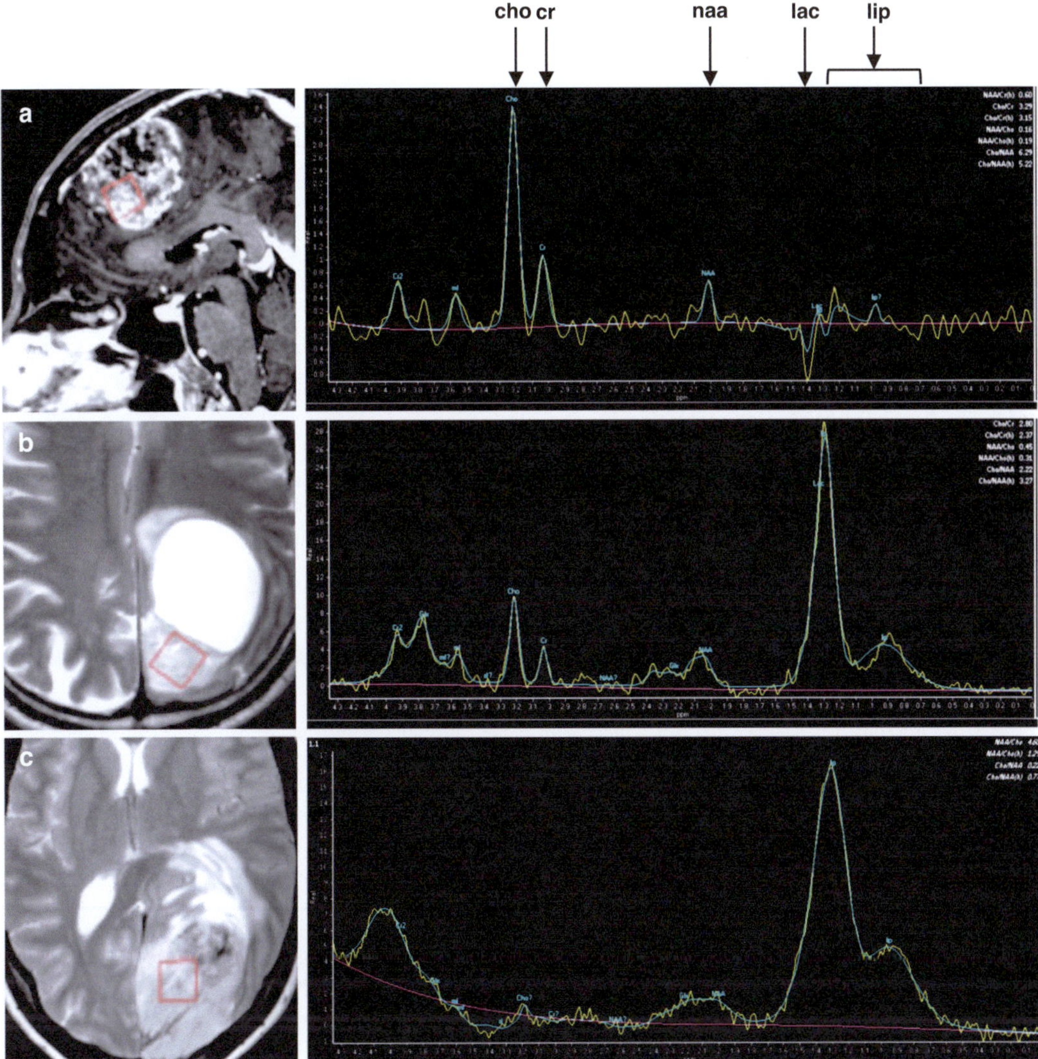

Fig. 2.28 MR spectroscopy in GBMs. A marked increase of Cho/NAA ratio is usually evident within the solid portion of the tumor (**a**), a variable amount of lactate and lipids can be found in the necrotic inhomogeneous part of the neoplasm (**b**, **c**)

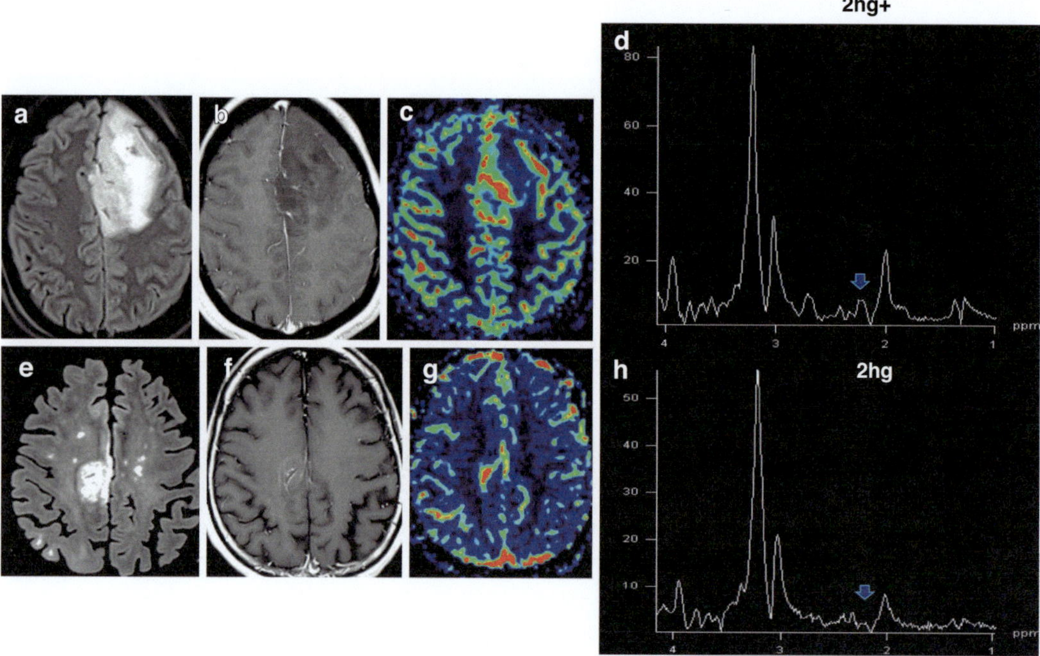

Fig. 2.29 MRI FLAIR (**a**), post-contrast T1WI (**b**), CBV (**c**), and spectroscopy at 97 ms TE (**d**) in a patient with oligodendroglioma grade 2, vs. MRI FLAIR (**e**), post-contrast T1WI (**f**), CBV (**g**), and spectroscopy at 97 ms TE (**h**) in a patient with GBM. The spectroscopy acquisition was a PRESS 97 ms with a postprocessing analysis performed through the LC model statistical evaluation. On conventional imaging the two lesions are quite similar, but a small peak of 2-hydroxyglutarate is detectable in D showing the presence of an IDH mutation in the oligodendroglioma case. (Courtesy Dr. R. Liserre, Brescia)

blastomas demonstrate apparent contiguous pathways of spread between different foci and should be differentiated from the so-called multicentric glioblastomas where different foci are widely separated (Figs. 2.27, 2.30, and 2.31). On careful histological evaluation however only a very small percentage of the multicentric glioblastomas are real independent tumors (WHO 2021).

The gliomatosis cerebri pattern refers to an extensive involvement of the brain at clinical diagnosis with involvement of at least three lobes in both hemispheres (Fig. 2.30), together with possible deep gray matter nuclei and/or brainstem and cerebellum involvement. This pattern can be encountered for any type of glioma and not only for glioblastoma.

Spread. The growth and spread of a glioblastoma could be extremely rapid as shown in Fig. 2.25, where the first histological diagnosis was an astrocytoma grade 2, but the MR follow-up studies at 4 and 5 months from the first MR study clearly showed a very rapid increase of the residual tumor with heterogeneous and infiltrative pattern and the final molecular diagnosis has been a glioblastoma IDH-wildtype.

Infiltrative spread is a typical feature of all types of diffuse gliomas, but this feature is expressed at its greatest level in case of glioblatomas. Infiltrative cells can be located both inside and outside the contrast-enhancing rim of glioblastoma and in some case infiltrative tumoral cells can be identified well far from the enhancing tumoral mass. This pattern of growth is one of the main obstacles to any therapy, being by definition impossible on the basis of neuroimaging to precisely define the real border and limit of the neoplasm.

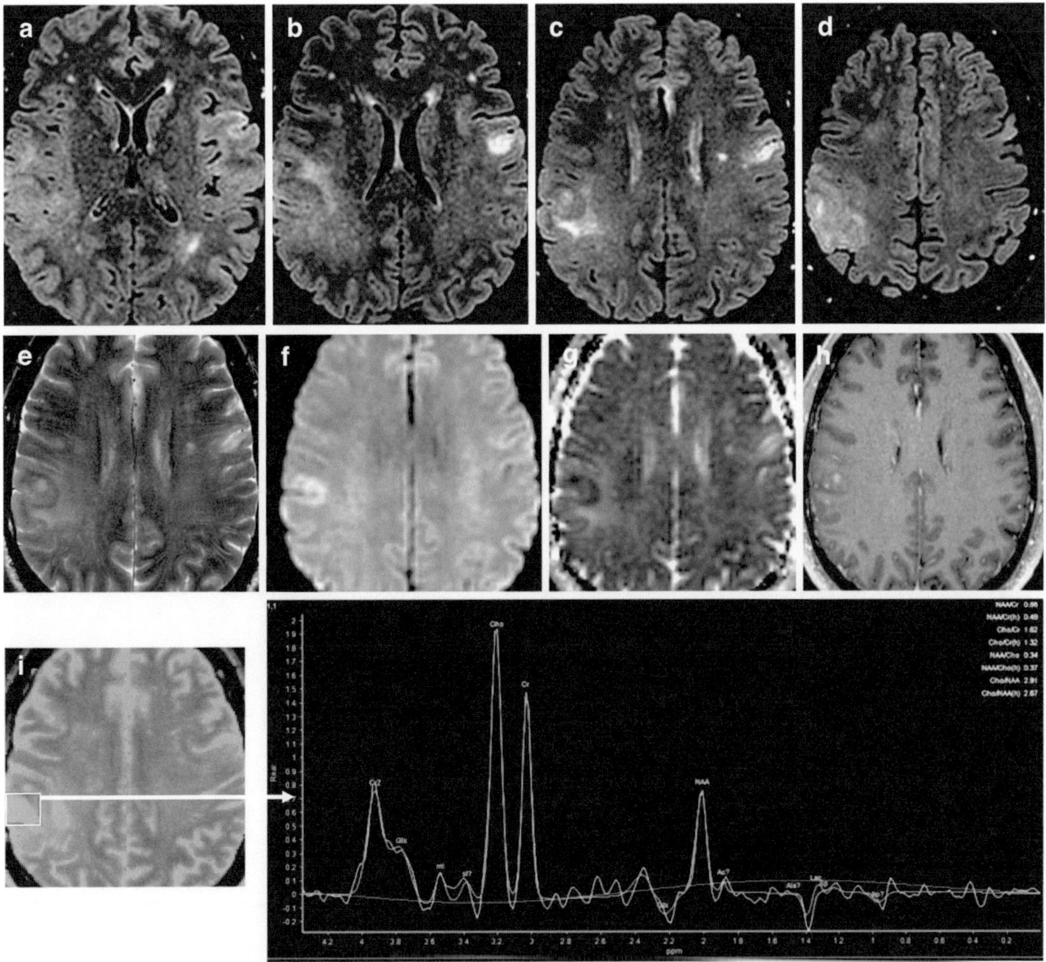

Fig. 2.30 Multicentric glioblastoma IDH-wildtype. MRI FLAIR images (**a–d**). On FLAIR images at least three localizations of the tumor are visible, in these four axial sections, at the level of right temporo-fronto-parietal lobes and in left frontal and frontomesial areas. MRI T2WI (**e**), FLAIR (**f**), ADC (**g**), post-contrast T1WI (**h**), and single voxel spectroscopy (**i**) at the level of the section in (**c**). The largest location of this tumor exhibits a more aggressive pattern with ADC restriction, contrast enhancement, and marked NAA reduction

Neoplastic cells grow primarily along white matter fiber, but they can also infiltrate gray matter, ependymal cells along the ventricular walls (Figs. 2.32 and 2.33) or the dural sheaths (Fig. 2.34).

Tumoral seeding within the cerebrospinal fluid is possible, but systemic metastases are exceedingly uncommon.

Differential diagnosis. Glioblastomas should be differentiated from a number of lesions both neoplastic and non-neoplastic. Abscesses are the main non-neoplastic differential diagnosis, whereas between the brain neoplasms the most frequent differential diagnosis is with: astrocytomas grade 3 or 4 (Figs. 2.11, 2.12, 2.13, and 2.14), lymphoma and metastases. Imaging features of glioblastoma are summarized in Table 2.8.

Post-treatment changes. Glioblastomas IDH-wildtype has a severe prognosis with a mean survival of 9–15 months even though some progress in survival has been achieved with combined

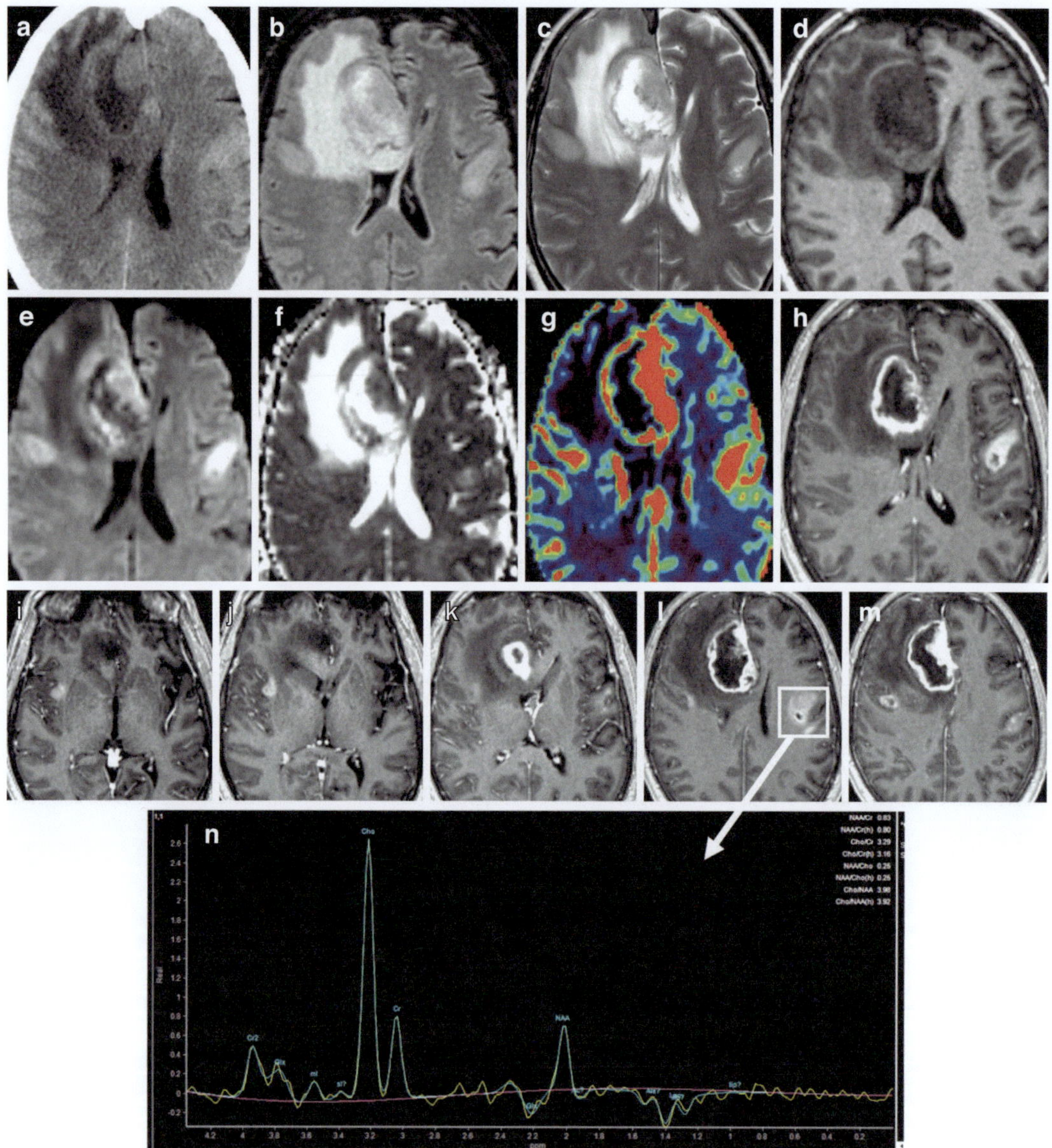

Fig. 2.31 Multifocal/multicentric glioblastoma IDH-wildtype. CT (**a**). MRI FLAIR (**b**), T2WI (**c**), T1WI (**d**), DWI (**e**), ADC (**f**), CBV (**g**), post-contrast T1WI (**h-m**), spectroscopy (**n**). A large inhomogeneous tumor is visible in right frontal region, but at least other two lesions are visible in the right insular region and in the left posterior and inferior fronto-insular area. All the lesions exhibit a clear CBV increase, and show an irregular enhancement after contrast administration. Spectroscopy of the left frontal lesion demonstrates a marked increase of Cho/NAA ratio

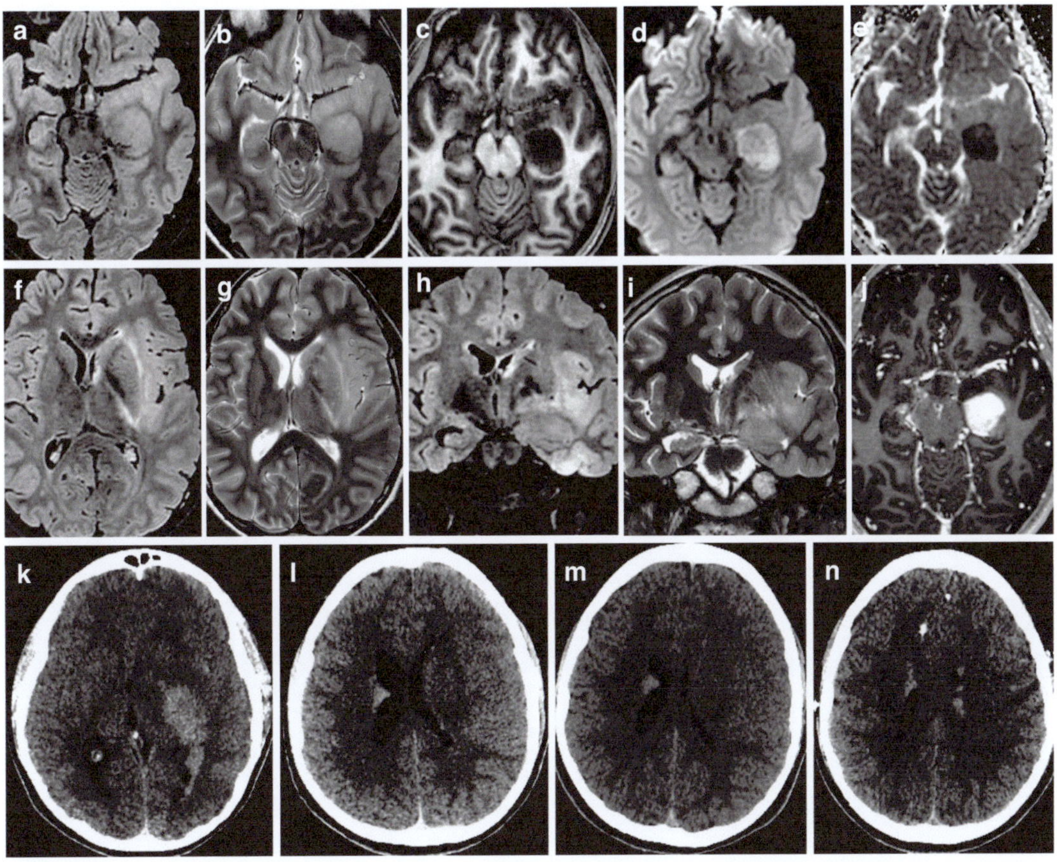

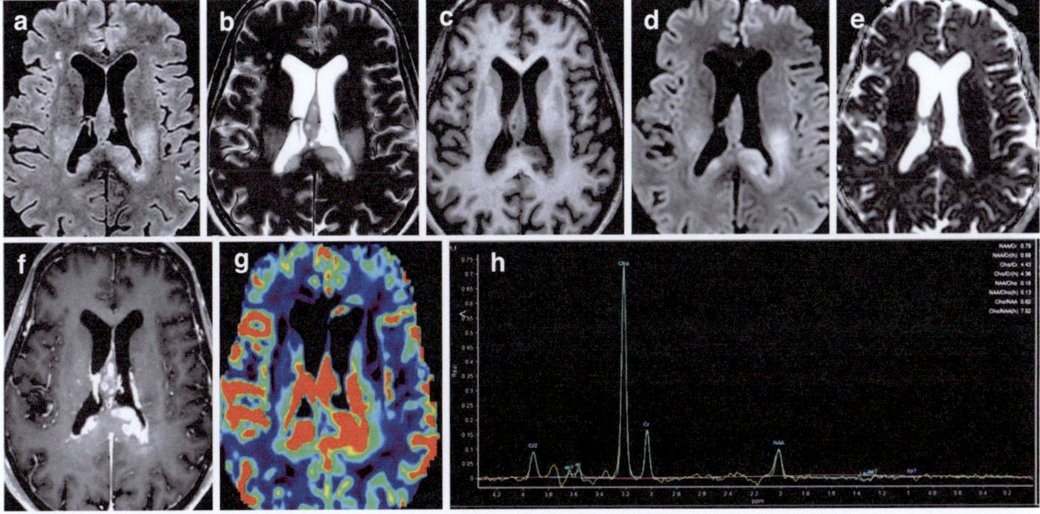

Fig. 2.32 Glioblastoma IDH-wildtype. MRI FLAIR (**a, f, h**), T2WI (**b, g, i**), T1WI (**c**), DWI (**d**), ADC (**e**), post-contrast T1WI (**j**). Large nodular lesion in left tempor-mesial region with a clear homogeneous diffusion restricton (**d, e**) and post-contrast enhancement (**j**). A diffuse infiltrative involvement of ipsilateral insular region is as well evident (**f–i**). The 1 month CT follow-up study demonstrates the rapid growth of the tumor and its diffusion along ventricular wall. CT (**k-n**)

Fig. 2.33 Glioblastoma IDH-wildtype. MRI FLAIR (**a**), T2WI (**b**), T1WI (**c**), DWI (**d**), ADC (**e**), post-contrast T1WI (**f**), CBV (**g**), spectroscopy (**h**). The neoplasm is primarily located within the splenium of the corpus callosum with a secondary spreading along the subependymal region of both lateral ventricles

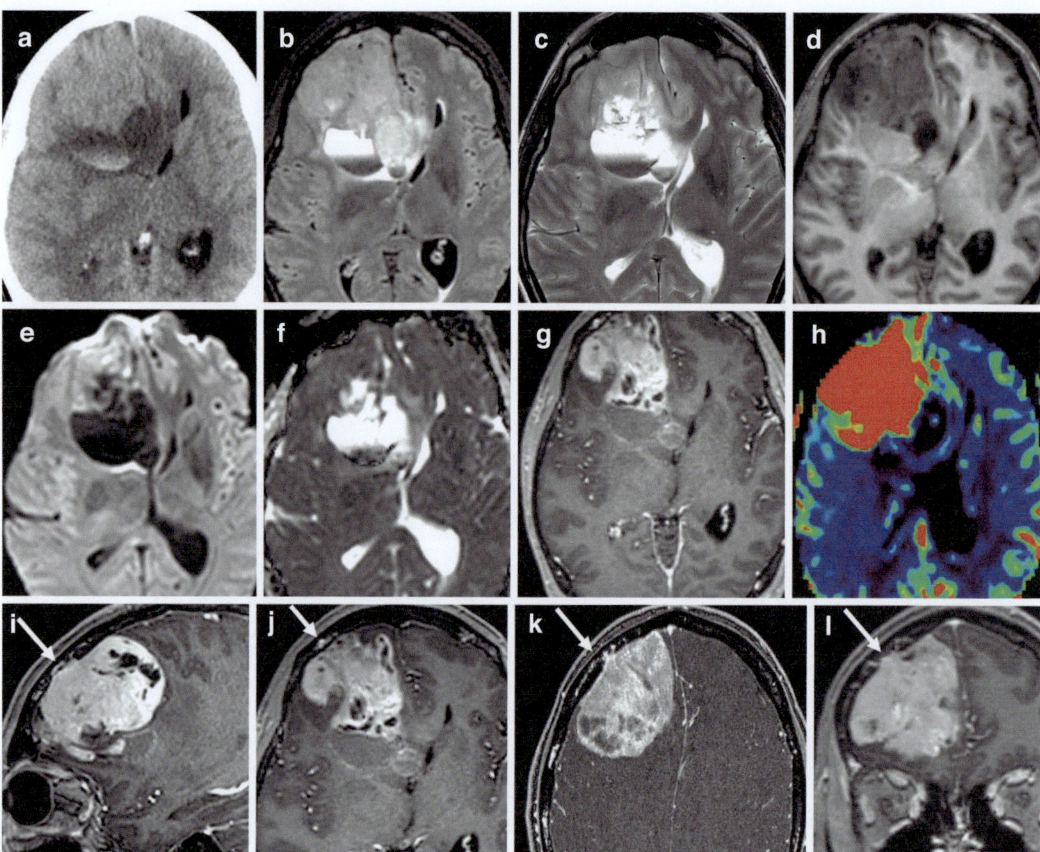

Fig. 2.34 Glioblastoma IDH-wildtype. CT (**a**). MRI FLAIR (**b**), T2WI (**c**), T1WI (**d**), DWI (**e**), ADC (**f**), post-contrast T1WI (**g, i-l**), CBV (**h**). A large inhomogeneous right frontal lesion with a marked increase of CBV. There is a diffuse invasion of the leptomeninges with an apparent infiltration of the diploic vessels (arrows **I-L**)

Table 2.8 Glioblastoma imaging features

Mass effect		Edema	Inhomogeneity		Cysts	Necrosis		Hemorrhage		Calcifications
+/+++		+/+++	+/+++		++	+++		++		0/+

CT	T1	T2	FLAIR	DWI	ADC	T1 Gd	CBV	Spec
○	◐	◐	○	○	◐	+++	●	↑↑↑Cho/NAA

therapy. In the original study of Stupp and colleagues [11] the two-year survival rate was 26.5% for patients with glioblastoma treated with radiotherapy plus temozolomide and 10.4% for patients treated with radiotherapy alone.

Recurrencies can however appear after few months after starting therapy either in the previous site of the original tumor (Fig. 2.35) or at a distance (Fig. 2.36).

Tumor recurrencies present all the MR features of the original tumor with diffusion restriction, CBV increase, and increased Cho/NAA ratio.

Radiotherapy alone, and more frequently combined therapy, can cause an acute reaction after a time interval of weeks to about 3 months with rupture of the blood–brain barrier that mimics tumor progression and for this reason called pseudoprogression. The pathophysiology of pseudoprogression is not completely understood, but this condition is exceedingly frequent in patients with glioblastoma IDH-wildtype and

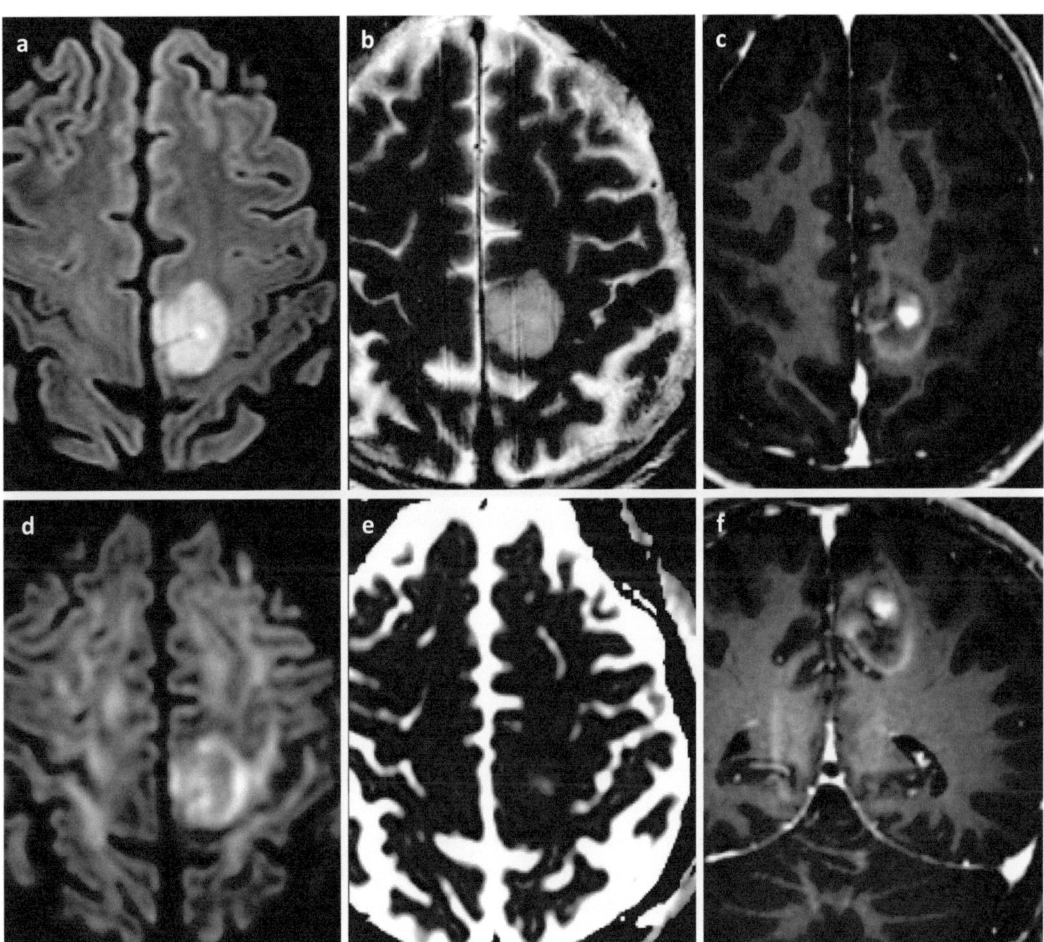

Fig. 2.35 Glioblastoma IDH-wildtype. MRI FLAIR (**a**), T2WI (**b**), post-contrast T1WI (**c**, **f**), DWI (**d**), ADC (**e**). Left rolandic tumor with mild diffusion restriction and irregular enhancement. 11 months follow-up after combined tratment. MRI FLAIR (**g**), T2WI (**h**), post-contrast T1WI (**i**), DWI (**j**) ADC (**k**), CBV (**l**). The MRI follow-up study shows a diffuse tumor recurrence spreading through the periventricular white matter and corpus callosum with marked increase in CBV and diffusion restriction

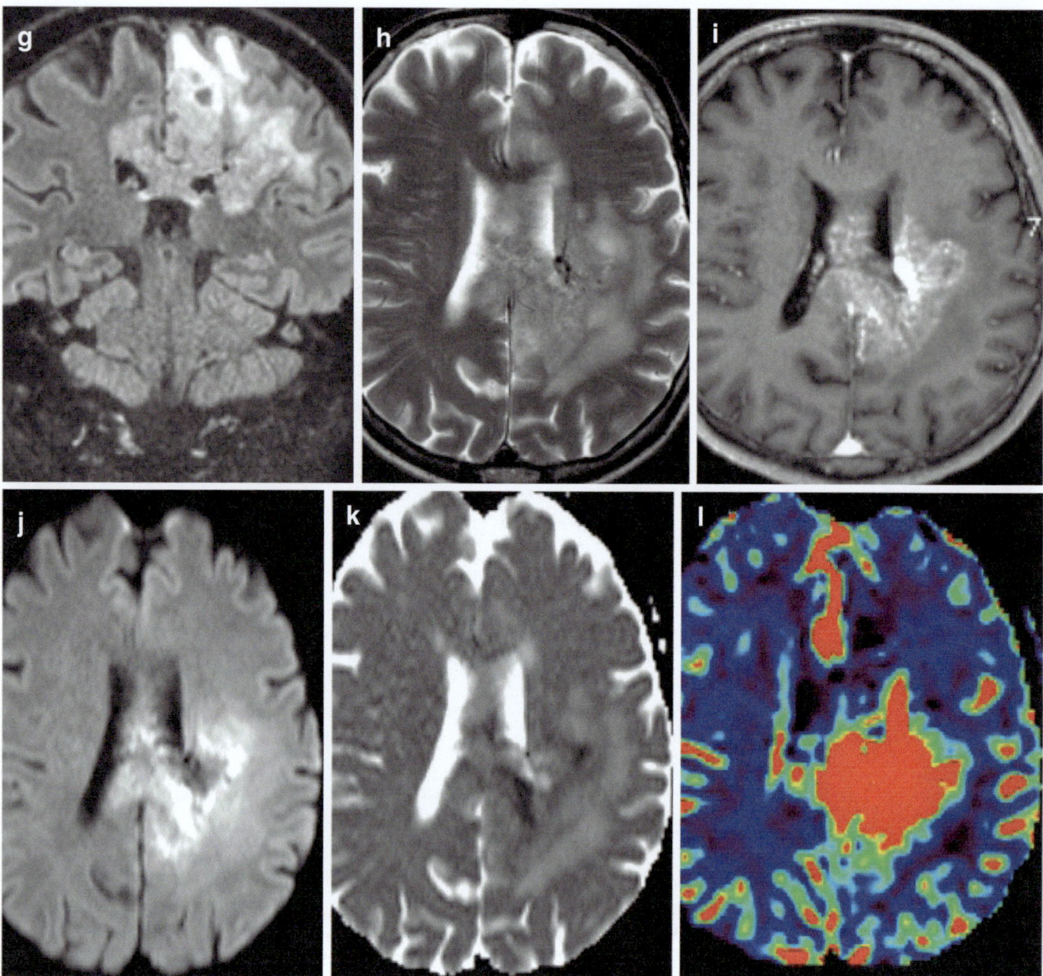

Fig. 2.35 (continued)

O(6)-methylguanine-DNA methyltransferase (MGMT) methylation status (Fig. 2.37).

Usually, pseudoprogression can be differentiated from true progression due to a normal o reduced CBV and a normal or reduced diffusion.

The other major consequence of therapy is *radionecrosis,* but differently from pseudoprogression it can be detected from at least 3 months after therapy to three, or sometimes more, years. Radionecrosis is a chronic inflammatory process with brain–blood barrier breakdown, vascular ectasia, and/or telangiectasia, and it can be progressive and sometimes difficult to treat. Similarly with pseudoprogression the differential diagnosis with a tumor recurrence is related to the presence of a normal or reduced CBV and a normal diffusion, even spectroscopy does not show an increase of Cho/NAA ratio (Fig. 2.38).

Sometimes radionecrosis can present as a large growing lesion with mass effect, but even in this case the diffusion is normal. In Fig. 2.39 a 6-year-old girl has been treated with combined therapy for an aggressive embryonal tumor. After 1 year she developed a large frontal lesion near the original tumor with mass effect and progressive enhancement. On DWI the lesion did not show any restriction and it slowly decreased after steroid therapy.

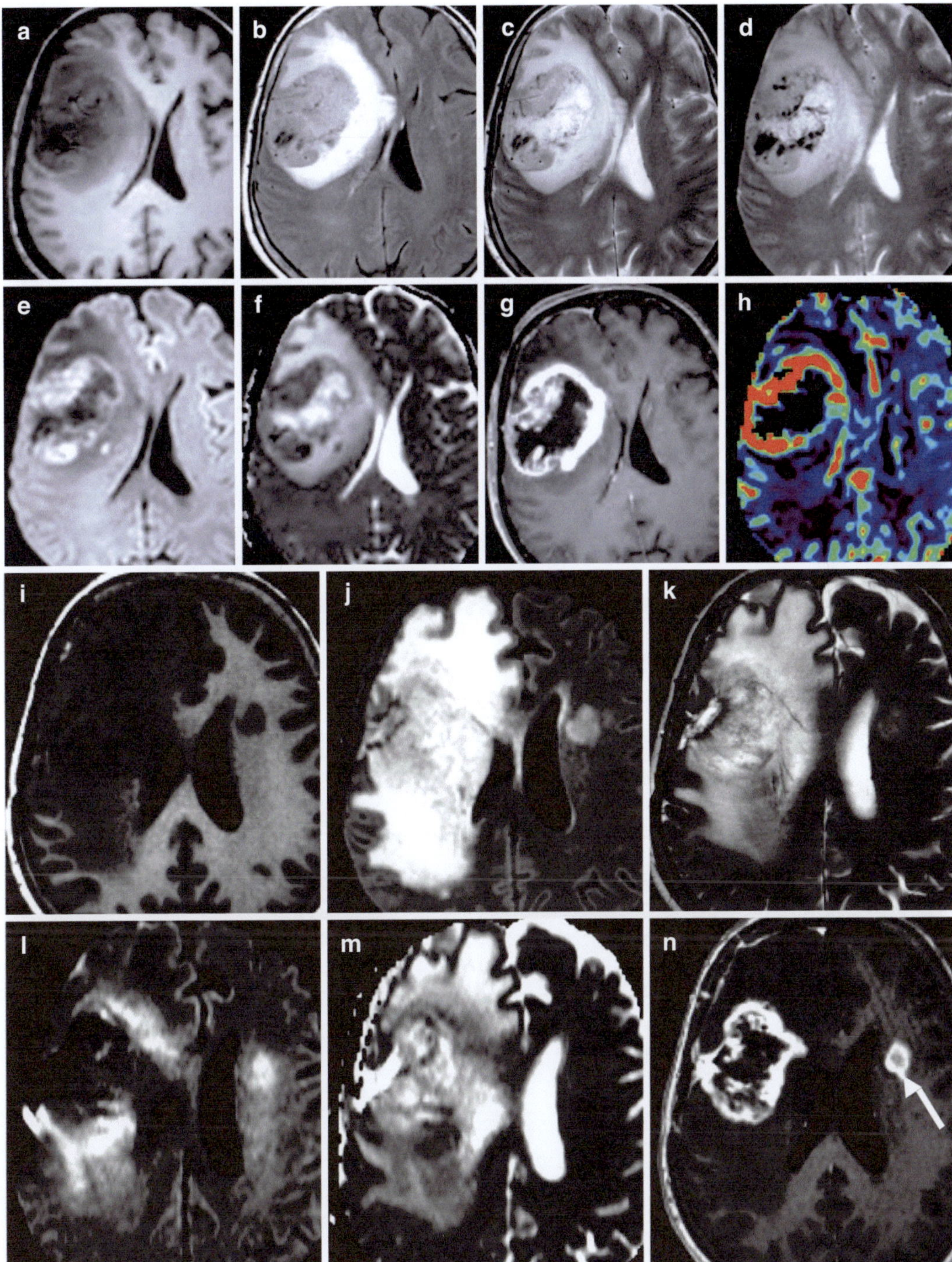

Fig. 2.36 Glioblastoma IDH-wildtype. MRI T1WI (**a**), FLAIR (**b**), T2WI (**c**), T2*WI (**d**) DWI (**e**), ADC (**f**), post-contrast T1WI (**g**), CBV (**h**). Large right frontal aggressive neoplasm, with diffusion restriction, irregular enhancement, and increased CBV. Six months follow-up after surgery and combined therapy. MRI T1WI (**i**), FLAIR (**j**), T2WI (**k**), DWI (**l**) ADC (**m**), post-contrast T1WI (**n**). In the site of the original tumor an irregular but nonspecific enhancement is visible; however, another lesion with restriction diffusion and post-contrast enhancement (arrow **n**) is visible in the left hemisphere

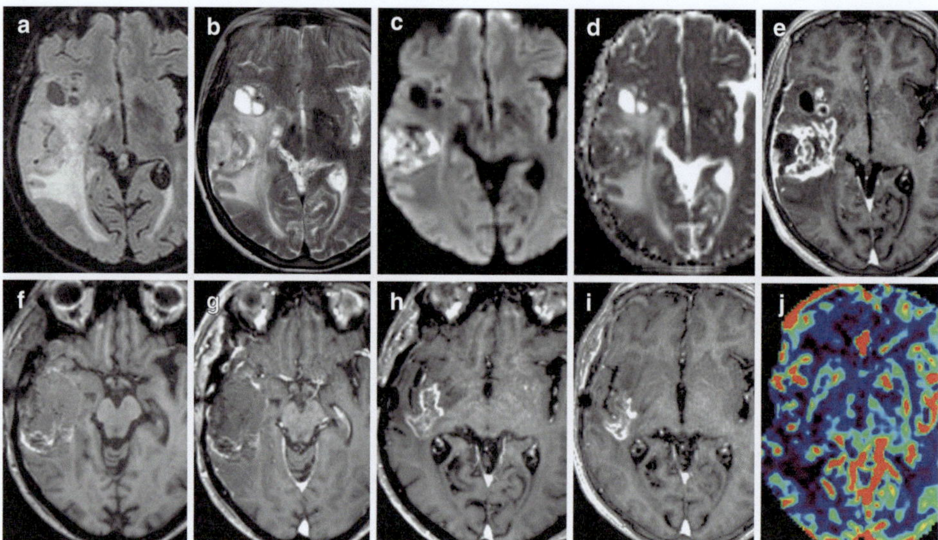

Fig. 2.37 Glioblastoma IDH-wildtype, with MGMT methylation. MRI FLAIR (**a**), T2WI (**b**), DWI (**c**), ADC (**d**), post-contrast T1WI (**e**). Large left temporal heterogeneous tumor with irregular enhancement. MRI T1W1 (**f**), post-contrast T1WI (**g**). MR study 5 days after surgery resection does not show residual enhancement. MRI post-contrast T1WI (**h**) 3 months follow-up after combined therapy shows a diffuse enahcement in the left temporo-insular region. MRI post-contrast T1WI (**i**), CBV (**j**) 7 months after combined therapy the enhancing lesion is less evident and CBV is reduced

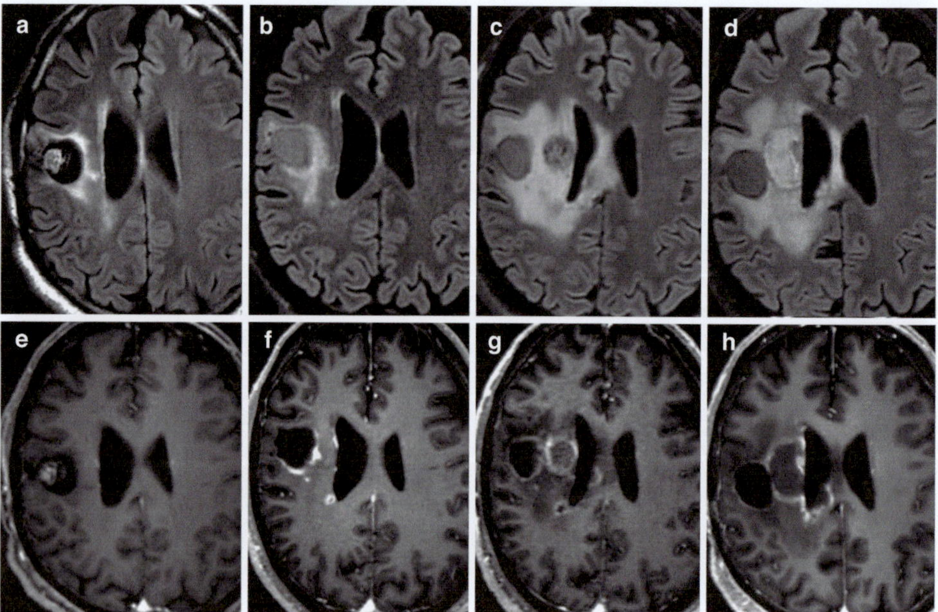

Fig. 2.38 Radionecrosis. MRI FLAIR (**a–d**), post-contrast T1WI (**e–h**). A lesion diagnosed as glioblastoma IDH-wildtype was operated and treated with combined therapy in 2016 (**a, e**). Three years later an irregular area of post-contrast enhancement appeared (**b, f**) and progressively grow in the subsequent follow-up studies (**c, g** and **d, h**). Last follow-up study at 9 months. MRI FLAIR (**i**), post-contrast T1WI (**j**), CBV (**k**), k-trans (**l**), SWI (**m**), spectroscopy (**n**). The lesion seems stabilized and shows a CBV reduction and low k-trans, the spectroscopy is almost normal and SWI demonstrates multiple microhemorrhagic foci

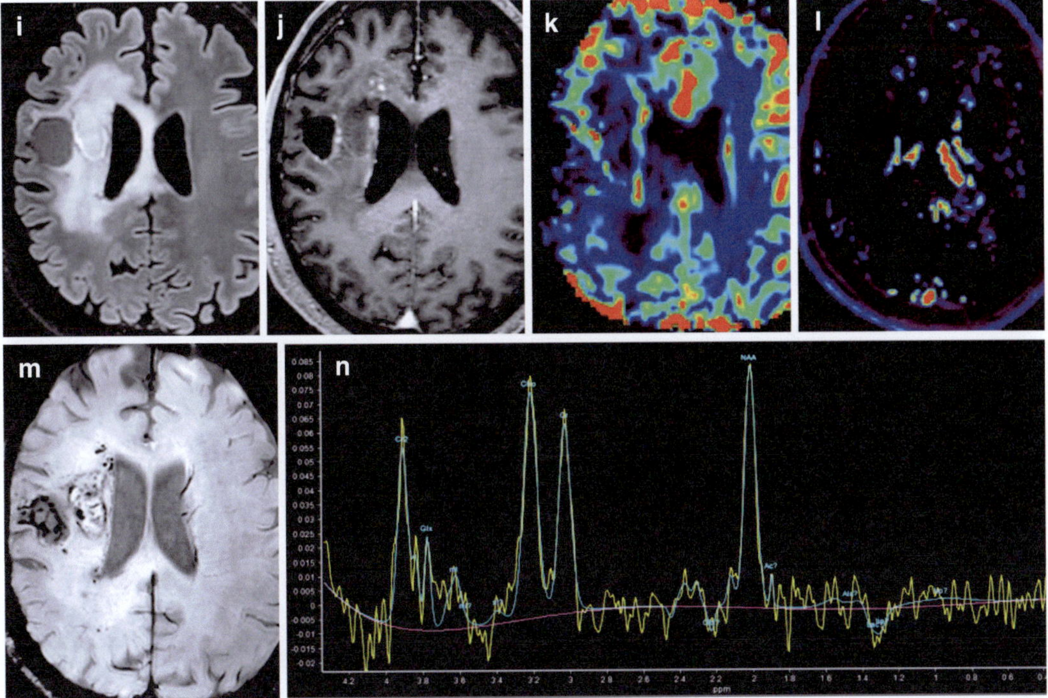

Fig. 2.38 (continued)

Other late effects of radiotherapy are:

- A progressive nonspecific leukoencephalopathy (Fig. 2.39).
- The development of vascular lesions and anomalies: microhemorrhages (Fig. 2.38), mineralizing vasculopathy, telangiectasias, a progressive moyamoya pattern, and cavernous angiomas (Fig. 2.40).
- The development of secondary tumors mainly: meningiomas, gliomas, and sarcomas.

The imaging features of pseudoprogression and radionecorsis are summarized in Table 2.9

2.1.4 Gliosarcoma

WHO definition. The designation of gliosarcoma should be reserved for tumors showing prominent mesenchymal differentiation, characterized by a biphasic pattern with alternating areas displaying glial and mesenchymal differentiation.

Metaplastic changes in glioblastoma may be mesenchymal (gliosarcoma) or epithelial (epithe-lioid glioblastoma) being the latter quite more rare.

Sarcomatous metaplasia is encountered most often in glioblastoma; however, it is rarely possible also in IDH-mutant astrocytomas or in oligodendrogliomas (oligosarcoma).

Gliosarcoma can also arise secondarily after conventional adjuvant treatment of high-grade glioma.

Gliosarcoma is an aggressive WHO grade 4 tumor.

Epidemiology. It is a rare tumor which, acorrding to WHO 2021 represents 2% of all glioblastomas. It occurs usually in the same age group of glioblastoma.

Location. The cerebral hemispheres are the more frequent location with a prevalence in temporal region, a dural component is possible.

Clinical features. As for the other intracranial tumors symptoms depend on the clinical location and vary from epileptic seizures, to focal neurological deficits to behavioral and cognitive symptoms.

Prognosis. Prognosis is similar to glioblastoma.

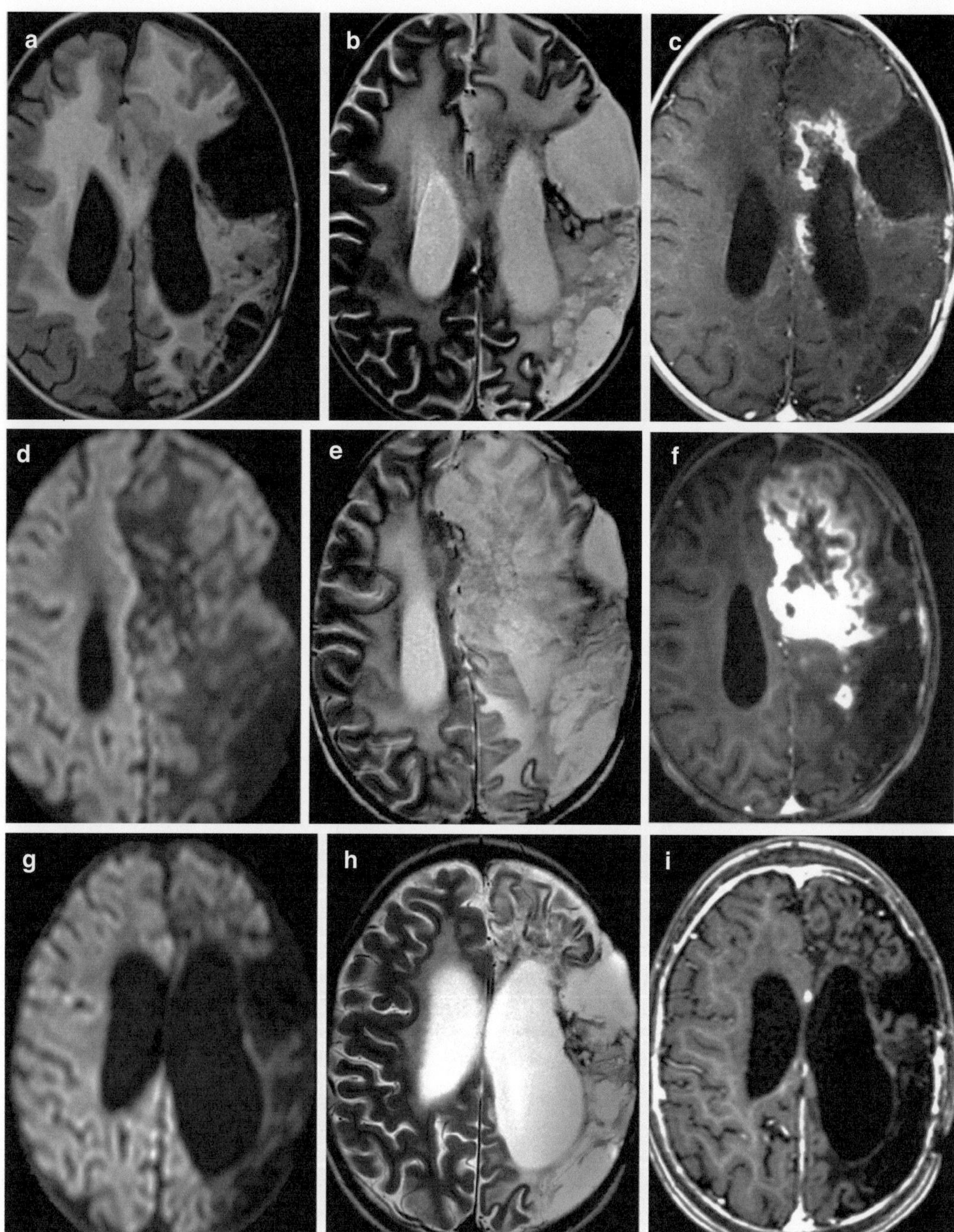

Fig. 2.39 Radionecrosis. MRI FLAIR (**a**), T2WI (**b**, **e**, **h**), DWI (**d**, **g**) post-contrast T1WI (**c**, **f**, **i**). After 1 year from combined therapy for an aggressive embryonal tumor this 6-year-old girl showed an area of diffuse enhancement near the previous lesions (**a**, **b**, **c**). In the 3 months follow-up the enhancing area was strikingly increased involving all the left frontal pole, (**d**, **e**, **f**), but diffusion is normal or increased (**d**). After 2 years the lesions decrease with a progressive shrinking of the frontal pole. White matter is diffusely hyperintense due to a post-radiation leukoencephalopathy

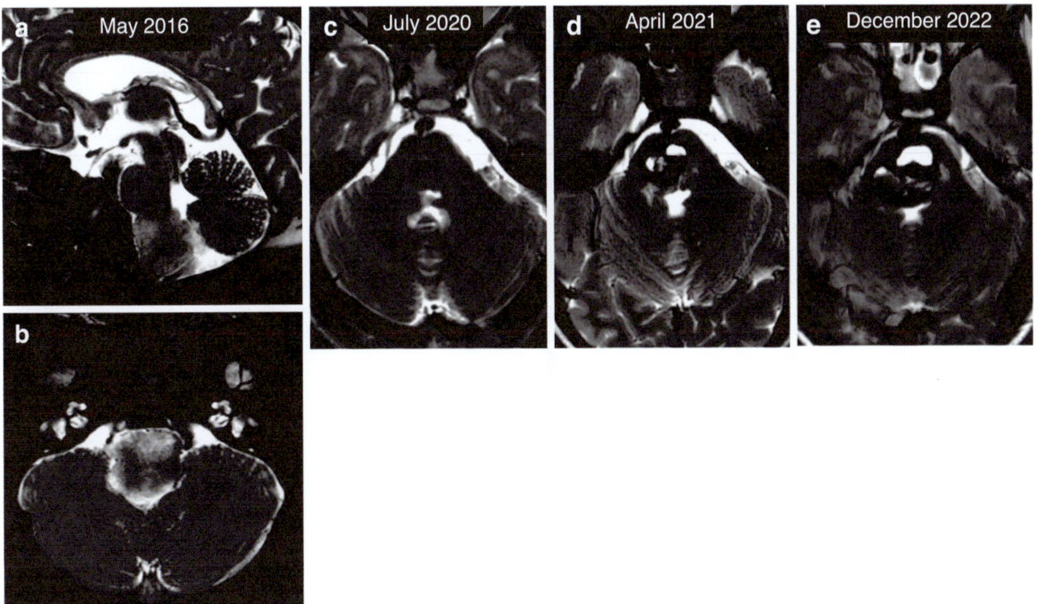

Fig. 2.40 Post-radiotherapy cavernous angioma in a 6-year-old boy. MRI T2WI at diagnosis (**a**, **b**) and in three different follow-up studies (**c-e**). This brainstem infiltrative glioma was treated with combined therapy. After 4 years a small cavernous angioma becomes evident within the pons and rapidly enlarges in the subsequent follow-up studies

Table 2.9 Pseudoprogression and radionecrosis imaging features

Mass effect	Edema	Inhomogeneity	Cysts	Necrosis	Hemorrhage	Calcifications
+/++	+/++	++	0	+/++	0	0/+

CT	T1	T2	FLAIR	DWI	ADC	T1 Gd	CBV	Spec
◉	◉	○	◯	◉	○	+/+++	●	↑ = Cho/NAA

Imaging. Differentiating a gliosarcoma from a glioblastoma is almost impossible. In both tumors there are inhomogeneous lesions with irregular enhancement necrotic cyst with possible hemorrhagic component. Some differences such as a greater degree of thickening of the cystic wall in gliosarcoma, with a higher rate of hemorrhage, or the presence of an eccentric cystic region are reported [12]. In a series of 25 cases all lesions contacted a dural, pial, or ependymal surface [13] and the presence of dural components could be another more specific feature of gliosarcoma (Fig. 2.41).

Diffusion is predominantly restricted; perfusion is increased, and spectroscopy shows a clear increase of Cho/NAA ratio (Fig. 2.41). Imaging features of Gliosarcoma are summarized in Table 2.10.

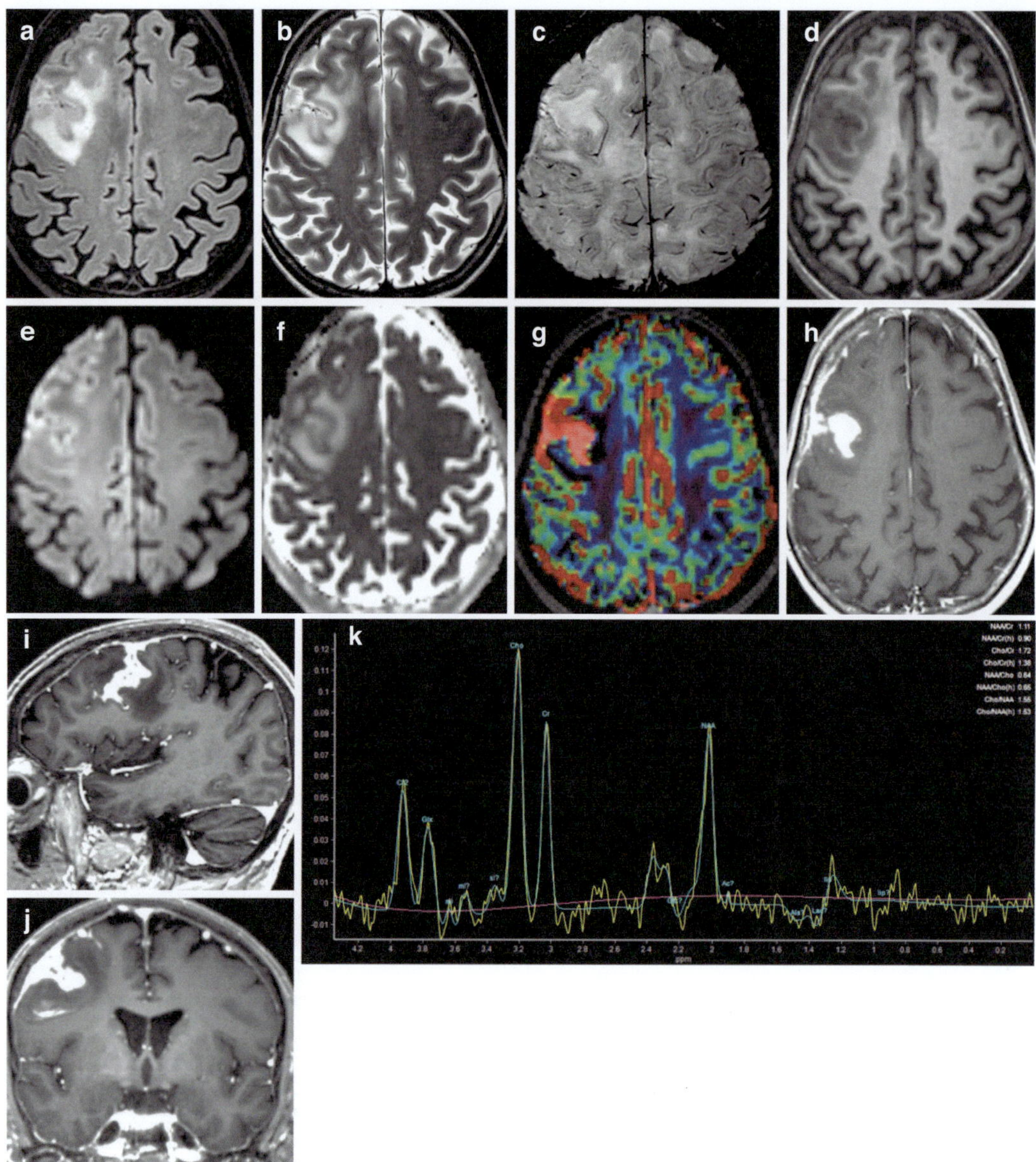

Fig. 2.41 Primary gliosarcoma. MRI FLAIR (**a**), T2WI (**b**), SWI (**c**), T1WI (**d**), DWI (**e**), ADC (**f**), CBV (**g**), post-contrast T1WI (**h, j**), spectroscopy (**k**). MRI study shows an inhomogeneous right frontal lesion predominately affecting the leptomeninges with an apparent dural tail. CBV is greatly increased and the enhancement is intense. No hemorrhagic components are visible on (**c**). Coronal and sagittal post-contrast studies well documented the extracerebral extension of the lesion, spectroscopy shows an increase of Cho/NAA ratio

Table 2.10 Gliosarcoma imaging features

Mass effect		Edema	Inhomogeneity		Cysts	Necrosis		Hemorrhage	Calcifications
+/+++		+/+++	+++		++	+++		++	0/+

CT	T1	T2	FLAIR	DWI	ADC	T1 Gd	CBV	Spec
○	●	●	○	○	●	+++	●	↑↑↑Cho/NAA

References

1. Patel SH, Laila M, Poisson LM, Brat DJ, et al. T2–FLAIR mismatch, an imaging biomarker for IDH and 1p/19q status in lower-grade gliomas: a TCGA/TCIA project. Clin Cancer Res. 2017;23:6078–85.
2. Pinto C, Noronha C, Taipa R, Ramos C. T2-FLAIR mismatch sign: a roadmap of pearls and pitfalls. Br J Radiol. 2021;95:20210825.
3. Do YA, Cho SJ, Choi BS, et al. IDH-mutant, 1p/19q noncodeleted low-grade glioma: an updated systematic review and meta-analysis. Neurooncol Adv. 2022;4(1):vdac010. https://doi.org/10.1093/noajnl/vdac010.
4. Park SI, Suh CH, Guenette JP, Huang RK, Kim HS. The T2-FLAIR mismatch sign as a predictor of IDH-mutant, 1p/19q-noncodeleted lower-grade gliomas: a systematic review and diagnostic meta-analysis. Eur Radiol. 2021;31:5289–99.
5. Deguchi S, Oishi T, Mitsuya K, et al. Clinicopathological analysis of T2-FLAIR mismatch sign in lower- grade gliomas. Sci Rep. 2020;10:10113.
6. Autry AW, Lafontaine M, Jalbert L, et al. Spectroscopic imaging of D-2-hydroxyglutarate and other metabolites in pre-surgical patients with IDH-mutant lower-grade gliomas. J Neurooncol. 2022;159:43–52.
7. Branzoli F, Di Stefano AL, Capelle L, et al. Highly specific determination of *IDH* status using edited in vivo magnetic resonance spectroscopy. Neuro Oncol. 2018;20:907–16.
8. Corell A, Ferreyra Vega S, Hoefling N, et al. The clinical significance of the T2-FLAIR mismatch sign in grade II and III gliomas: a population-based study. BMC Cancer. 2020;20:450.
9. Central Brain Tumor Registry od the United States. CBTRUS 2020. https://cbtrus.org/.
10. POLA – National POLA Network for the Treatment of High-Grade Oligodendroglial Tumors; update 2015. https://epidemiologie-france.aviesan.fr/fr/content/view/full/87575.
11. Stupp R, Mason WP, van den Bent MJ, et al. N Engl J Med. 2005;352:987–96.
12. Yi X, Cao H, Tang H, et al. Gliosarcoma: a clinical and radiological analysis of 48 cases. Eur Radiol. 2019;29:429–38.
13. Peckham ME, Osborn AG, Palmer CA, Tsai A, Salzman KL. Gliosarcoma: neuroimaging and immunohistochemical findings. J Neuroimaging. 2019;29:126–32.

Gliomas, Glioneuronal Tumors, and Neuronal Tumors: Pediatric and Circumscribed Gliomas

3

3.1 Pediatric-Type Diffuse Low-Grade Gliomas

3.1.1 Diffuse Astrocytoma *MYB*-or *MYBL1*-Altered

WHO definition. Diffuse astrocytoma *MYB*- or *MYBL1*-altered is a diffusely infiltrative astroglial neoplasm composed of monomorphic cells with genetic alterations in *MYB* or *MYBL1*.

It is a WHO grade 1 tumor.

Epidemiology. It is a rare pediatric tumor with apparently no sex prevalence, the largest series contains 20 patients.

Location. It is mainly located in the cerebral hemispheres with both cortical and subcortical components.

Clinical features. It is typically associated with drug-resistant epileptic seizures.

Prognosis. Data on long-term follow-up are scarce, but the prognosis is considered to be favorable. The tumor presents an extremely slow growth and a very low recurrence rate if completely resected.

Imaging: These tumors are hyperintense both on FLAIR and T2WI and hypointense on T1WI, contrast enhancement is never observed [1]. Most lesions are well confined with a sharp margin. The case in Fig. 3.1 shows a well-delimited cortical and subcortical lesion with increased diffusion, decreased CBV, and increased Cho/NAA ratio. Imaging features of diffuse astrocytoma

MYB- or *MYBL1*-altered are summarized in Table 3.1.

3.1.2 Angiocentric Glioma

WHO definition. Angiocentric glioma is a diffuse glioma composed mainly of thin cytological bland, bipolar cells aggregating are least partly in perivascular spaces. This tumor has a *MYB::QKI* gene fusion.

It is a WHO grade 1 tumor.

Epidemiology. Is a rare tumor with no clear epidemiological data, most cases occur in children and young adults with a median age of 13 years.

Location. It is typically a cortical tumor even though some brainstem locations are reported.

Clinical features. It is mainly associated with intractable partial epilepsy.

Prognosis. If completely resected the prognosis is favorable.

Imaging. It is usually located in the frontal or temporal lobe and well circumscribed even though some inhomogeneous aspects could be present.

It is hyperintense on FLAIR and T2WI and the most typical appearance is a T1WI hyperintensity which is not related to either the presence of calcification or the presence of hemorrhages (Fig. 3.2). A stalk-like extension to the adjacent ventricle has been reported. There is no enhancement after the

© The Author(s), under exclusive license to Springer Nature Switzerland AG 2023
F. M. Triulzi, *Neuroradiology of Brain Tumors*, https://doi.org/10.1007/978-3-031-38153-9_3

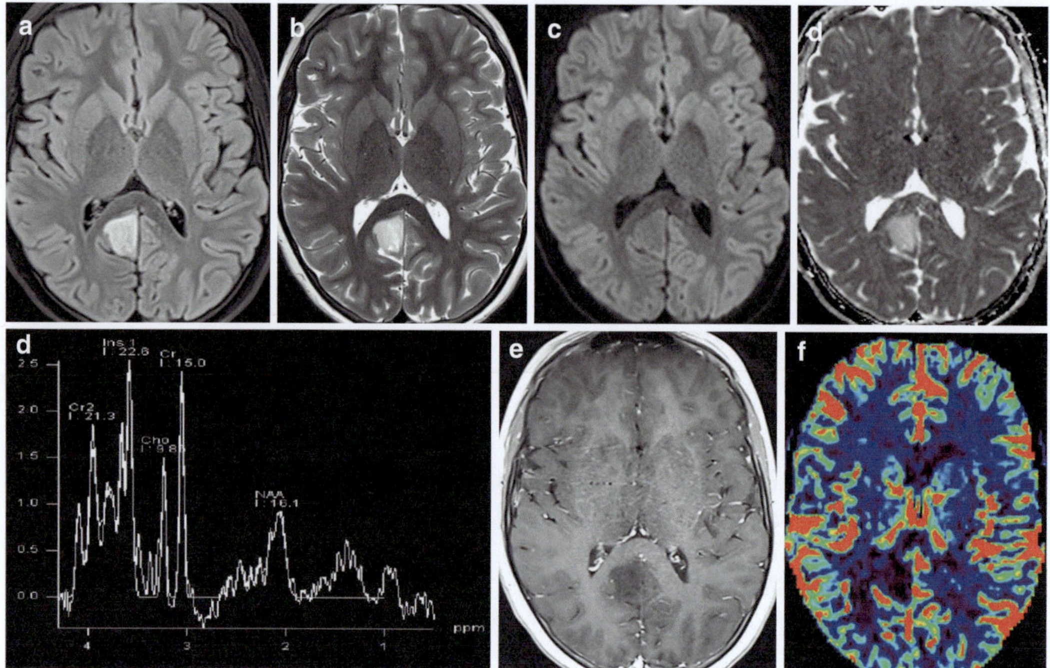

Fig. 3.1 Diffuse astrocytoma *MYB/MYBL1*-altered in a 10-year-old boy with epileptic seizures. MRI FLAIR (**a**), T2WI (**b**), DWI (**c**), ADC (**d**), spectroscopy (**e**), post-contrast T1WI (**f**), CBV (**g**). A well-delimited cortical–subcortical lesion hyperintense on T2WI/FLAIR sequences and hypointense on T1Wi is visible in the right occipito-mesial region. There is no enhancement after contrast administration (**f**), the CBV is reduced (**g**), and the spectroscopy shows an increase of Cho/NAA ratio (Courtesy Dr. S. Colafati, Rome)

Table 3.1 Diffuse astrocytoma *MYB*- or *MYBL1*-altered imaging features

Mass effect	Edema	Inhomogeneity	Cysts	Necrosis	Hemorrhage	Calcifications
0/+	0/+	0	0	0	0	0

CT	T1	T2	FLAIR	DWI	ADC	T1 Gd	CBV	Spec
◉	◉	○	○	◉	○	0	●	↑Cho/NAA

administration of contrast [2, 3]. Diffusion is usually increased. Spectroscopy shows the pattern of a slow growing tumor. Imaging features of angiocentric glioma are summarized in Table 3.2.

3.1.3 Polymorphous Low-Grade Neuroepithelial Tumor of the Young

WHO definition. Polymorphous low-grade neuroepithelial tumor of the young (PLNTY) is a slow growing tumor strongly associated with seizures in young individuals, frequent presence of oligodendroglioma-like components, calcification, CD34 immunoreactivity, and MAPK pathway-activating genetic abnormalities.

It is a WHO grade 1 tumor.

Epidemiology. It is a rare neoplasm with scarce epidemiological data. It is most frequently reported in the second and third decades with a median age at diagnosis of 16 years.

Location. It is a cortical–subcortical tumor with a predominant location in the temporal lobes (roughly 80% of cases), mostly in the medial and postero-inferior structures.

Clinical features. This tumor typically causes refractory epilepsy.

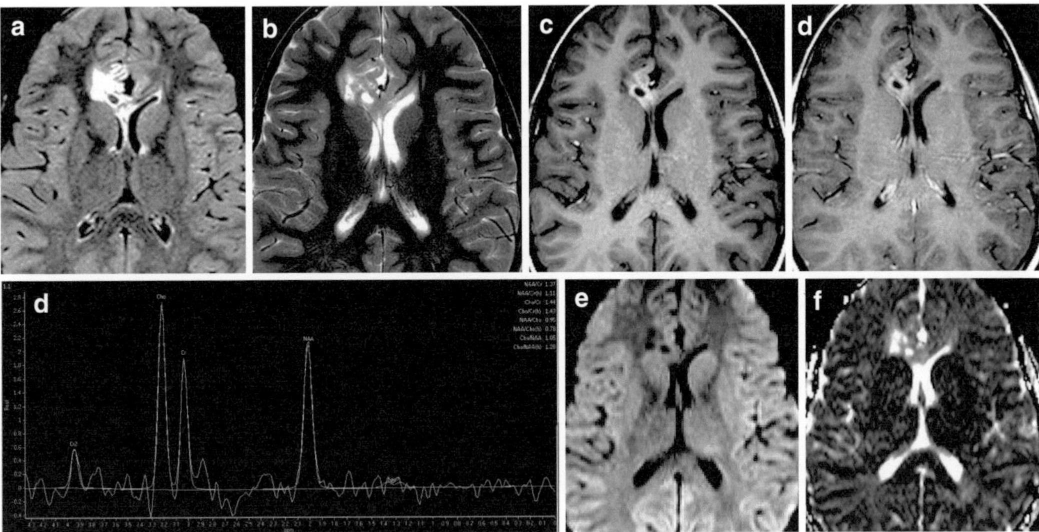

Fig. 3.2 Angiocentric glioma in a 12-year-old boy with epileptic seizures. MRI FLAIR (**a**), T2WI (**b**), T1WI (**c**), post-contrast T1WI (**d**), spectroscopy (**e**), DWI (**f**), ADC (**g**). An irregular lesion is visible in right frontomesial cortical area, it is mainly hyperintense on FLAIR and T2WI and presents a central aspect of spontaneous hyperintensity on T1WI (**c**), there is no enhancement after contrast (**d**) and the spectroscopy shows a pattern of a slow growing tumor with a slight increase of Cho/NAA ratio. (Courtesy Dr. L. Pinelli, Brescia)

Table 3.2 Angiocentric glioma imaging features

Mass effect	Edema	Inhomogeneity	Cysts	Necrosis	Hemorrhage	Calcifications
0/+	0/+	+/++	0/+	0	0	0/+

CT	T1	T2	FLAIR	DWI	ADC	T1 Gd	CBV	Spec
◓	○	○	○	●	◔	0	NA[a]	↑Cho/NAA

[a]NA (not available) = incomplete or sporadic reports

Prognosis. PLNTY is a grade 1 tumor and if completely resected the prognosis is good with complete or at least partial resolution of the seizures.

Imaging. Like other benign cortical–subcortical tumor PLNTY can show, cystic, solid, and calcific components.

The solid portion exhibits a T2WI/FLAIR hyperintensity and a T1 hypointensity.

Calcifications are frequent (Fig. 3.3) as well as cystic components (Fig. 3.4) even not specific for the diagnosis [4].

PLNTYs do not show enhancement after contrast administration.

Diffusion is normal or increased. PLNTY imaging feature are reported in Table 3.3.

3.1.4   Diffuse Low-Grade Glioma MAPK Pathway-Altered

WHO definition. Diffuse low-grade glioma MAPK pathway-altered is a low-grade glioma with diffuse astrocytic or oligodendroglial morphology that generally occurs in childhood and is characterized by a pathogenic alteration in a gene that codes for a MAPK pathway protein.

WHO 2021 considered three molecular subtypes:

(a) Diffuse low-grade glioma *FGFR1* tyrosine kinase domain-duplicated.
(b) Diffuse low-grade glioma *FGFR1*-mutant.
(c) Diffuse low-grade glioma *BRAF* p.V600E-mutant.

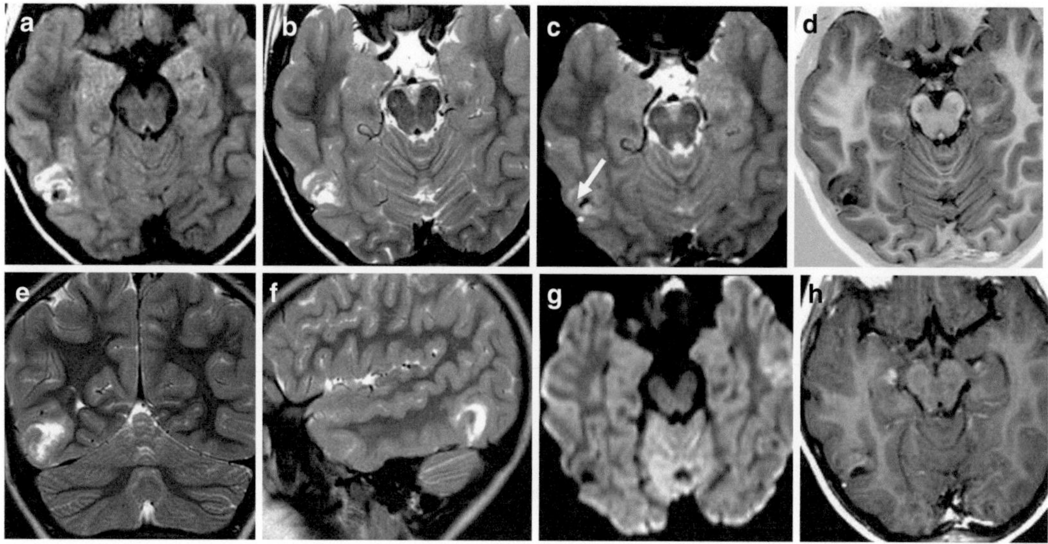

Fig. 3.3 PLNTY in a 7-year-old girl with epileptic seizures. MRI FLAIR (**a**), T2WI (**b**, **e**, **f**), T2*GRE (**c**), T1WI-IR (**d**), DWI (**g**), post-contrast T1WI (**h**). A cortico-subcortical lesion is present in the temporo-occipital right region with a parenchymal component hyperintense on T2 and FLAIR and a small calcification hypointense in all sequences (arrow C). No enhancement is visible after contrast administration (**h**). (Courtesy Dr. N. Colombo, Milan)

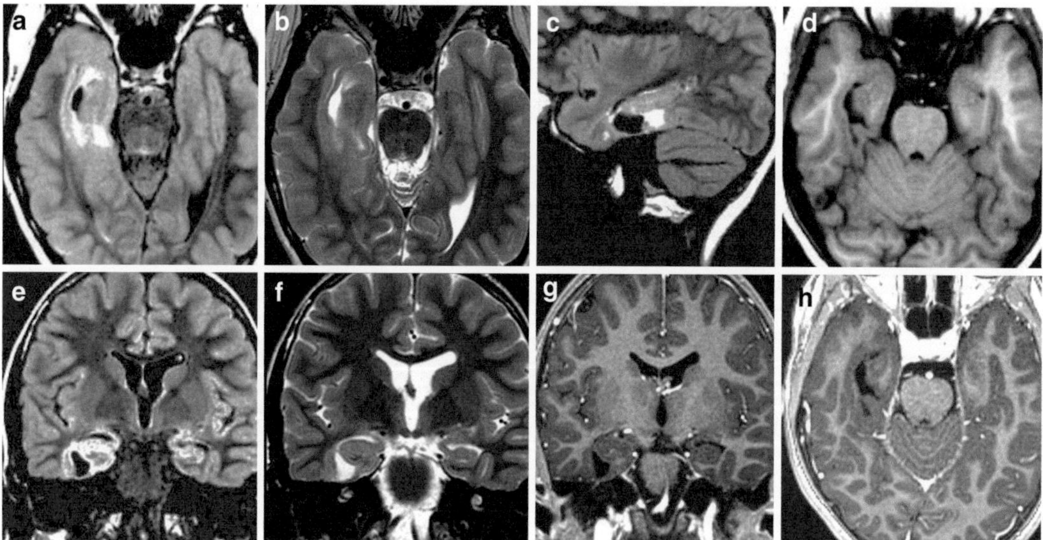

Fig. 3.4 PLNTY in a 10-year-old boy with epileptic seizures. MRI FLAIR (**a**, **c**, **e**), T2WI (**b**, **f**), T1WI (**d**), post-contrast T1WI (**g**), post-contrast T1WI-IR (**h**). A cortico-subcortical right temporo-mesial lesion with a cystic component is evident in the fusiform gyrus. Lesion borders are not clearly defined and the FLAIR hyperintensity can be related both to the solid portion and to a small amount of perilesional edema. (Courtesy Dr. N. Colombo, Milan)

Table 3.3 PLNTY imaging features

Mass effect	Edema	Inhomogeneity	Cysts	Necrosis	Hemorrhage	Calcifications
0/+	0/+	+/++	+/++	0	0	+/++

CT	T1	T2	FLAIR	DWI	ADC	T1 Gd	CBV	Spec
◐	◐	○	○	●	○	0	NAᵃ	↑Cho/NAA

ᵃNA (not available) = incomplete or sporadic reports

Epidemiology. There are no epidemiological data both due to the rarity of this neoplasm and to the previous confounding terminology such as *diffuse astrocytoma, pediatric-type oligodendroglioma,* etc.

Location. The most frequent location are the cerebral hemispheres.

Clinical features. It is frequently associated with epilepsy, but other signs and symptoms may be present.

Prognosis. There are no data on prognosis, even though these tumors show a very slow progression and the overall prognosis is favorable.

Imaging. Data on imaging are few and ambiguous due to the confused terminology. These are benign tumors with an hyperintense aspect on T2WI/FLAIR and hypointense aspect on T1WI, enhancement after contrast may be present [5, 6].

The case in Fig. 3.5 shows a reduced CBV, a slightly increased diffusion. and a quite normal Cho/NAA ratio, with a relatively high lipid-lactate peak, enhancement after contrast administration is absent. Imaging features of diffuse low-grade lioma MAPK pethway altered are summarized in Table 3.4.

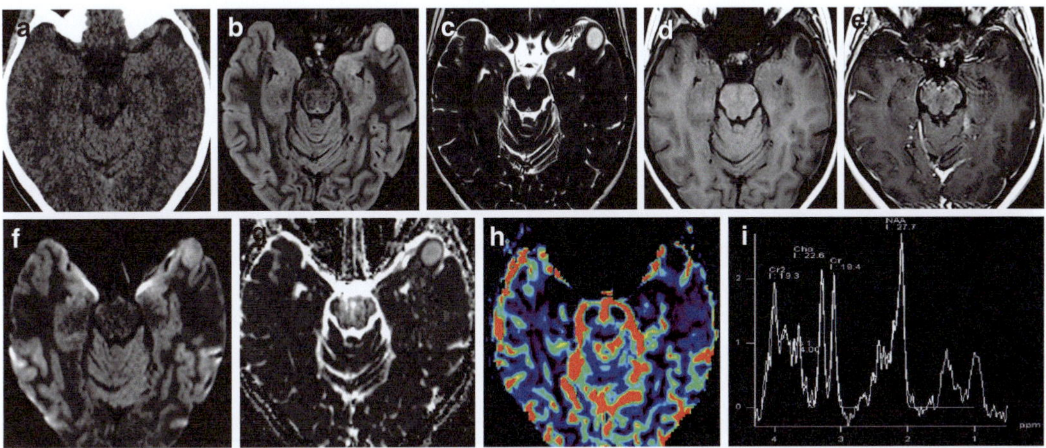

Fig. 3.5 Diffuse low-grade glioma MAPK pathway-altered in a 15-year-old girl. CT (**a**). MRI FLAIR (**b**), T2WI (**c**), T1WI (**d**), post-contrast T1WI (**e**), DWI (**f**), ADC (**g**), CBV (**h**), spectroscopy (**i**). A cortico-subcortical focal lesion is present in left temporal pole. It is a well demarcated lesion hyperitnesense on T2WI/FLAIR images (**b**, **c**) and hypointense on T1WI (**d**). Post-contrast enhancement seems to be absent (**e**), ADC is slightly increased (**g**), and CBV is clearly reduced (**h**). A lactate-lipid peak is evident (**i**).(Courtesy Dr. S. Colafati, Rome)

Table 3.4 Diffuse low-grade glioma MAPK pathway-altered imaging features

Mass effect	Edema	Inhomogeneity	Cysts	Necrosis	Hemorrhage	Calcifications
0/+	0/+	0	0/+	0	0	0

CT	T1	T2	FLAIR	DWI	ADC	T1 Gd	CBV	Spec
◐	◐	○	○	◐	○	0/+	●	NA[a]

[a]NA (not available) = incomplete or sporadic reports

3.2   Pediatric-Type Diffuse High-Grade Gliomas

3.2.1   Diffuse Midline Glioma H3 K27-Altered

WHO definition. Diffuse midline glioma (DMG) H3 K27-altered is an infiltrative midline glioma with loss of H3 pK28me3 (K27me3) and usually either an H3 c.83A > T p.K28M (K27K) substitution in one of the histone H3 isoform, aberrant overexpression of EZHIP, or an EGFR mutation.

It is a WHO grade 4 tumor.

Epidemiology. Diffuse intrinsic pontine gliomas (DIPGs) are 10–15% of all pediatric tumor and 75% of all pediatric brainstem tumor. They occur in 2.3 cases per one million person-years under 20 years of age with no sex prevalence and are rare in people >20 years of age.

Location. The diffuse midline gliomas (DMGs) arise most frequently in the pons (DIPG) and less frequently in the thalamus and the spinal cord. In thalamus DMGs are bithalamic in children and predominantly unilateral in adolescents or adults.

Clinical features. Due to the infiltrative behavior this tumor causes clinical symptoms later in its development and when diagnosed it is usually of large size. For DIPGs more typical clinical signs are related to cranial nerve neuropathies, whereas for thalamic tumors signs of increased intracranial pressure are the most common.

Prognosis. The presence of K27 M H3 mutation in any type of diffuse midline gliomas is related to a worse prognosis than that of wildtype cases, the survival rate at 2 years is less than 10% and it is even worst for DIPGs.

Imaging. DIPGs are centered on the pons and when diagnosed they typically involve more than 50% of its surface. Exophytic components may be present with possible basilar artery encasement. They appear as hypodense on CT, predominantly hypointense on T1WI, and hyperintense on T2. On FLAIR sequence the lesion could present an aspect similar to the mismatch T2-FLAIR sign reported in astrocytomas IDH-mutant grade 2 or 3 with areas of iso-hypointensity (Fig. 3.6). In DIPG the presence of mismatch T2-FLAIR sign has been reported to be associated with a

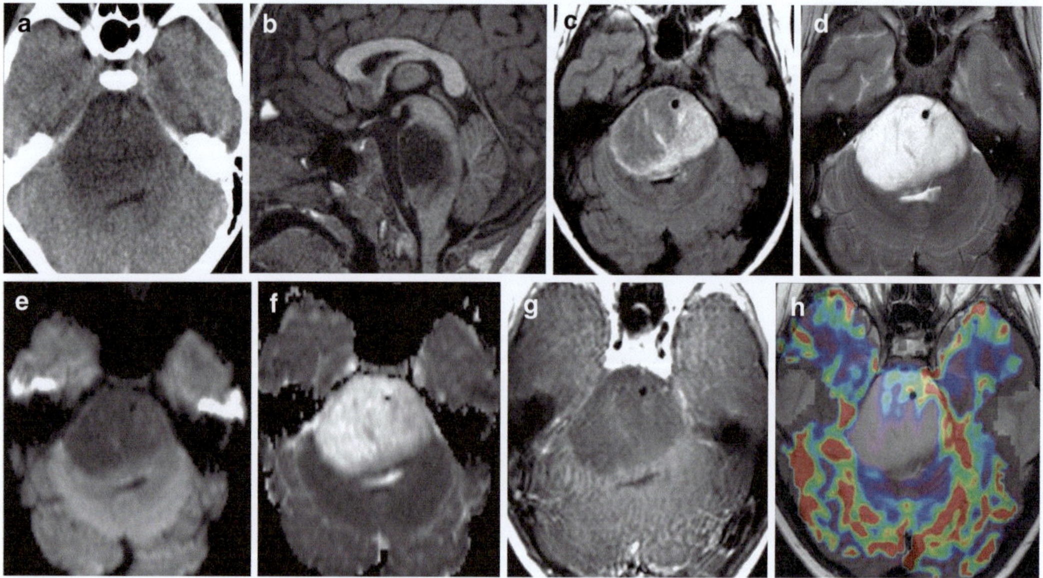

Fig. 3.6 DIPG in a 7-year-old boy. CT (**a**). MRI T1WI (**b**), FLAIR (**c**), T2WI (**d**), DWI (**e**), ADC (**f**), post-contrast T1WI (**g**), CBV (**h**). A large DIPG involves great part of the pons encasing anteriorly the basilar artery. After contrast administration no enhancement is visible (**g**), diffusion is quite homogeneously increased (**e, f**). A mismatch T2-FLAIR sign is visible

better response to radiotherapy [7] and to a slight better survival in patients under 18 years of age.

The absence of mismatch T2-FLAIR sign is however more frequent (Figs. 3.7 and 3.8) and a more inhomogeneous pattern can be present and can correlate with modification in contrast enhancement and diffusion. Enhancement may be present or not, but this does not correlate with the prognosis that remains poor in any case.

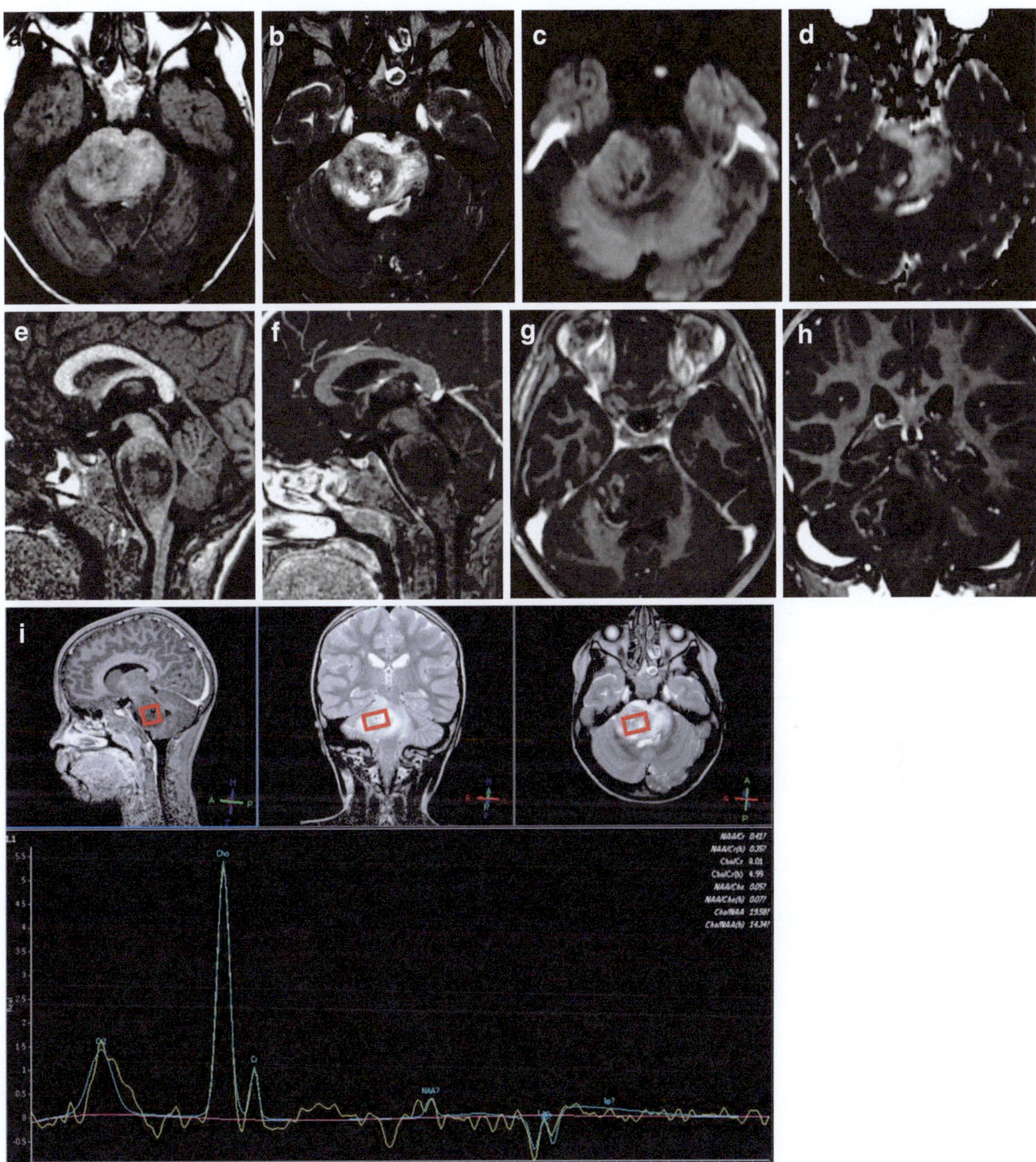

Fig. 3.7 DIPG in a young boy. MRI FLAIR (**a**), T2WI (**b**), DWI (**c**), ADC (**d**), T1WI (**e**), post-contrast T1WI (**f–h**). spectroscopy (**i**). A large inhomogeneous DIPG involves great part of the pons encasing the basilar artery. Same small areas of diffusion restriction are present in the right part of the tumor (**c, d**) where an irregular enhance-ment is visible after contrast administration (**f–h**). For the spectroscopyc study the voxel has been placed in the more inhomegeneous part of the tumor showing a typical aggressive pattern with a NAA peak barely visible and presence of lactate

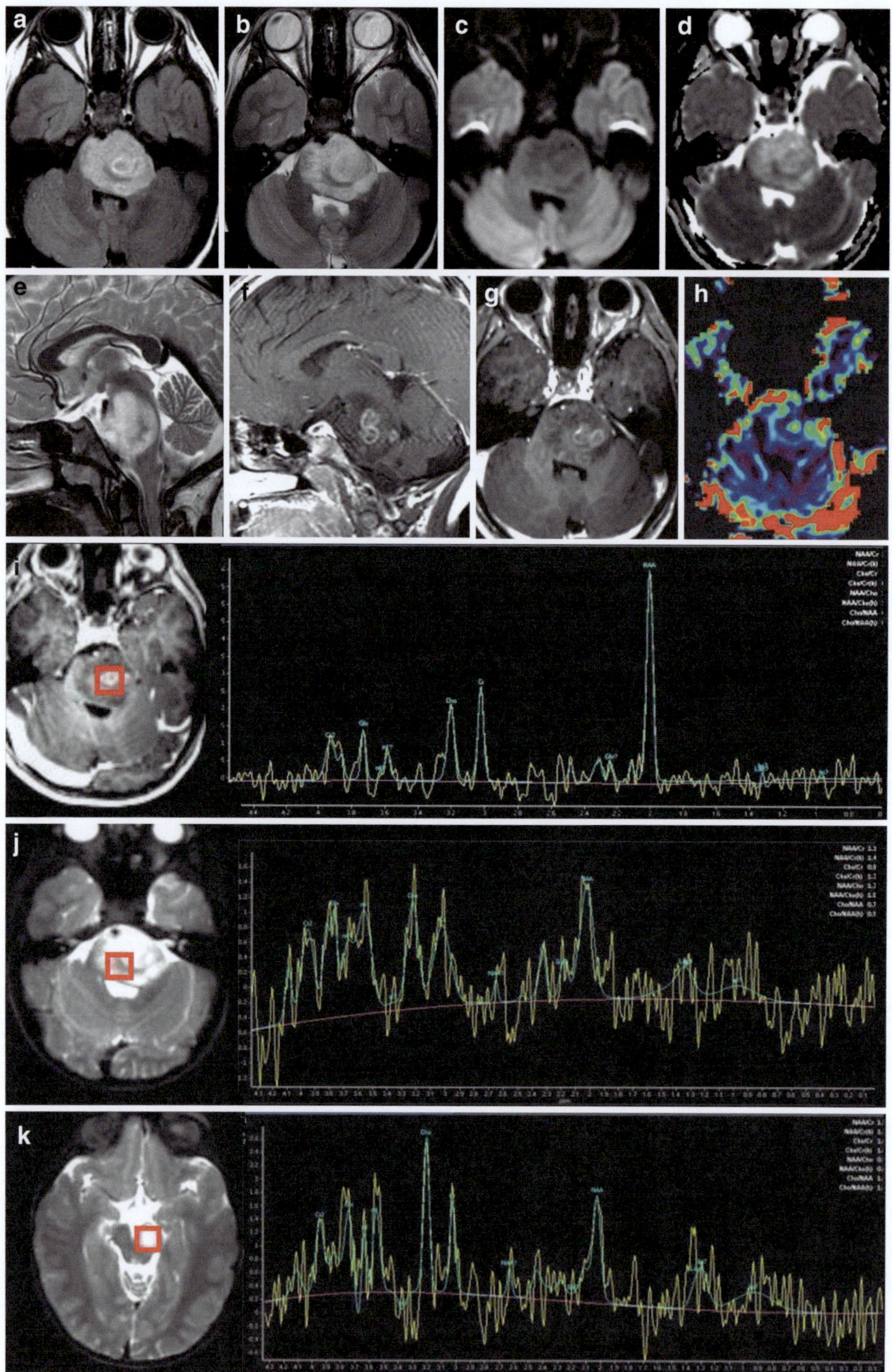

Fig. 3.8 DIPG in a young girl. MRI FLAIR (**a**), T2WI (**b**, **e**), DWI (**c**), ADC (**d**), T1WI (**e**), post-contrast T1WI (**f**, **g**), CBV (**h**), spectroscopy (**i-k**). Another large inhomogeneous DIPG involves great part of the pons and encasing the basilar artery. Same small areas of irregular enhancement are visible after contrast administration (**f–h**). An irregular CBV is visible as well (**h**). The voxels of the spectroscopic studies have been placed in two different areas of the tumor (**i**, **j**) and its superior margin (**k**) showing a completely different spectrum profile

Diffusion. The diffusion is usually increased in the case of homogeneous tumor (Fig. 3.6), but irregular area of diffusion restriction can be present in more inhomogeneous tumors (Figs. 3.7 and 3.8).

Spectroscopy. MR spectroscopy is variable and the presence of a lactate peak has been associated with worst prognosis [7] (Fig. 3.7). The spectrum profile can however change significantly in different areas of the tumor (Fig. 3.8).

Perfusion. As for diffusion and spectroscopy even perfusion and/or permeability can change accordingly to the inhomogeneity of the tumor (Fig. 3.8).

DIPG differential diagnosis. Astrocytomas IDH-mutant can be present anywhere within the brain. In Fig. 3.9 a 28-year-old man presented with a neoplasm quite similar to the case of Fig. 3.6, with mismatch T2-FLAIR, involvement of more than 50% of pons surface and basilar artery encasement. On biopsy the tumor resulted to be an astrocytoma IDH-mutant grade 2, it was treated with temozolomide and the tumor progressively decreased.

Thalamic DMG. Thalamic DMG appears usually more homogeneous than DIPG with diffuse hypodensity on CT, hypointensity on T1WI, and hyperintensity on both T2WI and FLAIR.

Diffusion is increased and CBV is reduced (Figs. 3.10 and 3.11).

As previously reported bithalamic lesion is usually more frequent in children (Fig. 3.10) and monothalamic lesion in adolescent and adult (Fig. 3.11). The DMG/DIPG image features are summarized in Table 3.5.

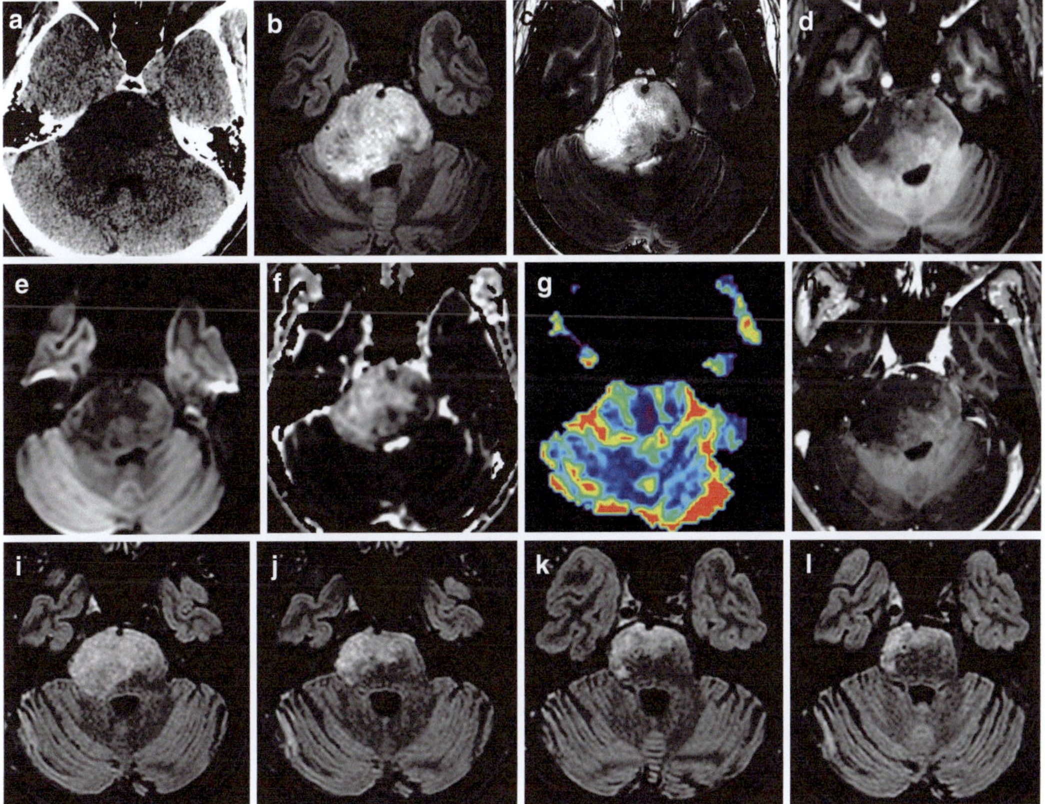

Fig. 3.9 Pontine astrocytoma IDH-mutant grade 2 in a 28-year-old man. CT (**a**). MRI FLAIR (**b and i-l**), T2WI (**c**), T1WI (**d**), DWI (**e**), ADC (**f**), CBV (**g**), post-contrast T1WI (**h**). A large infiltrating tumor involves great part of the pons encasing anteriorly the basilar artery. After contrast administration no enhancement is visible (**h**), diffusion is quite homogeneously increased (**e, f**). A mismatch T2-FLAIR sign is visible. The tumor progressively reduces its volume in the 1 year (**i**), 2 years (**j**), 3 years (**k**), and 4 years (**l**) follow-up

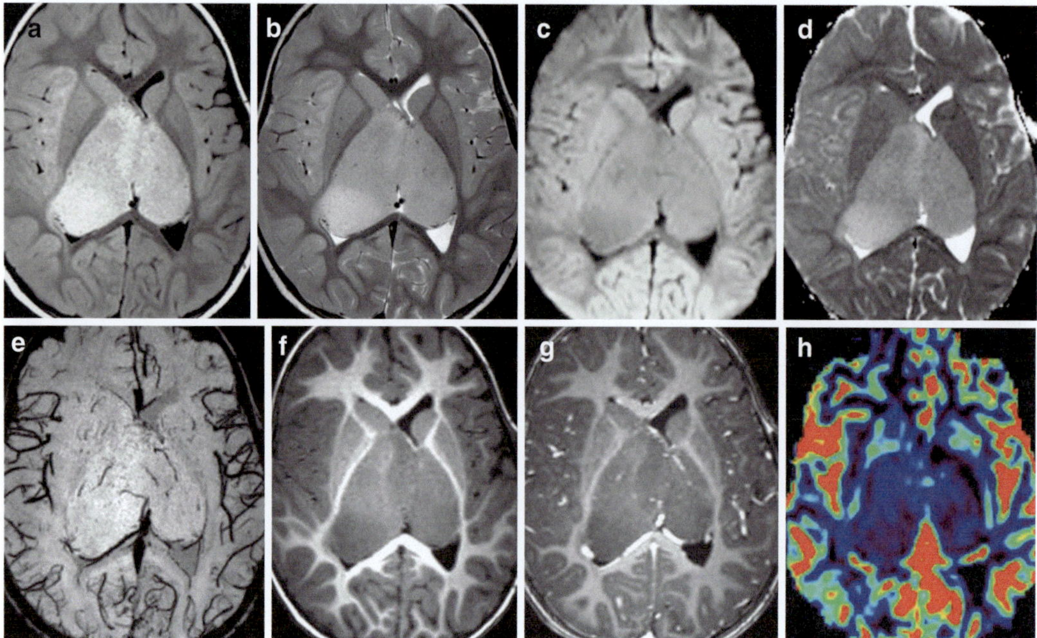

Fig. 3.10 Bithalamic DMG in a 3-year-old girl. MRI FLAIR (**a**), T2WI (**b**), DWI (**c**), ADC (**d**), SWI (**e**), T1WI (**f**), post-contrast T1WI (**g**), CBV (**h**). A large homogeneous infiltrating bithalamic tumor with quite similar signal intensity on both T2 and FLAIR sequences, absence of enhancement after contrast administration and low CBV

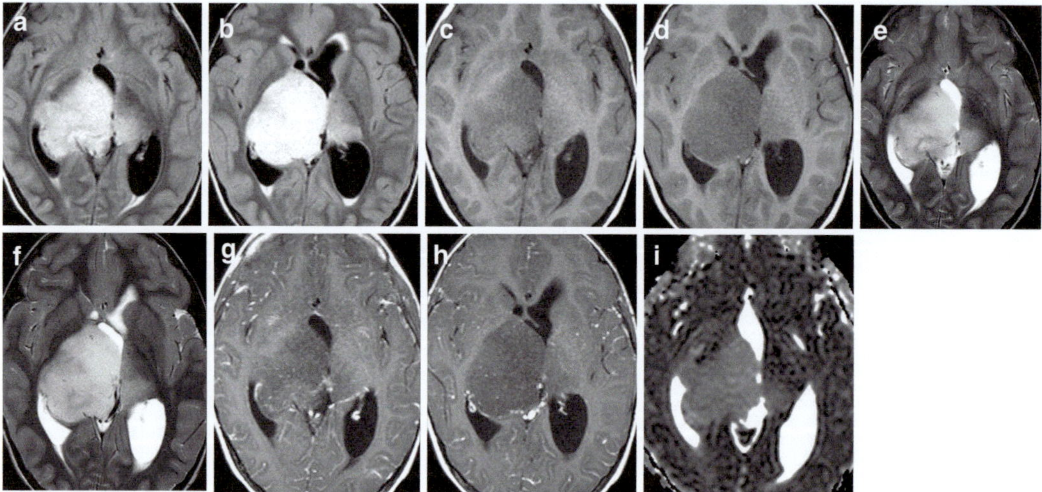

Fig. 3.11 Thalamic DMG in an adolescent. MRI FLAIR (**a, b**), T1WI (**c, d**), T2WI (**E,F**) post-contrast T1WI (**g, h**), ADC (**i**). A large right thalamic tumor with a relatively homogeneous pattern, no enhancement after contrast adminnistration and slight ADC increase. An initial involvement of the postero-mesial aspect of the left thalamus is evident as well

Table 3.5 DMG/DIPG imaging features

Mass effect	Edema	Inhomogeneity	Cysts	Necrosis	Hemorrhage	Calcifications
+/+++	0/++	0/++	0	0/+	0/+	0/+

CT	T1	T2	FLAIR	DWI	ADC	T1 Gd	CBV	Spec
●	●	○	○●	●○	○●	0/++	●●	↑Cho/NAA, ↑ lac,

3.2.2 Diffuse Hemispheric Glioma H3 G34-Mutant

WHO definition. Diffuse hemispheric glioma H3 G34-mutant is an infiltrative glioma involving the cerebral hemisphere with a missense mutation of the H3–34 gene.

It is a WHO grade 4 tumor.

Epidemiology. Epidemiological data are scarce, according to some authors these tumors account for 16% of pediatric hemisphere tumor, but other authors reported lower percentage. It affected mainly adolescents with a median age of 15–19 years.

Location. This is a hemispheric tumor that can spread to the midline or leptomeninges.

Clinical features. Seizures or sensory-motor deficits are the most significant clinical feature.

Prognosis. It is a highly aggressive tumor with a median overall survival of less than 2 years.

Imaging. Imaging features are nonspecific and quite similar to the other high-grade non-midline tumors. On CT it has been reported as possible hyperdense, whereas on MRI it appears as a cortical–subcortical mass mainly in parietal or temporal lobes with possible leptomeningeal dissemination, both necrosis and hemorrhages are possible as well as calcifications. Post-contrast enhancement is usually present. It is iso- to hyperintense on T2WI/FLAIR images and iso- to hypointense on T1WI. Diffusion is mainly restricted and perfusion increased. On spectroscophy an increase of Cho/NAA ratio is present as well as a lipid-lactate peak (Fig. 3.12) [2, 3]. Imaging features of diffuse hemospheric glioma H3 G34-mutant are summarized in Table 3.6.

3.2.3 Diffuse Pediatric-Type High-Grade Glioma H3-Wildtype and IDH-Wildtype

WHO definition. Diffuse pediatric-type high-grade glioma (pHGG) H3-wildtype and IDH-wildtype is a diffuse glioma with histological features of malignancy, typically occurring in children, adolescents, or young adults, which is wildtype for histone H3, *IDH1*, and *IDH2*.

It is a WHO grade 4 tumor.

Three subtypes are reported in WHO 2021

- Diffuse pediatric-type high-grade glioma RTK2.
- Diffuse pediatric-type high-grade glioma RTK1.
- Diffuse pediatric-type high-grade glioma MYCN.

Epidemiology. Epidemiological data are still not available. This tumor is rare and usually encountered in children, but its occurrence in adult population is still not clear.

Location. Tumor location is predominantly supratentorial, even brainstem and cerebellar pHGG are reported.

Clinical features. Signs and symptoms vary depending on the tumor's location. Seizures, and signs of cranial hypertension are the most commonly observed.

Prognosis. These tumors are aggressive with an unfavorable prognosis and the reported 2 years survival rate is only something between 20 and 25%.

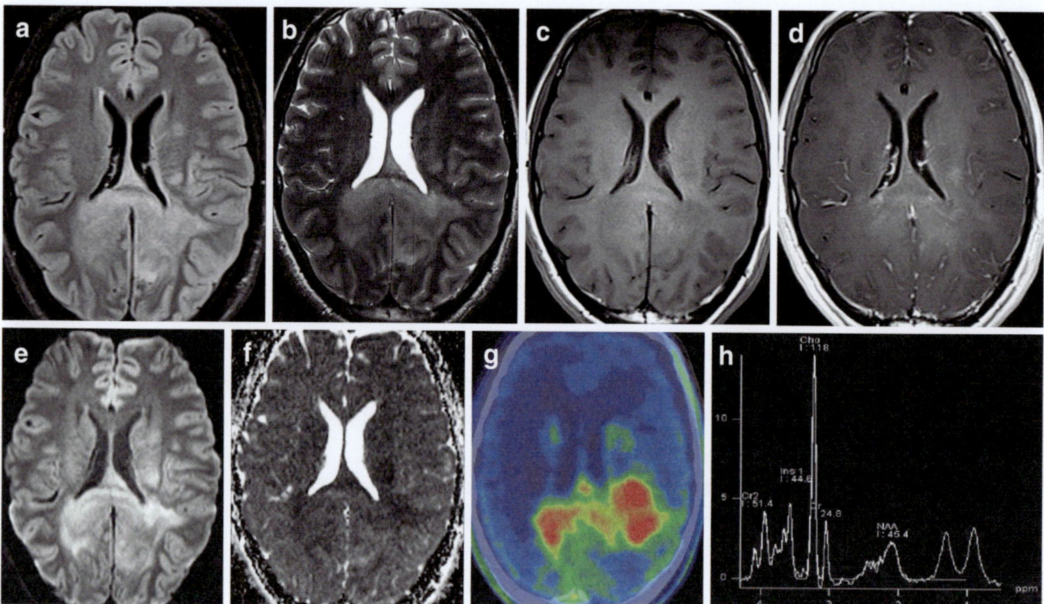

Fig. 3.12 Diffuse hemispheric glioma H3 G34-mutant in a 20-year-old male. MRI FLAIR (**a**), T2WI (**b**), T1WI (**c**), post-contrast T1WI (**d**), DWI (**e**), ADC (**f**), spectroscopy (**h**). PET-CT with an amino acid tracer (**g**). This is a huge infiltrative tumor involving large parts of the left hemi- sphere with a contralateral spread through the splenium of the corpus callosum, with areas of diffusion restriction and marked radiotracer uptake. On spectroscopy a marked decrease in NAA peak with a lipid-lactate peak is evident. (Courtesy Dr. S. Colafati, Rome)

Table 3.6 Diffuse hemispheric glioma H3 G34-mutant imaging features

Mass effect	Edema	Inhomogeneity	Cysts	Necrosis	Hemorrhage	Calcifications
+/+++	0/++	+/++	0	0/+	0/+	0/+

CT	T1	T2	FLAIR	DWI	ADC	T1 Gd	CBV	Spec
○	○	○	○	○	●	0/++	◯	↑Cho/NAA, ↑ lac,

Imaging. This tumor presents all the typical characteristics of an aggressive tumor: inhomogeneity, necrosis, irregular enhancement, and diffusion restriction.

On T2 and FLAIR, as well as on T1WI the signal intensity is inhomogeneous. The post-contrast enhancement is irregular and almost always present.

Diffusion is restricted and the spectroscopy shows a high Cho/NAA ratio (Figs. 3.13 and 3.14) [8]. Imaging features of pHHG H-3 wildtype and K27-wildtype are summarized in Table 3.7.

3.2.4 Infant-Type Hemispheric Glioma

WHO definition. Infant-type hemispheric glioma is a cerebral hemispheric, high-grade cellular astrocytoma that arises in early childhood, typically with receptor tyrosine kinase (RTK) fusions including those in the NTRK family or in *ROS1, ALK,* or *MET.*

Epidemiology. These tumors occur early in childhood usually in the first 3 years of life, it can also be found in neonatal and fetal period (Fig. 6.9).

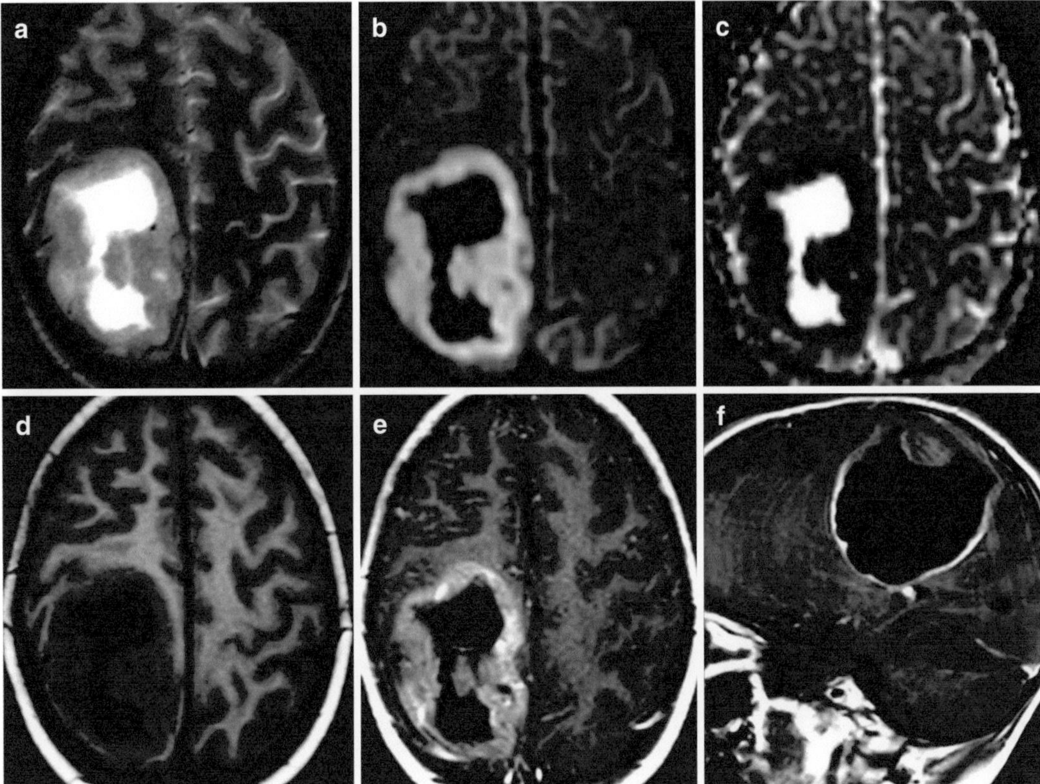

Fig. 3.13 pHGG H-3 wildtype and K27-wildtype in a 8-year-old boy. MRI T2WI (**a**), DWI (**b**), ADC (**c**), T1WI (**d**), post-contrast T1WI (**e**, **f**). A large inhomogeneous right parietal tumor is visible with a necrotic center and an irregular parenchymal portion showing diffusion restriction. (Courtesy Prof G. Morana, Turin)

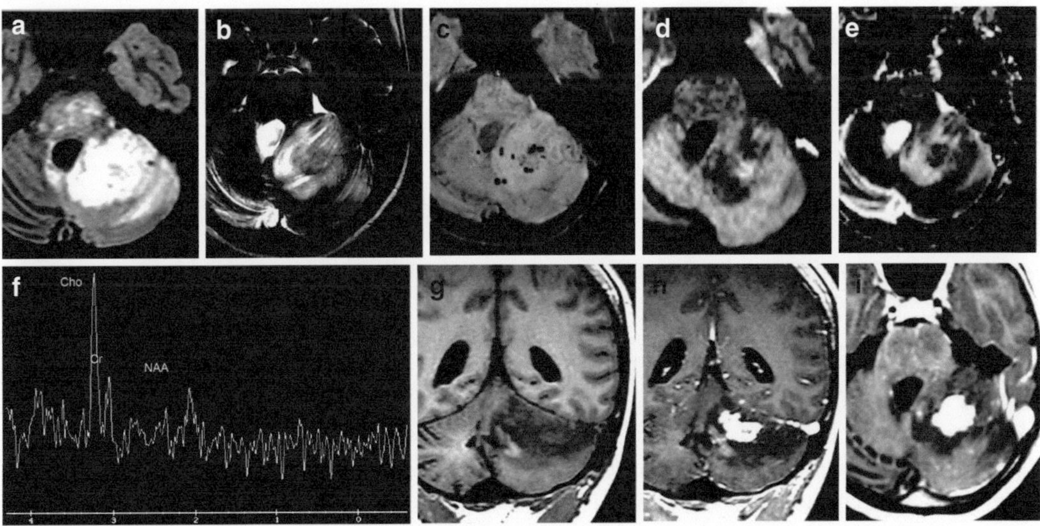

Fig. 3.14 Post-radiation pHGG H-3 wildtype and K27-wildtype in a 20-year-old woman with a previously treated ependymoma. MRI FLAIR (**a**), T2WI (**b**), SWI (**c**), DWI (**d**), ADC (**e**), spectroscopy (**f**), T1WI (**g**), post-contrast T1WI (**h**, **i**). An inhomogeneous left cerebellar tumor is visible with parenchymal portion showing diffu-sion restriction and enhancement after contrast adminis-tration. Some punctate hemorrhagies are evident on SWI (**c**). Spectroscopy shows a tipical pattern of an aggressive neoplasm with high Cho and low NAA. (Courtesy Prof G. Morana, Turin)

Table 3.7 pHGG imaging features

Mass effect	Edema	Inhomogeneity	Cysts	Necrosis	Hemorrhage	Calcifications
+/+++	+/+++	+/+++	0/++	+/+++	+/++	0/+

CT	T1	T2	FLAIR	DWI	ADC	T1 Gd	CBV	Spec
◯	◯	◯	◯	◯	⬤	+/+++	🔴	↑↑Cho/NAA, ↑ lac,

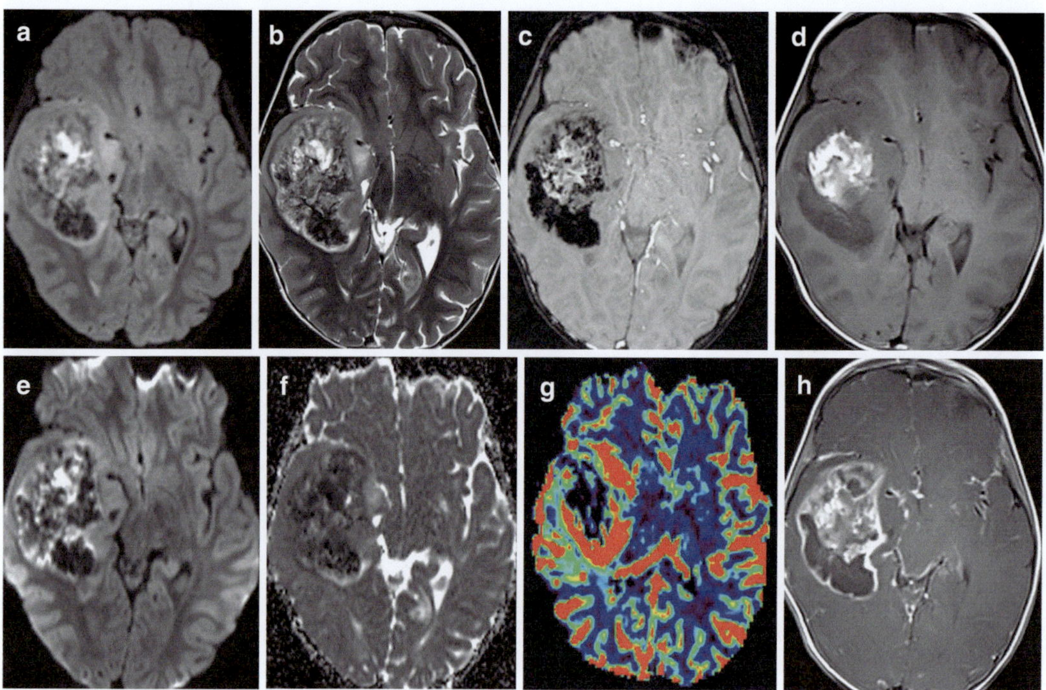

Fig. 3.15 Infant-type hemispheric glioma in a 3-year-old girl. MRI FLAIR (**a**), T2WI (**b**), SWI (**c**), T1WI (**d**), DWI (**e**), ADC (**f**), CBV (**g**), post-contrast T1WI (**h**). An inhomogeneous huge hemispheric mass is evident in the right temporo-insular region. Diffuse hemorrhagic components are evident, the enhancement is irregular, the diffusion is restricted and the CBV is decreased. (Courtesy Dr. S. Colafati, Rome)

Location. They are large supratentorial masses.

Clinical features. Signs and symptoms are not specific, usually characterized by a generic encephalopathy.

Prognosis. Data on prognosis are scarce, a possible overall better prognosis of high-grade gliomas in younger children is reported.

Imaging. Data on imaging are scarce and confused due to the changing terminology [9]. The case in Fig. 3.15 shows all the typical features of an aggressive glioma, with an inhomogeneous aspect with diffuse hemorrhagic component, irregular enhancement, diffusion restriction, and increased CBV. There is no specific patterns and the case reported in Fig. 6.9 was initially diagnosed as an ATRT: Imaging features of infant-type hemispheric glioma are summarized in Table 3.8.

Table 3.8 Infant-type hemispheric glioma imaging features

Mass effect	Edema	Inhomogeneity	Cysts	Necrosis	Hemorrhage	Calcifications
+/+++	+/+++	+/+++	0/++	+/+++	+/++	0/+

CT	T1	T2	FLAIR	DWI	ADC	T1 Gd	CBV	Spec
○	○	○	○	○	●	+/+++	●	NA[a]

[a]NA (not available) = incomplete or sporadic reports

3.3 Circumscribed Astrocytic Gliomas

3.3.1 Pilocytic Astrocytoma

WHO definition. Pilocytic astrocytoma is a neoplasm with a variable proportion of bipolar hairlike pilocytic cells, compact and loose or myxoid regions, rosenthal fibers, and eosinophilic granular bodies.

It is associated with MAPK pathway gene alterations, most often with *KIAA1549:BRAF* gene fusions. This kind of mutation can be found in all tumor locations but is most characteristic for cerebellar location (70% of cases). Alterations in MAPK pathway can be present in patients with *neurofibromatosis 1* (NF1) and pilocytic astrocytomas are the principal CNS neoplasm associated with NF1.

It is a WHO grade 1 tumor.

Epidemiology. Pilocytic astrocytomas account for more than 33% of all glioma in the 0–14 age group and represent 17,6% of all childhood primary tumors being the most frequent tumor in this age group. The incidence of pilocytic astrocytomas rapidly declined in adulthood and it is exceptionally reported in patients › 50 years.

Location. The most common and characteristic location is the cerebellum (50–70%) involving both the hemispheres and the vermis, but pilocytic astrocytoma can localized throughout the neuraxis with a preference for midline structures, such as optic chiasm and nerves, hypothalamus, and brainstem. Less frequent locations are cerebral hemispheres, spinal cord, and ventricles.

Clinical features. Being most frequently located in the cerebellum clinical symptoms can be typically related to a cerebellar syndrome with ataxia and/or vertigo, but frequently symptoms and signs of high intracranial pressure can overcome symptomatology.

Prognosis. The overall survival rate of pilocytic astrocytoma at 10 years is greater than 95% after total surgical removal. Cerebellar localization is related to an even better prognosis due to the most favorable surgical access.

Imaging. The typical imaging appearance of pilocytic astrocytoma is characterized by two components: a cyst with fluid aspect on both CT and MRI and a mural nodule. This aspect is exceedingly frequent in the cerebellar hemispheric location, but some changes can be encountered in extra-cerebellar locations.

The cyst exhibits the same density of CSF on CT images and on T1WI and T2WI, whereas on FLAIR images it can present a variable aspect from a slight hypointensity (Figs. 3.16 and 3.17) to a relative hyperintensity (Fig. 3.18) with respect to brain parenchyma. On DWI-ADC it presents diffusion values similar to CSF. The cyst wall can enhance or not, without any apparent relationship with its prognostic behavior.

The mural nodule is iso-hypodense on CT, iso-hypointense on MRI T1WI, hyperintense on T2WI, and FLAIR images (Figs. 3.16, 3.17, and 3.18) with a relatively homogeneous enhancement after contrast administration.

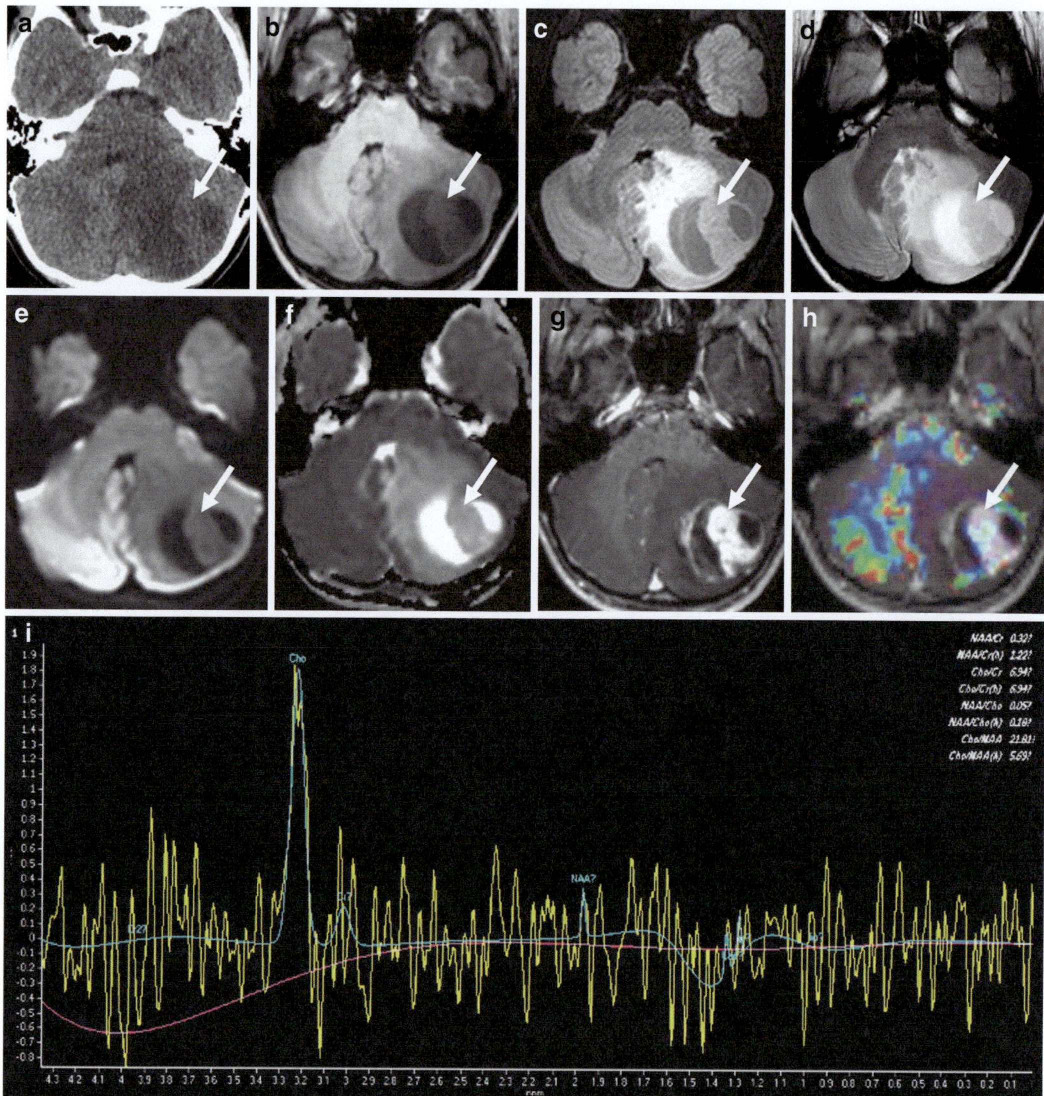

Fig. 3.16 Pilocytic astrocytoma in a 10-year-old boy. CT (**a**), MRI T1WI (**b**), FLAIR (**c**), T2WI (**d**), DWI (**e**), ADC (**f**), post-contrast T1WI (**g**), CBV (**h**), spectroscopy (**i**). A typical pilocytic astrocytoma is visible in the left cerebellar hemisphere with a discrete mass effect and perilesional edema. The cystic component is slightly hypointense on FLAIR image (**c**) and exhibits a wall enhancement after contrast administration (**g**). The mural nodule (arrow **a-h**) shows the characteristic appearance on both CT and MRI, most important for the differential diagnosis the iso-hypointensity on CT (**a**), the hyperintensity on T2WI (**d**), and the relative ADC increase (**f**). A minimal increase in CBV is visible as well (**h**). MR spectroscopy (**i**) centered on mural nodule reveals only the peak of choline, with Cr and Naa peaks undetectable. MR spectra baseline is partly artifacted due to the small size of the voxel

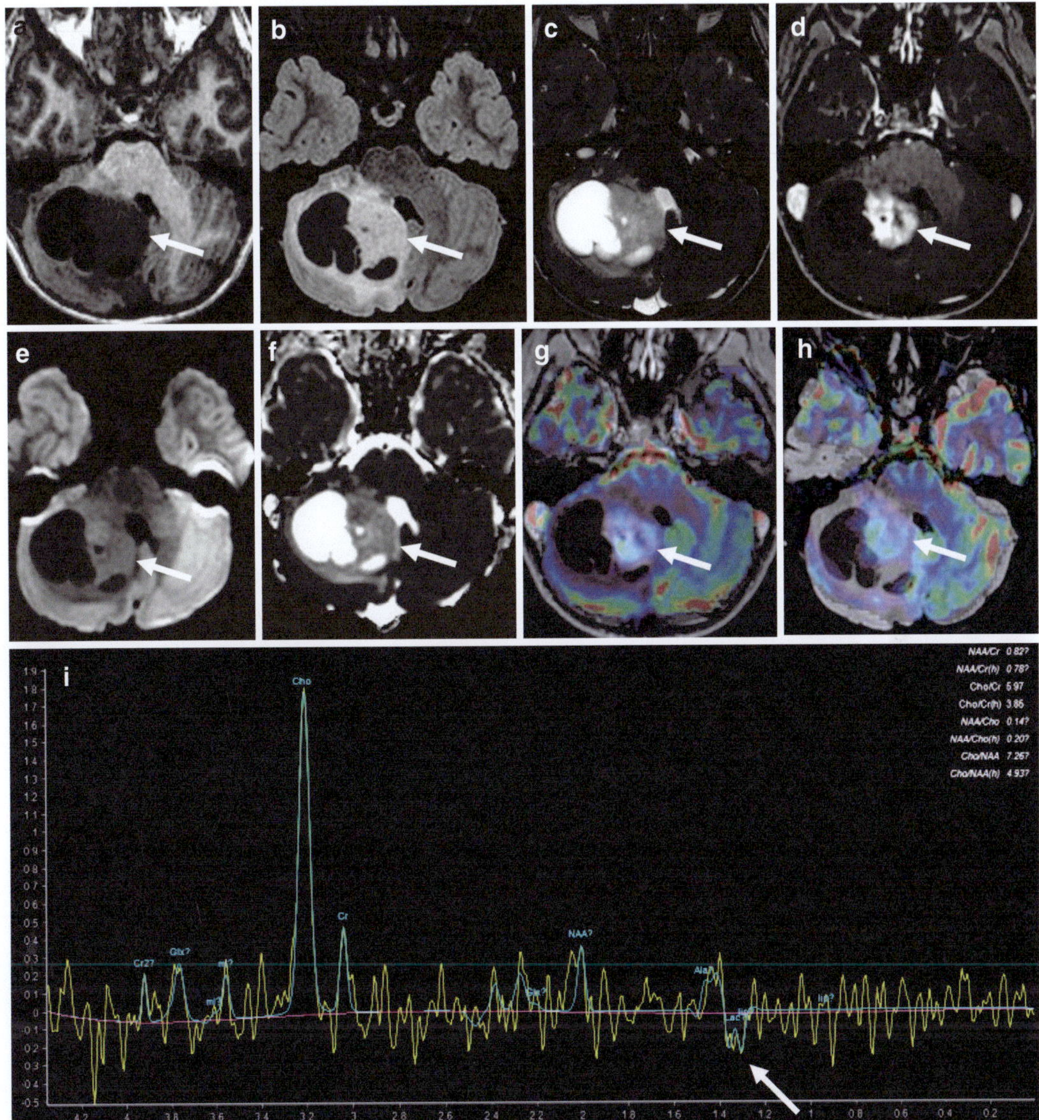

Fig. 3.17 Pilocytic astrocytoma in a 7-year-old boy. MRI T1WI (**a**), FLAIR (**b**), T2WI (**c**), post-contrast T1WI (**d**), DWI (**e**), ADC (**f**), CBF (**g**), CBV (**h**), spectroscopy (**i**). A typical pilocytic astrocytoma is detectable in the right cerebellar hemisphere with a discrete mass effect, but without significant perilesional edema. The cystic component is hypointense on FLAIR image (**b**) and without wall enhancement after contrast administration (**d**). The mural nodule (arrow **a-h**) shows the characteristic appearance on MRI, with an hyperintensity on T2WI (**C**) and a relative ADC increase (**f**). A minimal increase in both CBF and CBV is visible as well (**g**, **h**). MR spectroscopy (**i**) centered on mural nodule reveals a marked increase in Cho/Cr ratio with a scarcely detectable Naa. A small inverse lactate doublet is also visible (arrow)

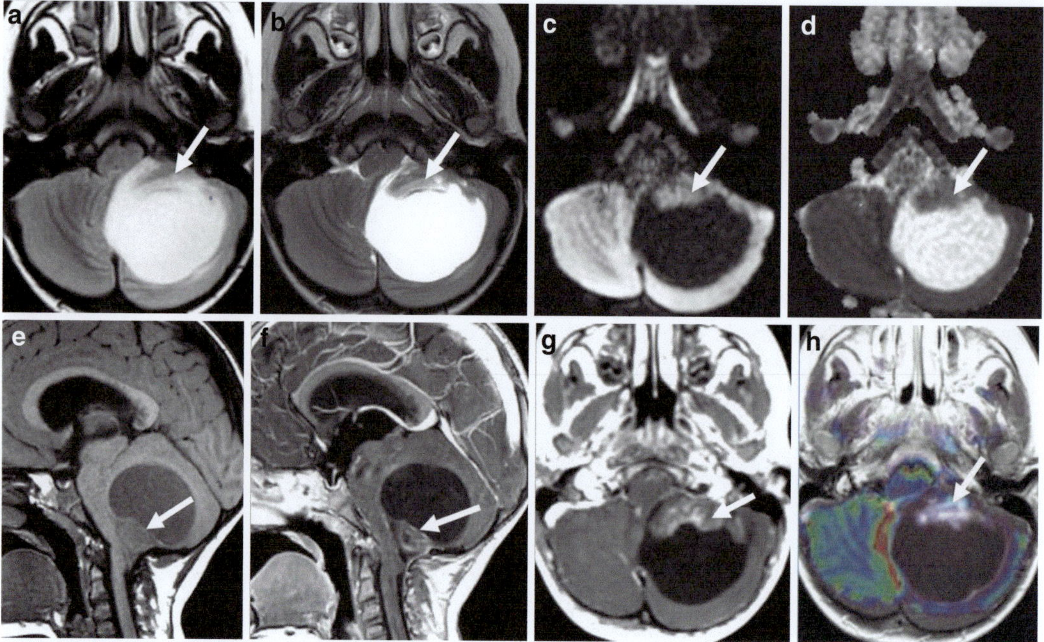

Fig. 3.18 Pilocytic astrocytoma in a 4-year-old boy. MRI FLAIR (**a**), T2WI (**b**), DWI (**c**), ADC (**d**),T1WI (**e**), post-contrast T1WI (**f, g**), CBV (**h**). A large pilocytic astrocytoma is detectable in the antero-inferior aspect of the left cerebellar hemisphere with a discrete mass effect, but without significant perilesional edema. The cystic component is huge, hyperintense on FLAIR image (**a**) and without wall enhancement after contrast administration (**f, g**). The mural nodule (arrow **a-h**) is small and with a relatively scarce enhancement (**f, g**) and normal to low CBV

Calcifications or hemorrhage within the nodule are rare even though not impossible (Figs. 3.21 and 3.22).

Diffusion. The parenchymal portion of pilocytic astrocytoma typically shows a diffusion increase and that is one of the most important features, together with T2WI hyperintensity, in the differential diagnosis with the other typical posterior fossa tumors in childhood (Figs. 3.16, 3.17, 3.18, 3.19, 3.20, 3.21, 3.22 and 3.23).

Spectroscopy. MR spectroscopy shows a sort of paradoxical spectral profile for a WHO grade 1 tumor, with a marked increase of Cho/Cr ratio and marked decrease of Naa peak, a typical profile of an aggressive tumor (Figs. 3.16 and 3.17). A lactate peak is reported as well making impossible a differentiation from a more aggressive tumor [10].

Myoinositol presence in pilocytic astrocytoma it also been reported, albeit more frequently associated with supratentorial location and with tumor recurrence [11].

Perfusion. CBF and CBV values of mural nodule are variable from normal to a slight increase (Figs. 3.16, 3.17, 3.18 and 3.22).

Locations other than in the cerebellar hemispheres.

Cerebellar hemispheres are the more typical location of pilocytic astrocytomas; however, they can be found everywhere within cerebellar structures even in vermis (Fig. 3.19). When pilocytic astrocytomas are located in the vermis compressing the fourth ventricle some difficulties can arise in differential diagnosis with the more typical midline cerebellar lesions, such as medulloblastoma and ependymoma. Diagnostic clues are

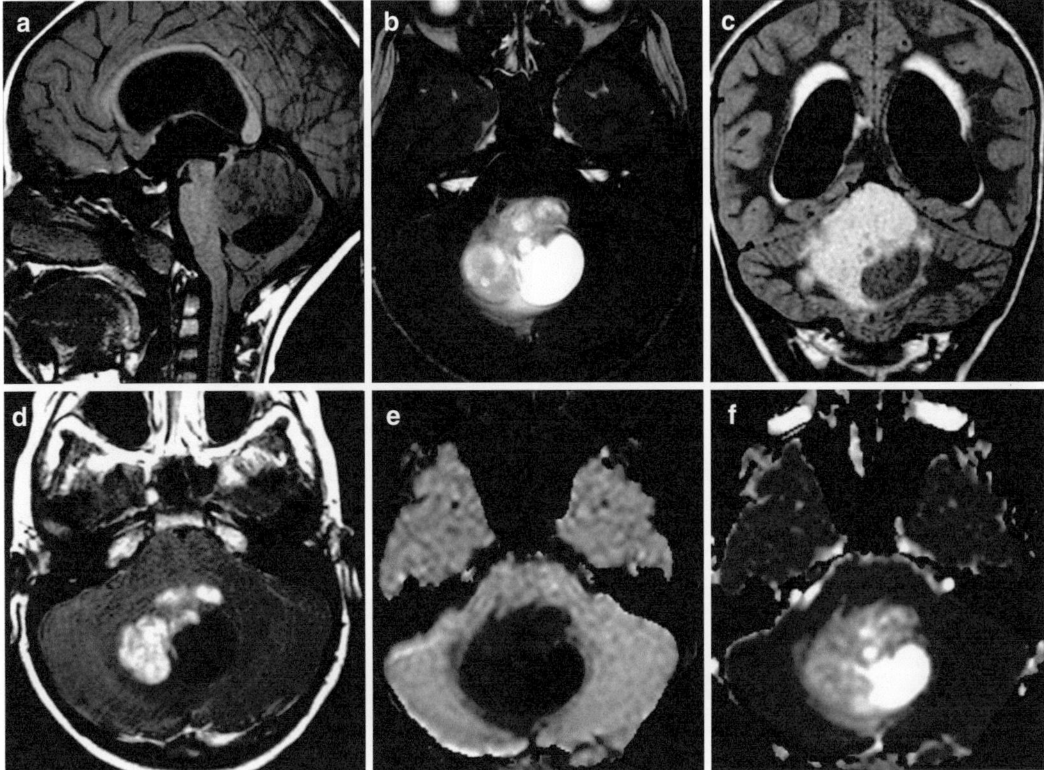

Fig. 3.19 Pilocytic astrocytoma in the cerebellar vermis in an 8-year-old girl. MRI T1WI (**a**), T2WI (**b**), FLAIR (**c**), post-contrast T1WI (**d**), DWI (**e**), ADC (**f**). The lesion is located in the superior vermis compressing the fourth ventricle and causing a supratentorial hydrocephalus (**a**, **c**). The solid portion is relatively large; however, the signal intensity remains largely hyperintense on T2WI and with an increased diffusion (**e**, **f**)

mostly related even in this case to the signal intensity of the solid portion of the tumor. It remains usually iso-hypodense on CT, frankly hyperintense on T2WI and with an increased ADC with respect to the brain parenchyma.

Less frequently pilocytic astyrocytos can localize supratentorially where the preferential location is in the chiasmatic-hypothalamic region (Figs. 3.20 and 3.21), followed by thalamus/basal ganglia location (Fig. 3.22) and cerebral hemispheric location. The spinal cord location is rare.

The majority of optic pathways gliomas in NF1 patients are actually pilocytic astrocytomas.

Tumor seeding along neuroaxis is rare and relatively more common in the histologic variant of pilocytic astrocytoma known as pilomyxoid astrocytoma. Histologically pilomyxoid astrocytomas are characterized by an angiocentric arrangement of monomorphous bipolar tumor cells in a prominent myxoid background. The typical location of pilomyxoid astrocytomas is the hypothalamic region and they usually occur in the first 2 years of life. Even if a definite grade

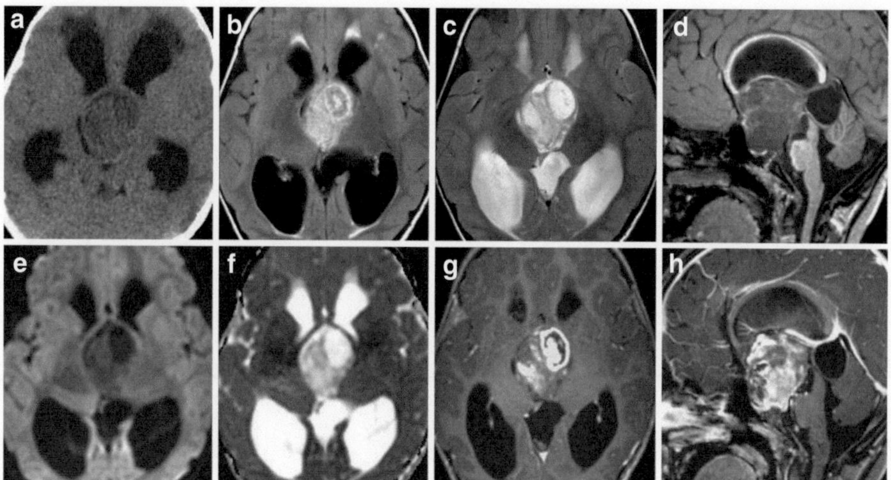

Fig. 3.20 Hypothalamic pilocytic astrocytoma in a 4-year-old girl. CT (**a**). MRI FLAIR (**b**), T2WI (**c**), T1WI (**d**), DWI (**e**), ADC (**f**), post-contrast T1WI (**g, h**). A large hypothalamic lesion occupying the third ventricle and causing an obstructive hydrocephalus is visible. The lesion is heterogeneous and it is not clearly separate into a solid and cystic portion, but it is, as expected, hyperintense on T2WI and with an increased diffusion

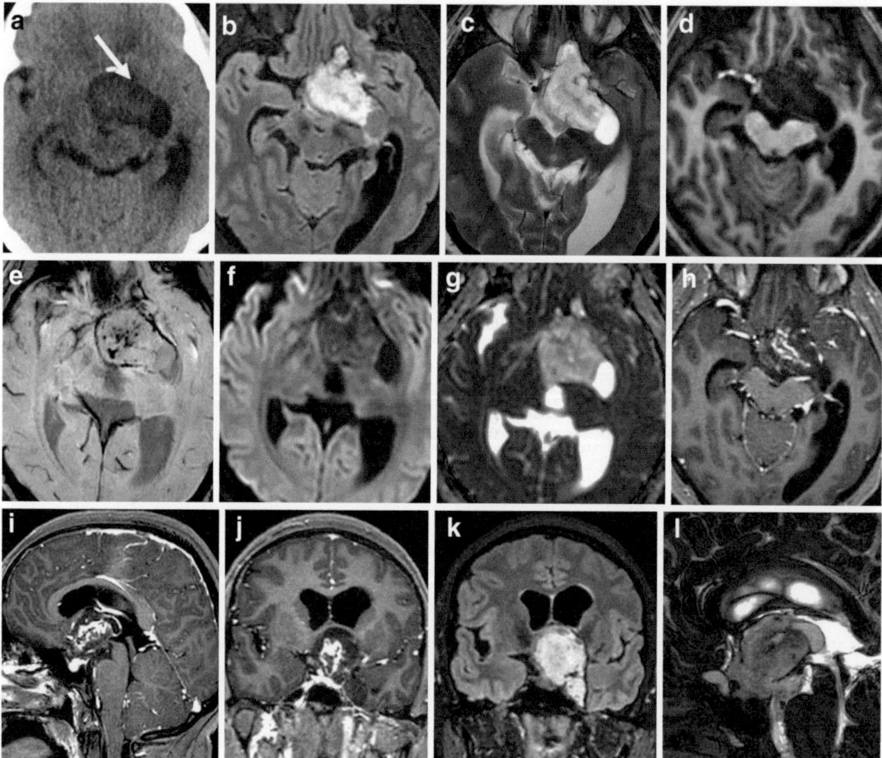

Fig. 3.21 Hypothalamic pilocytic astrocytoma in a 32-year-old woman. CT (**a**). MRI FLAIR (**b, k**), T2WI (**c**), T1WI (**d**), SWI (**e**), DWI (**f**), ADC (**g**) post-contrast T1WI (**h-j**), bSSFP (**l**). A large hypothalamic lesion occupies the third ventricle and apparently the left parasellar region. The lesion is heterogeneous with a posterior cyst and a calcification on CT (a arrow) and SWI (**e**), and it is hyperintense on T2WI, with a diffusion increase. The enhancement is extremely inhomogeneous and it is present only in the central portion of the lesion (**h**). In the coronal section it is evident the parasellar growth of the lesion. Due to the calcification, the age of the patient, and the location, the lesion has been erroneously diagnosed as a craniopharyngioma

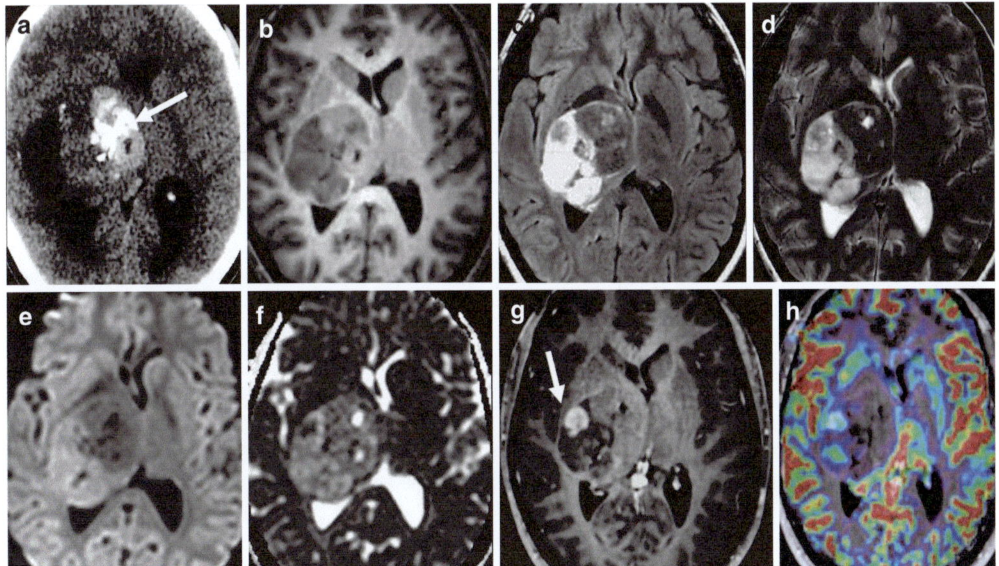

Fig. 3.22 Thalamic pilocytic astrocytoma in an 11-year-old girl. CT (**a**). MRI T1WI (**b**), FLAIR (**c**), T2WI (**d**), DWI (**e**), ADC (**f**) post-contrast T1WI (**g**), CBV (**h**). A large heterogeneous mass is detectable in the right thalamus with a lateral extension in the capsulo-lenticular region. Similar to the previous case it is challenging if not impossible to distinguish the solid and cystic components of the neoplasm. In this case a large calcification is visible on the basal CT scan (arrow, **a**), whereas the enhancing area is relatively small (arrow, **g**)

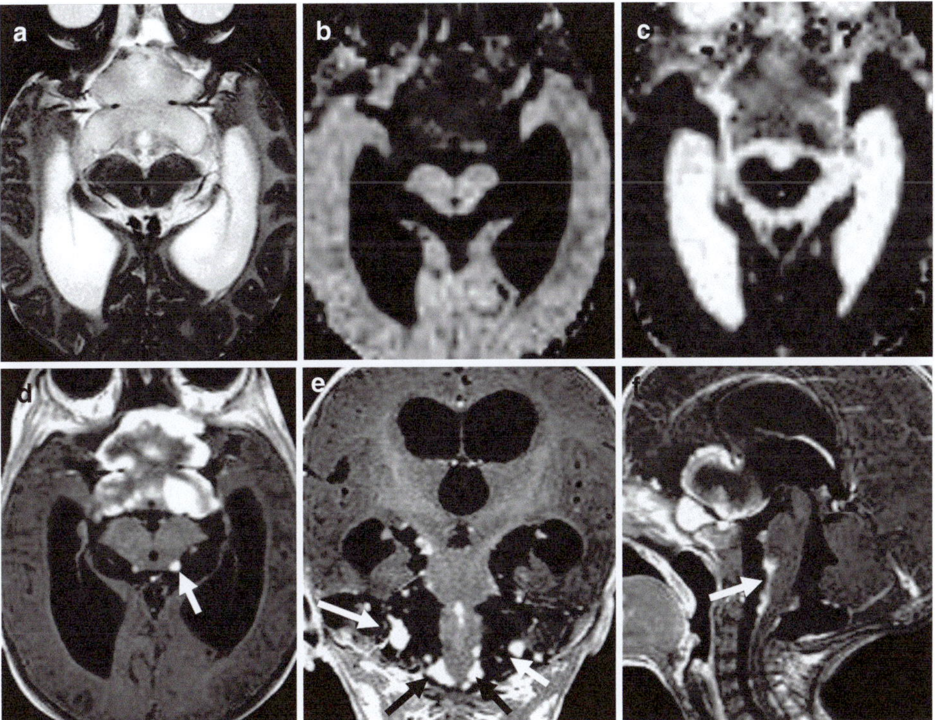

Fig. 3.23 Hypothalamic pilomyxoid astrocytoma in a 5-month-old girl. MRI T2WI (**a**), DWI (**b**), ADC (**c**), post-contrast T1WI (**d–f**). A large hypothalamic lesion occupies the third ventricle causing an hydrocephalus. The lesion is marked hyperintense on T2WI and with a diffusion increase, but after contrast a diffuse CSF neoplasm seeding is visible (**d**, **e**, **f** arrows)

assignment is still not obtained they are usually considered as WHO grade 2 tumors with a prognosis less favorable than pilocytic astrocytomas (Fig. 3.23).

In some rare cases cerebrospinal fluid dissemination can occur also in pilocytic astrocytoma, more frequently after radio- and chemotherapy (Fig. 3.24). Imaging features of pilocytic astrocytoma are summarized in Table 3.9.

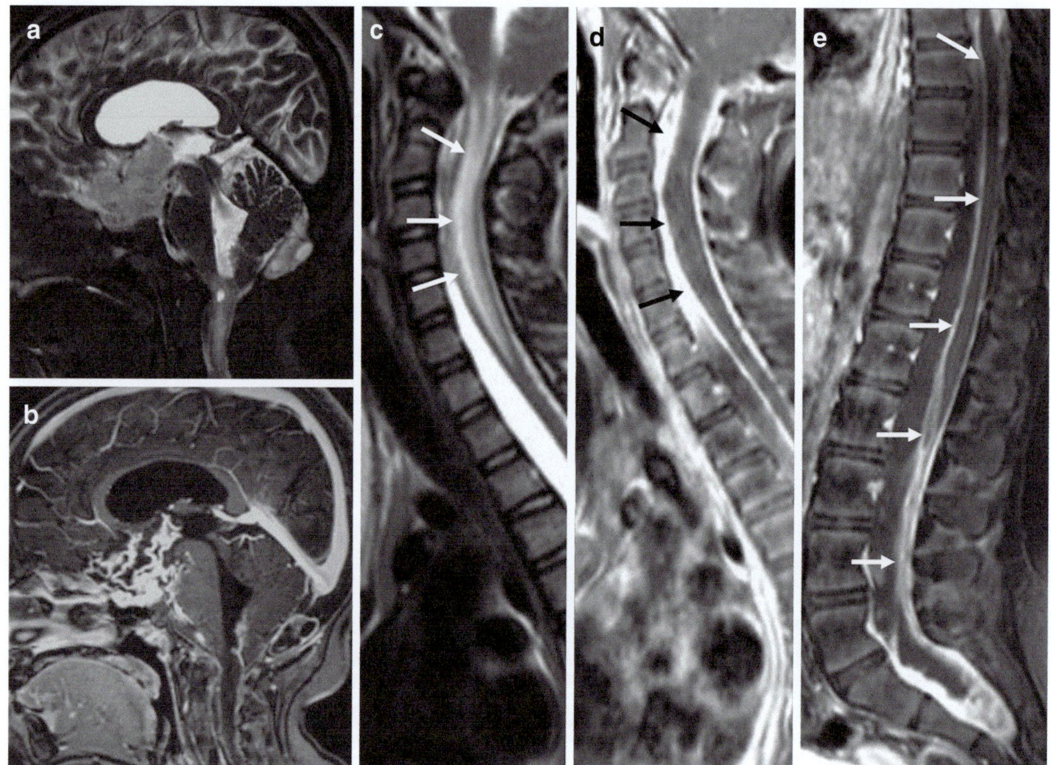

Fig. 3.24 Pilocityc astrocytoma cerebrospinal fluid dissemination in a 10-year-old girl. MRI bSSFP (**a**), T2WI (**c**), post-contrast T1WI (**b**, **d**, **e**). A large chiasmatic-hypothalamic lesion, previously partly removed, shows a diffuse tumor seeding along CSF with areas of diffuse enhancement along the pial surface of brainstem and spinal cord (B, D, E, arrows). Tumor spreading causes an initial cavitation of the cervical spinal cord (arrows C) and an hydrocephalus

Table 3.9 Pilocytic astrocytoma imaging features

Mass effect	Edema	Inhomogeneity	Cysts	Necrosis	Hemorrhage	Calcifications
+/+++	0/++	+/++	++	0	0/+	0/++

CT	T1	T2	FLAIR	DWI	ADC	T1 Gd	CBV	Spec
◔	◔	○	○	◕	○	++/+++	◉	Low Naa, ↑Cho, ↑lac, ↑Myo

3.3.2 High-Grade Astrocytoma with Piloid Features

WHO definition. High-grade astrocytoma with piloid features (HGAP) is an astrocytoma that shows a distinct DNA methylation profile, often with high-grade piloid and/or glioblastoma-like histological features. Alteration os MAPK pathway genes are often combined with homozygous deletion involving the CDKN2A and/or CDKN2B locus, and/or ATRX mutation or loss of nucelar ATRX expression.

Epidemiology. Epidemiological data are are currently unavailable. It is on the matter of fact an extremely rare tumor.

Location. It seems to be more frequent in the posterior fossa, even though it can be found everywhere in the CNS.

Clinical features. They depend on tumor location.

Prognosis. WHO 2021 reported only a single retrospective study with a survival rate of 5 years nearly 50%.

Imaging. According to one of the greatest available series on 6 subjects lesions can be both sharp and infiltrating with a prevalent heterogeneous texture. They are hyperintense on T2WI and hypo- to isointense on T1WI. Post-contrast enhancement was always present and diffusion is not restricted [12]. Imageing features of HGAP are summarized in Table 3.10.

3.3.3 Pleomorphic Xanthoastrocytoma

WHO definition. Pleomorphic xanthoastrocytoma is an astrocytic glioma with large pleomorphic and frequently multinucleated cells, spindle cells often with numerous eosinophilic granular bodies, and reticulin deposition with *BRAF*p. V600E mutation and homozygous *CDKN2A* and/or *CDKN2B* deletion.

It is a WHO grade 2 or 3 tumor.

Epidemiology. It is a relatively rare tumor with an incidence rate < 0.7 cases for 100.000 population per year. It is more frequent in adolescents and young adults with incidence peak around 20 years (15–25 years). The estimated ratio between grade 2 and grade 3 is approximately 7/3.

Location. The typical location of this tumor is in the most superficial part of the cortex involving both leptomeninges and cerebrum. The majority of these tumors occur supratentorially, and most often in temporal lobe.

Clinical features. Seizures are the typical sign of this slow growing tumor.

Prognosis. The estimated 5-year survival rate in patients with a grade 2 tumor is between 80 and 90% and significantly higher than the survival rate in patients with a grade 3 tumor (50–60%).

Grade 2 tumor may recur, disseminate, and progress to a higher grade, consequently a complete surgical resection is critical in defining the final prognosis.

Table 3.10 HGAP imaging features

Mass effect	Edema	Inhomogeneity	Cysts	Necrosis	Hemorrhage	Calcifications
+/++	0/++	+/++	0	0	0	0

CT	T1	T2	FLAIR	DWI	ADC	T1 Gd	CBV	Spec
◉	◉	○	○	◉	◉	+/++	NA[a]	NA[a]

[a]NA (not available) = incomplete or sporadic reports

Imaging. Pleomorphic xanthoastrocytoma is a superficially located tumor frequently in temporal region and with a cystic component that often includes a diffuse infiltrating component. Calcification can be present and the solid portion may enhance after contrast. Mass effect is usually scarce. Diagnostic clues are related to the particular location of the tumor and to the double component cystic and solid.

CT appearance is variable from slight hyperdensity to hypodensity.

MRI features of the solid portion are similar to a slow growing infiltrative tumor, but with the possibility of enhancement after contrast. Contrast enhancement is usually present in the superficial pial component (Figs. 3.25 and 3.26).

Diffusion is normal or slightly decreased with mean value usually inferior to pilocytic astrocytomas [13].

Spectroscopy is indicative of a slow growing tumor with a slight increase of Cho/NAA ratio (Figs. 3.25 and 3.26).

Perfusion is normal or sometimes increased in the superficial component (Fig. 3.26). Imaging features of pleomorphic xanthoastrocytoma are summarized in Table 3.11.

3.3.4 Subependymal Giant Cell Astrocytoma

WHO definition. Subependimal giant cell astrocytoma (SEGA) is a periventricular tumor composed partly of large ganglionic-like astrocytes and strongly associated with tuberous sclerosis (TS) (Figs. 3.27).

It is a WHO grade 1 tumor.

Epidemiology. Is the most common CNS tumor in patient with TS where it can be present in 5–15% of cases. It occurs in the first two decades of life and it is unknown if it can be present even in patients without TS.

Location. The location of SEGA is quite typical, as it arises in nearly all cases within the subependymal region of the foramen of Monro.

Clinical features. The most frequent signs are related to the increased intracranial pressure due to the block of CSF circulation at the level of the foramen of Monro. The tumor growth is usually very slow and it is evident in the first two decades of life.

Prognosis. When a complete resection of the tumor is obtained the prognosis is favorable.

Imaging. Like the other subependymal tubers of TS, SEGA appears on CT as a solid calcified nodular lesion in the region of the foramen of Monro. Actually the only feature that can differentiate a SEGA from a simple tuber is the progressive increase in size.

On MRI the lesion is usually heterogeneous on T1WI, T2WI, and FLAIR images. It clearly enhances after contrast administration.

On spectroscopy it has been reported a high Cho/Cr ratio as a predictive sign of transformation of a simple subependymal tuber in a SEGA [14] (Table 3.12).

3.3.5 Chordoid Glioma

WHO definition. It is a well circumscribed glial tumor that arises in the anterior part of the third ventricle. It is histologically characterized by clusters and cords of GFAP-expressing epitheliod cells and exhibits a recurrent p. D463H missense mutation in the *PRKCA* gene.

It is a WHO grade 2 tumor.

Epidemiology. Is a rare tumor that accounts for <0.1% of all primary CNS tumor with a median age of approximately 45 years.

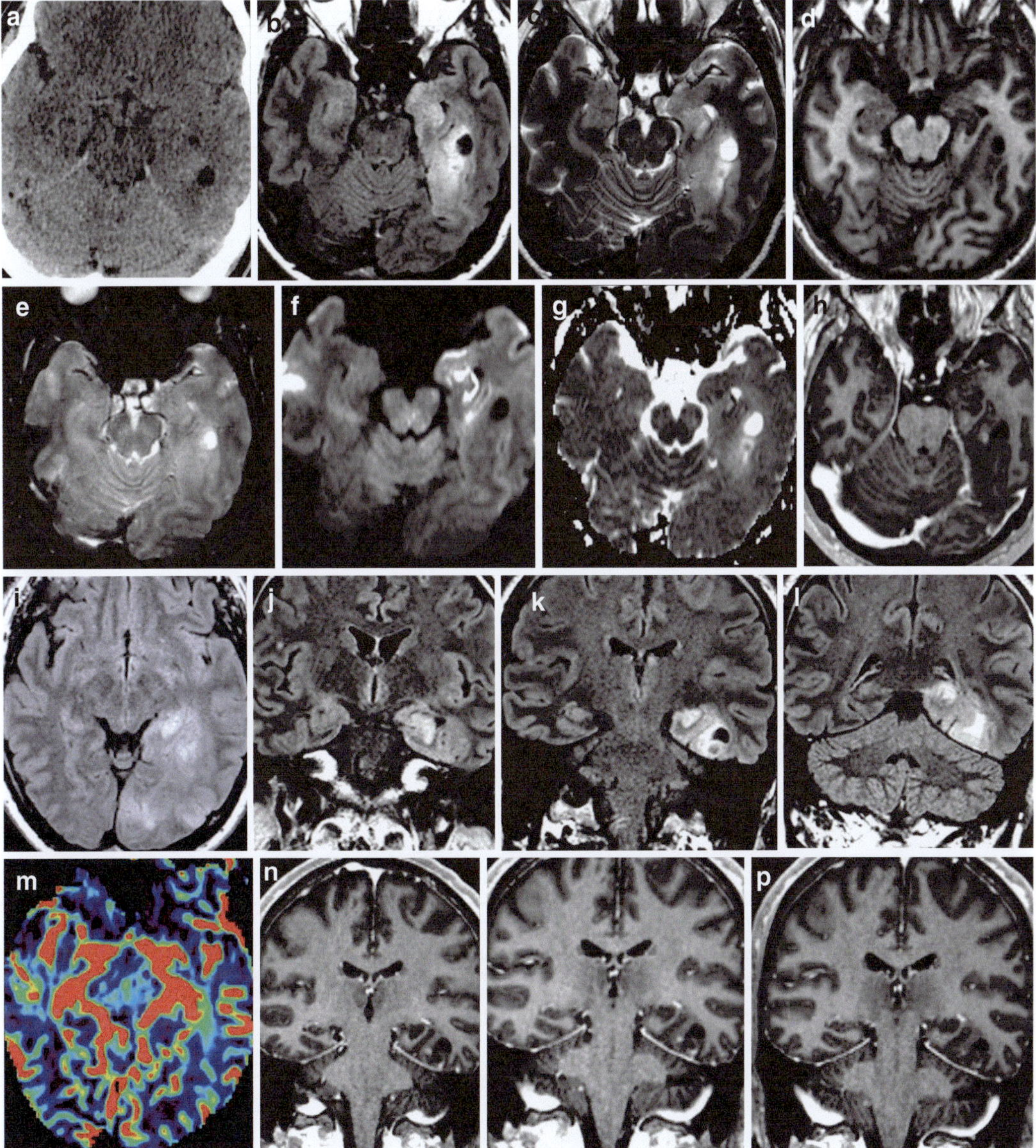

Fig. 3.25 Pleomorphic xanthoastrocytoma. CT (**a**). MRI FLAIR (**b, i-l**), T2WI (**c**), T1WI (**d**), T2*GRE (**e**), DWI (**f**), ADC (**g**), post-contrast T1WI (**h, n-p**), CBV (**m**), spectroscopy (**q**). A small cystic lesion is visible in the inferior part of the left temporal lobe. A slight hyperintense area on FLAIR and T2WI surrounds the cyst. No calcifications are visible on both CT and T2 GRE, the enhancement is doubtfull. (**b**) On coronal FLAIR images (**j-l**) the tumor exhibits a diffuse infiltrative component with an extension through temporo-occipital lobes in the basal and mesial regions. CBV seems to be normal or slightly increased, the enhancement remains doubtful or minimal and it is limited to the superficial areas. Spectroscopy shows a pattern compatible with a slow growing astrocytic tumor

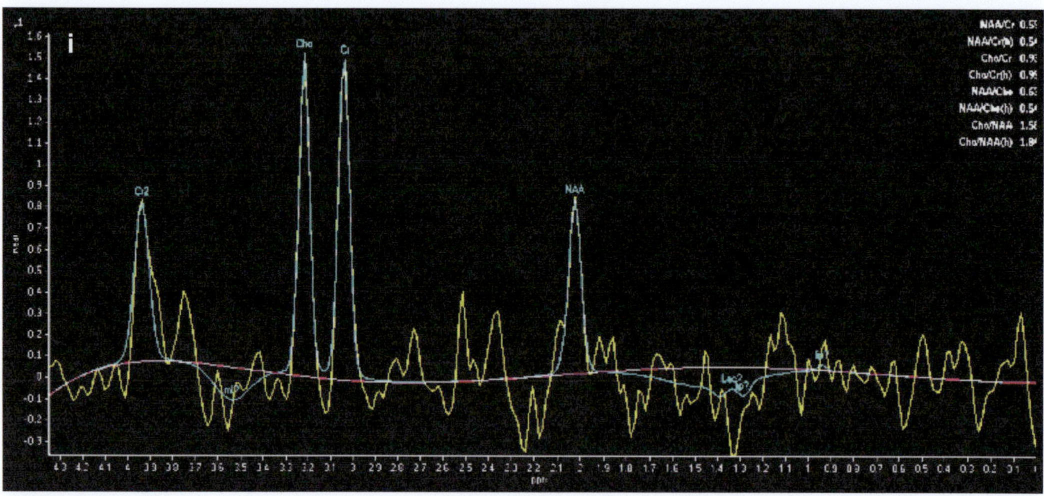

Fig. 3.25 (continued)

(c)

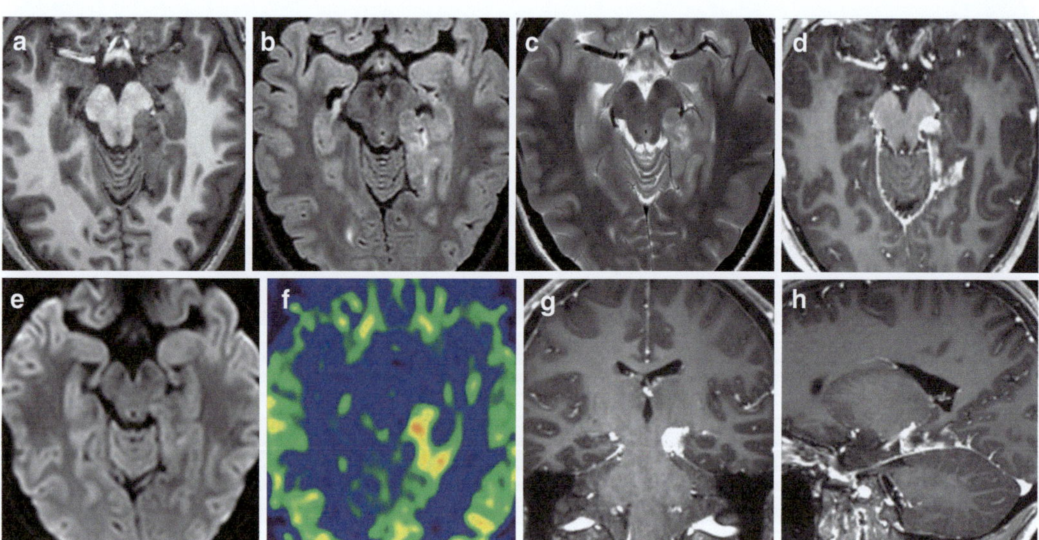

Fig. 3.26 Pleomorphic xanthoastrocytoma in a 24-year-old woman with epileptic seizures. MRI T1WI (**a**), FLAIR (**b**), T2WI (**c**), post-contrast T1WI (**d, g, h**), DWI (**e**), ASL-CBF (**f**), spectroscopy (**i**). A cortico-pial lesion is detectable in the left temporo-mesial region with an evident enhancement after contrast administration of the superficial component reaching posteriorly the occipital region. On ASL sequence (**f**) a perfusion increase is visible in the superficial part of the lesion as well. As for the previous case spectroscopy shows a pattern compatible with a slow growing tumor

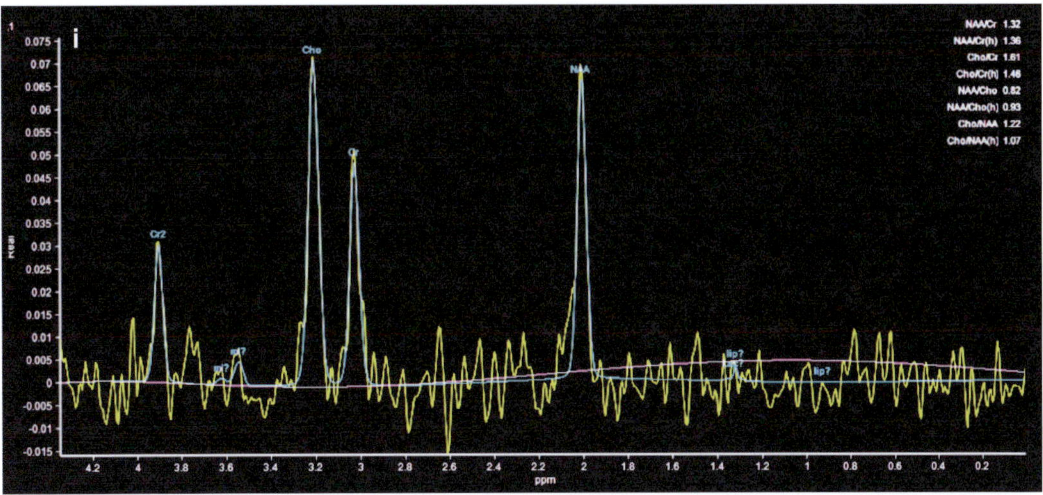

Fig. 3.26 (continued)

Table 3.11 Pleomorphic xanthoastrocytoma imaging features

Mass effect	Edema	Inhomogeneity	Cysts	Necrosis	Hemorrhage	Calcifications
0/+	0/+	++	0/+++	0	0	0/++

CT	T1	T2	FLAIR	DWI	ADC	T1 Gd	CBV	Spec
○	◉	○	○	◉	◉	0/++	●	↑Cho/NAA

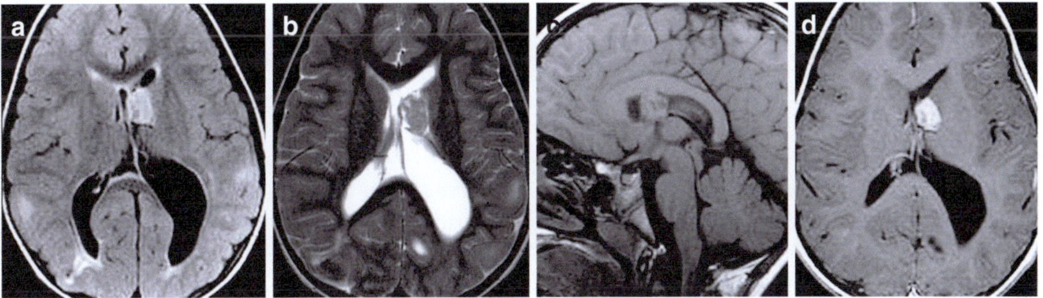

Fig. 3.27 SEGA in a patient with TS. MRI FLAIR (**a**), T2WI (**b**), T1WI (**c**), post-contrast T1WI (**d**). The lesion is typically located near the left foramen of Monro, it is an inhomogeneous lesion with evident calcification on CT study and with a clear enhancement after contrast administration. (Courtesy Dr. A. Righini, Milan)

Table 3.12 SEGA imaging features

Mass effect	Edema	Inhomogeneity	Cysts	Necrosis	Hemorrhage	Calcifications
0/++	0	++	0	0	0	+/++

CT	T1	T2	FLAIR	DWI	ADC	T1 Gd	CBV	Spec
○	○	○	○	○	○	++	NA[a]	↑Cho/Cr

[a]NA (not available) = incomplete or sporadic reports

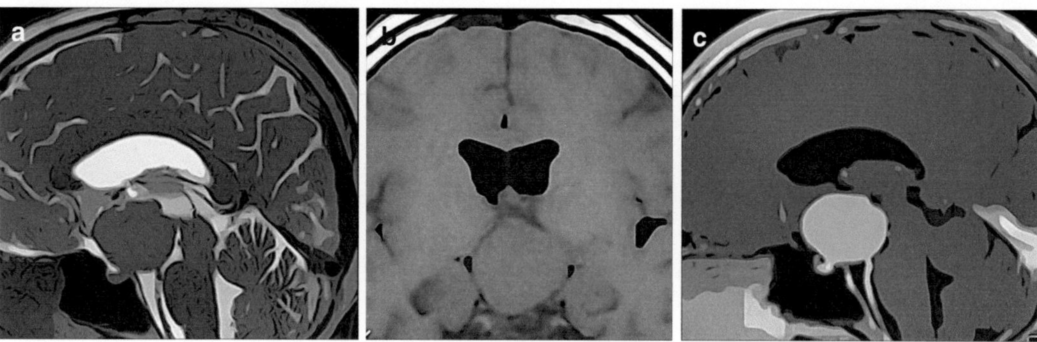

Fig. 3.28 A computer drawing of a typical chordoid glioma. MRI T2WI (**a**), T1WI (**b**), post-contrast T1WI (**c**). The location in the anterior part of the third ventricle in the hypothalamic region is quite typical for chordoid glioma and is similar to granular cell tumor of the sellar origin (Fig. 10.8)

Table 3.13 Chordoid glioma imaging features

Mass effect	Edema	Inhomogeneity	Cysts	Necrosis	Hemorrhage	Calcifications
0/++	0/+	0	0	0	0/+	0/+

CT	T1	T2	FLAIR	DWI	ADC	T1 Gd	CBV	Spec
○	○	○	○	○	○	+++	NA[a]	NA[a]

[a]NA (not available) = incomplete or sporadic reports

Location. The location is typically the anterior portion of the third ventricle. Chordoid gliomas are hypothesized to originate from the specialized tanycytic cells of the organum vasculosum of the lamina terminalis.

Clinical features. Clinical signs and symptoms are strictly related to the particular location of the tumor and they include: intracranial hypertension due to an obstructive hydrocephalus, endocrine or visual field disturbances due to the compression of the hypothalamic-chiasmatic areas.

Prognosis. Prognosis depends on the tumor size and its resectability.

Imaging. It is a well circumscribed mass in the anterior part of the third ventricles. On CT it may appear as slightly hyperdense, whereas on MRI it is characterized by an iso-hypointense signal on T2WI and in lesser way on FLAIR images. On T1WI it can be iso- or slightly hypointense (Fig. 3.28).

Chordoid gliomas homogeneously enhance after contrast administration [15].

The more complex differential diagnosis is with granular cell tumor of the sellar origin (Fig. 10.8). Imaging features of chordoid glioma are summarized in Table 3.13.

3.3.6 Astroblastoma *MN1*-Altered

WHO definition. Astroblatoma, *MN1*-altered, is a circumscribed glial neoplasm with *MN1* alteration that is composed of round, cuboidal, or columnar cells with variable pseudopapillary or perivascular growth, perivascular anucleate zones, and vascular and pericellular hyalinization.

Epidemiology. It is a rare tumor occurring in children to young adults with a strong female prevalence.

Location. It mainly occurs in cerebral hemispheres.

Clinical features. They are usually related to the increased intracranial pressure.

Prognosis It is a tumor with a good survival rate at 5 and 10 years, but with frequent recurrence.

Imaging. These tumors are predominantly hyperdense on pre-contrast CT, but they can be also iso- to slightly hypodense, calcifications are possible.

On MRI they appear as inhomogeneous tumors with possible cysts and a prevalent hyperintense aspect on T2WI/FLAIR images. Contrast enhancement is almost always present [16].

The case in Fig. 3.29 shows a slight diffusion restriction and an increase of Cho/NAA ratio with a lipid-lactate peak on spectroscopy. Imaging features of astroblastoma MN1-altered are summarized in Table 3.14.

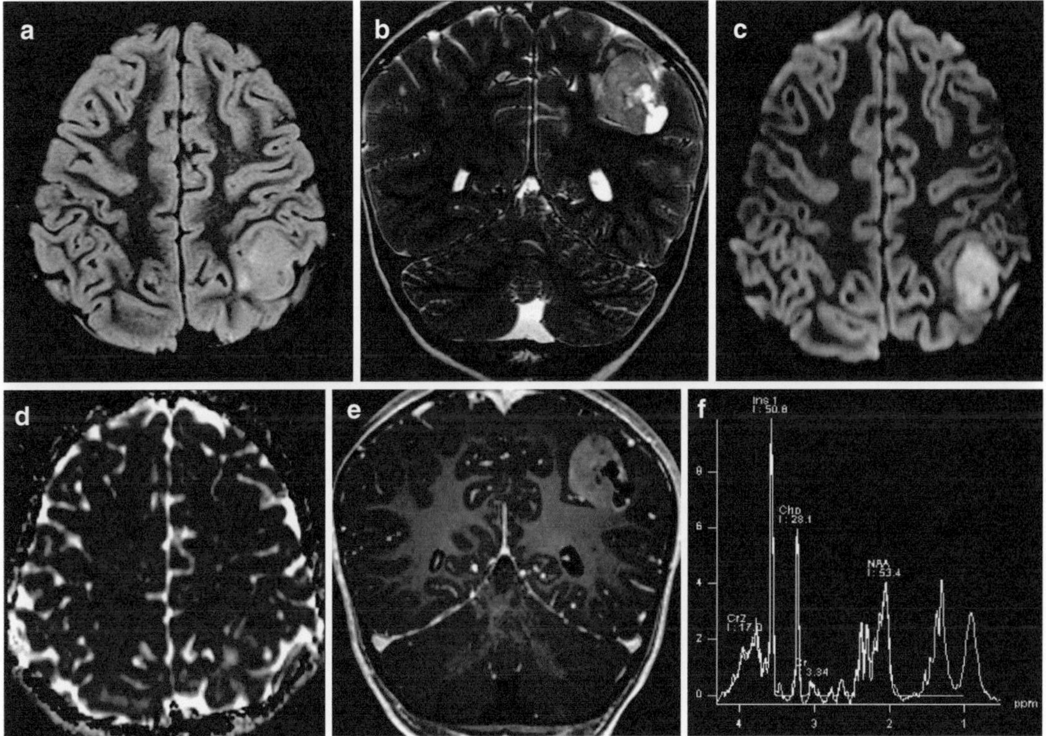

Fig. 3.29 An astroblastoma MN1-altered in a 4-year-old girl. MRI FLAIR (**a**), T2WI (**b**), DWI (**c**), ADC (**d**), post-contrast T1WI (**e**), spectroscopy (**f**). A solid and partly cystic lesion with no perilesional edema is visible in left retrorolandic cortical–subcortical region. Diffusion is slightly reduced, enhancement is minimal, and there is an increase in the Choo/NAA ratio with a lipid-lactate peak evident on spectroscopy. (Courtesy D. S. Colafati, Rome)

Table 3.14 Astroblastoma *MN1*-altered imaging features

Mass effect	Edema	Inhomogeneity	Cysts	Necrosis	Hemorrhage	Calcifications
+/++	0/+	+/++	+/++	0	0/+	0/++

CT	T1	T2	FLAIR	DWI	ADC	T1 Gd	CBV	Spec
○	◔	◔	◔	○	◕	0/++	NA[a]	↑Cho/NAA, ↑lipid-lac

[a]NA (not available) = incomplete or sporadic reports

References

1. Annika K, Wefers Damian, Stichel Daniel, et al. Isomorphic diffuse glioma is a morphologically and molecularly distinct tumour entity with recurrent gene fusions of MYBL1 or MYB and a benign disease course Acta Neuropathologica. 2020;139(1):193–209. https://doi.org/10.1007/s00401-019-02078-w.
2. Kurokawa R, Akira Baba A, Emile P, et al. Neuroimaging features of angiocentric glioma: a case series and systematic review. J Neuroimaging. 2022a;32:389–99.
3. Kurokawa R, Baba R, Kurokawa M, et al. Neuroimaging features of diffuse hemispheric glioma H3 G34-mutant: a case series and a systematic review. J Neuroimaging. 2022b;32:17–27.
4. Johnson DR, Giannini C, Jenkins RB, Kim DK, Kaufmann TJ. Plenty of calcification: imaging characterization of polymorphous low-grade neuroepithelial tumor of the young. Neuroradiology. 2019;61:1327–32.
5. Fabbri VP, Caporalini C, Asioli S, Buccoliero A. Paediatric-type diffuse low-grade gliomas: a clinically and biologically distinct group of tumours with a favourable outcome. Pathologica. 2022;114:410–21.
6. Ryall S, Zapotocky M, Fukuoka K, et al. Integrated molecular and clinical analysis of 1,000 pediatric low-grade gliomas. Cancer Cell. 2020;37:569–83.
7. Yamasaki F, Nishibushi I, Karakawa S, et al. T2-FLAIR mismatch sign and response to radiotherapy in diffuse intrinsic pontine glioma. Pediatr Neurosurg. 2021;56:1–9.
8. Tauziède-Espariat A, Debily M-A, Castel D, et al. The pediatric supratentorial MYCN amplified high-grade gliomas methylation class presents the same radiological, histopathological and molecular features as their pontine counterparts. Acta Neuropathol Commun. 2020;8:104.
9. Goncalves FG, Viaene AN, Vassough A. Advanced magnetic resonance imaging in pediatric glioblastoma. Front Neurol. 2021;12:733323.
10. Hwang JH, Egnaczyk GF, Ballard E, Scott Dunn R, Holland SK, Ball WS Jr. Proton MR spectroscopic characteristics of pediatric pilocytic astrocytomas. AJNR Am J Neuroradiol. 1998;19:535–40.
11. Harris LM, Davies NP, Macpherson L, Lateef S, Natarajan K, Sgouros S, English MW, Arvanitis TN, Grundy RG, Peet AC. Magnetic resonance spectroscopy in the assessment of pilocytic astrocytomas. Eur J Cancer. 2008;44:2640–7.
12. Bender K, Perez E, Chirica M, et al. High-grade astrocytoma with piloid features (HGAP): the Charité experience with a new central nervous system tumor entity. J Neuro-Oncol. 2021;153:109–20.
13. Moore W, Mathis D, Gargan L, Bowers DC, Klesse LJ, Margraf L, Koral K. Pleomorphic Xanthoastrocytoma of Childhood: MR Imaging and Diffusion MR Imaging Features. AJNR Am J Neuroradiol. 2014;35(11)2192–2196. https://doi.org/10.3174/ajnr.A4011.
14. de Carvalho NA, Gasparetto EL, Bruck I. Subependymal giant cell astrocytoma with high choline/creatine ratio on proton MR spectroscopy. Arch Neuropsiquiatr. 2006;64:877–80.
15. Pomper MG, Passe TJ, Burger PC, Sheithauer BW, Brat DJ. Chotdoid glioma: a neoplasm unique to the hypothalamus and anterior third ventricle. AJNR Am J Neuroradiol. 2001;22:464-9.
16. Bell J W, Osborn A G, Salzman K L, Blaser S I, Jones B V, Chin S S. Neuroradiologic characteristics of astroblastoma. Neuroradiology. 2007;49(3):203–9. https://doi.org/10.1007/s00234-006-0182-0.

4.1 Glioneuronal and Neuronal Tumors

4.1.1 Ganglioglioma

WHO definition. Ganglioglioma is a well-differentiated slow growing tumor composed by dysplastic ganglionic cells and neoplastic glial cells, which is molecularly characterized by genetic alterations that cause MAPK pathway activation.

It is a WHO grade 1 tumor.

Epidemiology. It can affect any age, but the majority of cases can be found in the first and second decade of life, a slight male prevalence was reported.

Location. Ganglioglioma can occur everywhere throughout the CNS even though the temporal lobe accounts for the vast majority of cases (> 70%).

Clinical features. Symptoms vary according to the location of the ganglioglioma. However since the temporal region is a frequent site, the most common clinical presentation is the presence of focal seizure.

Prognosis. Prognosis is good and the free recurrence survival rate after surgery is high.

Imaging. Ganglioglioma may typically present with three different components: a solid portion with frequent and variable enhancement, a cystic component, and calcifications (Fig. 4.1); however, this latter component is reported in only 30% of cases and sometimes even the cystic portion can be scarcely visible. The solid component presents with variable density and signal intensity, usually with increase in T2WI/FLAIR signal and hypointensity on T1WI. Enhancement of the solid portion is frequently seen and CBV can slightly increase (Fig. 4.2).

Small ganglioglioma can however present with very nonspecific aspects such in the case of Fig. 4.3.

Scarce and not conclusive data are at present available on spectroscopy. Imaging features of ganglioglioma are summarized in Table 4.1.

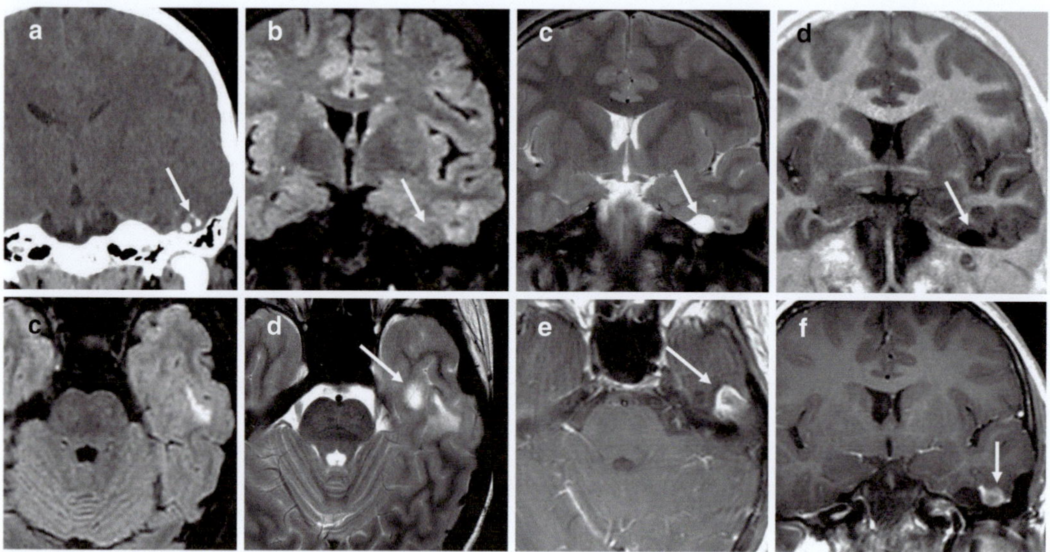

Fig. 4.1 Ganglioglioma in a 14-year-old girl with epileptic seizures. CT (**a**), MRI FLAIR (**b**, **e**), T2WI (**c**, **f**), T1WI inversion recovery (**d**), post-contrast T1WI (**g**, **h**). The lesion in the left temporal lobe shows all the three characteristic components of a ganglioma: calcifications (arrows **a**), cyst (arrow in **b**–**f**), and the solid portion that enhances after contrast (**g**, **h**)

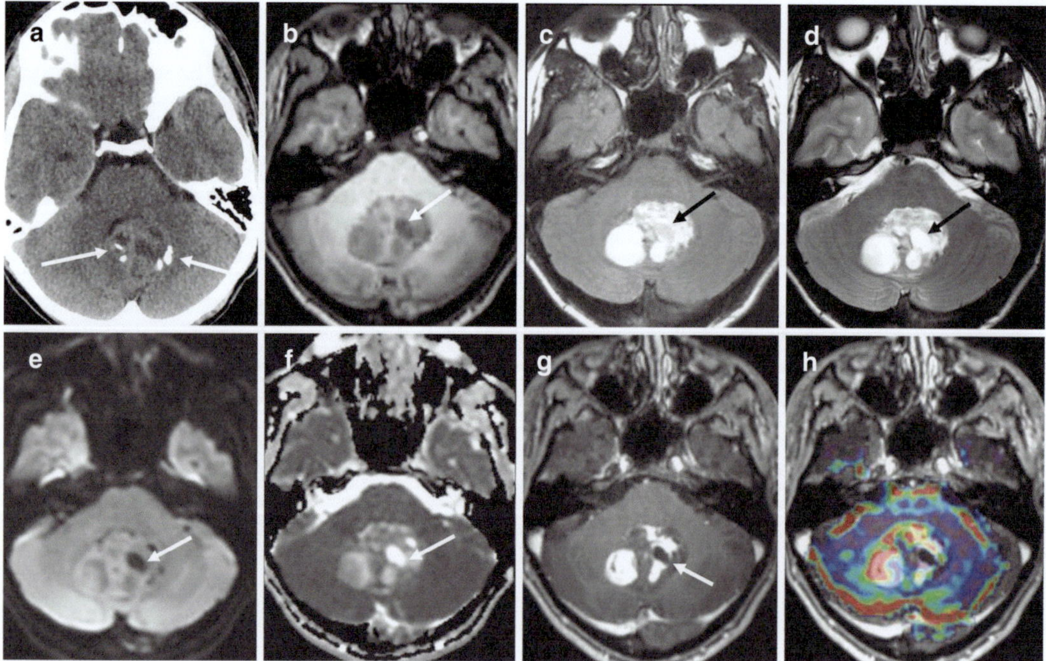

Fig. 4.2 Cerebellar ganglioglioma. CT (**a**), MRI T1WI (**b**), FLAIR (**c**), T2WI (**d**), DWI (**e**), ADC (**f**), post-contrast T1WI (**g**), CBV (**h**). Cerebellar gangliogliomas are rare, but also this lesion shows all the three characteristic components of the tumor: calcifications (arrows **a**), cysts, the largest pointed out by the arrow in (**b**-**g**), and the solid portion that partly enhances after contrast (**g**). CBV is slightly increased (**h**)

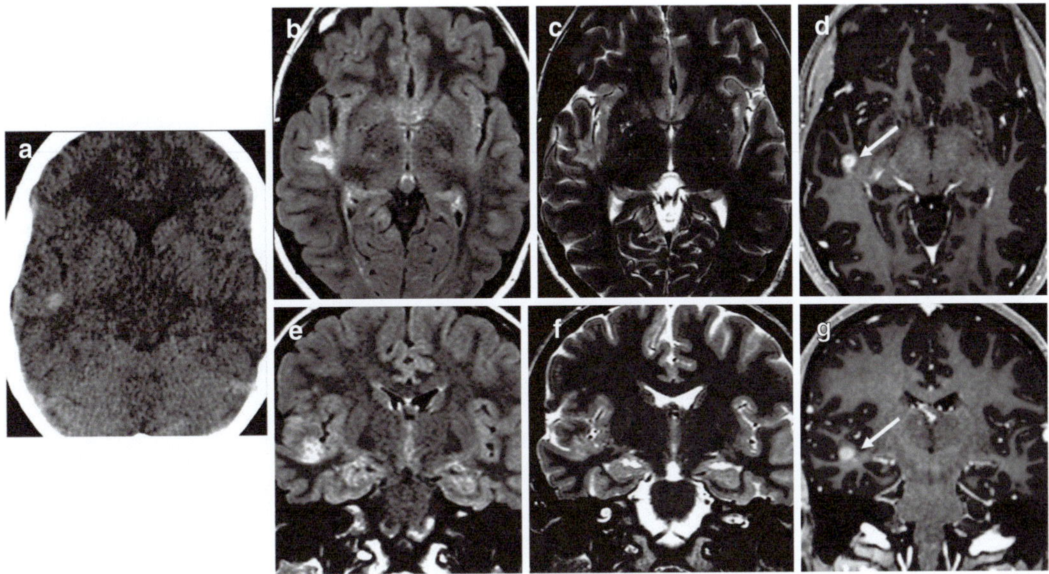

Fig. 4.3 Ganglioglioma. CT (**a**), MRI FLAIR (**b,e**), T2WI (**c, f**), post-contrast T1WI (**d, g**). Subcortical right temporal ganglioglioma presents with a slight hyper-dense nodule on CT (**a**) and hyperintensity on MRI FLAIR/T2 images (**b, c, e, f**), with enhancement after contrast (**d, g**)

Table 4.1 Ganglioglioma imaging features

Mass effect	Edema	Inhomogeneity	Cysts	Necrosis	Hemorrhage	Calcifications
0/+	0/+	0/++	0/++	0	0	0/++

CT	T1	T2	FLAIR	DWI	ADC	T1 Gd	CBV	Spec
◉○	◑	○	○	○	○	0/++	◉	NA[a]

[a]NA (not available) = incomplete or sporadic reports

4.1.2 Gangliocytoma

WHO definition. Gangliocytoma is a rare well-differentiated slow growing tumor composed by ganglionic cells often with dysplastic features.

It is a WHO grade 1 tumor.

Epidemiology. As for ganglioglioma, gangliocytoma can affect any age but the majority of cases can be found in young adults, it is definitely more rare than ganglioglioma.

Location. As for ganglioglioma also gangliocytoma can occur everywhere even though it is more frequently found in the cerebral hemispheres.

Clinical features. The most frequent clinical presentation are seizures.

Prognosis. If completely resected the prognosis is favorable.

Imaging. Gangliocytoma is very rare and the imaging presentation is aspecific, a small cortical nodule with a potential enhancement, as shown in the case of Fig. 4.4, can be a relatively typical presentation. Imaging features of gangliocytoma are summarized in Table 4.2.

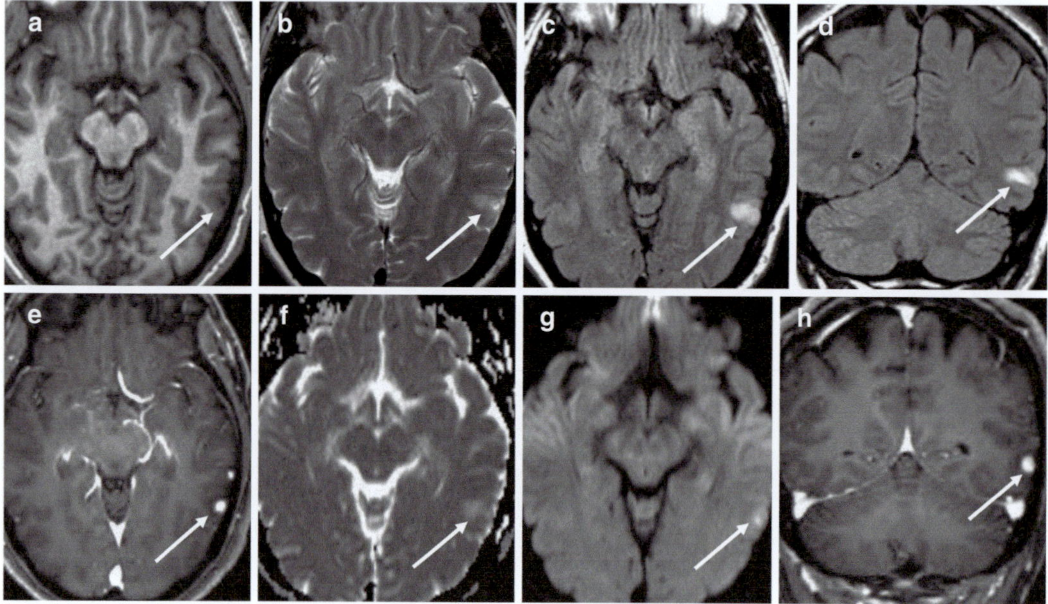

Fig. 4.4 Gangliocytoma. MRI T1WI (**a**), T2WI (**b**), FLAIR (**c**, **d**), T2WI (**d**), post-contrast T1WI (**e**, **h**), ADC (**f**), DWI (**g**). Gangliocytoma presents as a cortical left temporo-occipital lesions (arrows A-H), better seen before contrast on FLAIR images and with a clear enhancement after contrast (**e**, **h**). Patient suffers from seizures. This case is quite similar to ganglioglioma of Fig. 4.3

Table 4.2 Gangliocytoma imaging features

Mass effect	Edema	Inhomogeneity	Cysts	Necrosis	Hemorrhage	Calcifications
0/+	0/+	0/+	0/++	0	0	0/+

CT	T1	T2	FLAIR	DWI	ADC	T1 Gd	CBV	Spec
⬤◯	◯	◯	◯	◯	⬤	+/++	◯	NA[a]

[a]NA (not available) = incomplete or sporadic reports

4.1.3 Desmoplastic Infantile Ganglioglioma and Desmoplastic Infantile Astrocytoma

WHO definition. Desmoplastic infantile ganglioglioma (DIG) and desmoplastic infantile astrocytoma (DIA) are benign glioneuronal and glial tumor occurring mainly in the cerebral hemisphere of infants. They are composed by a mixed neuronal-glial component, or an astrocytic component only, embedded in an extensive desmoplastic stroma.

They are WHO grade 1 tumors.

Epidemiology. DIG and DIA are very rare childhood tumors that very rarely appear after 20 years of age.

Location. The location is almost exclusively in the cerebral hemispheres, involving the cerebral cortex and the leptomeninges.

Clinical features. The most frequent symptoms and signs are related to increased intracranial pressure.

Prognosis. The prognosis is very good when a total removal is achieved.

Imaging. The imaging features are quite characteristic for both tumors that appear as a large superficial hemispheric cyst with a solid nodule with a clear enhancement after contrast administration. In some way this aspect may be resembling a pilocytic astrocytoma even though the mural nodule of DIG/DIA is not clearly hyperintense on T2WI/FLAIR images (Figs. 4.5 and 4.6).

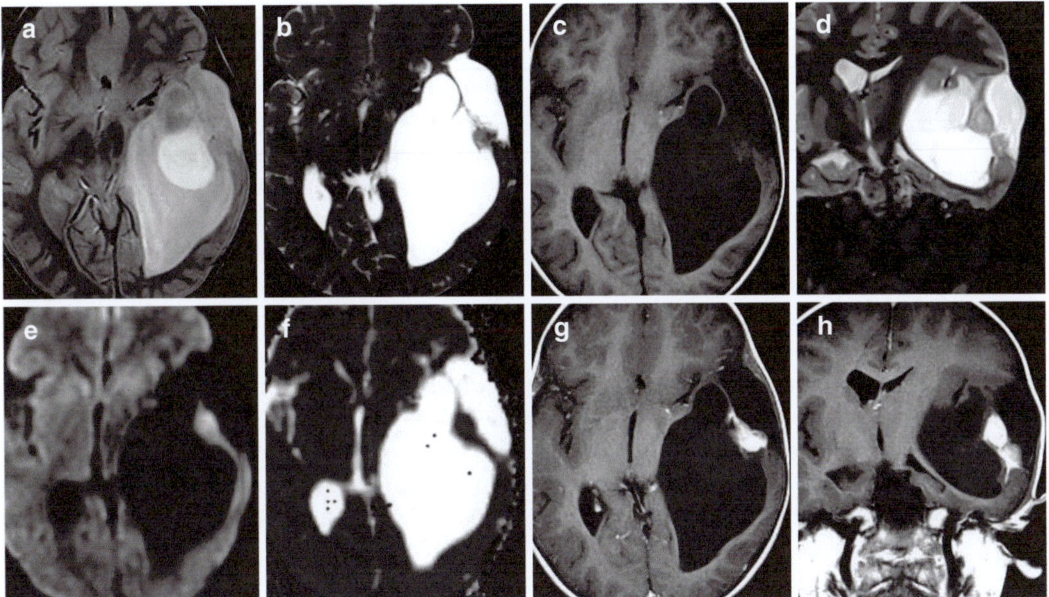

Fig. 4.5 Desmoplastic infantile ganglioglioma in a 8-year-old girl. MRI PDWI (**a**), T2WI (**b,d**), T1WI (**c**), DWI (**e**), ADC (**f**), post-contrast T1WI (**g, h**). DIG typically presents as a huge superficial hemispheric cystic lesion with an enhancing nodule

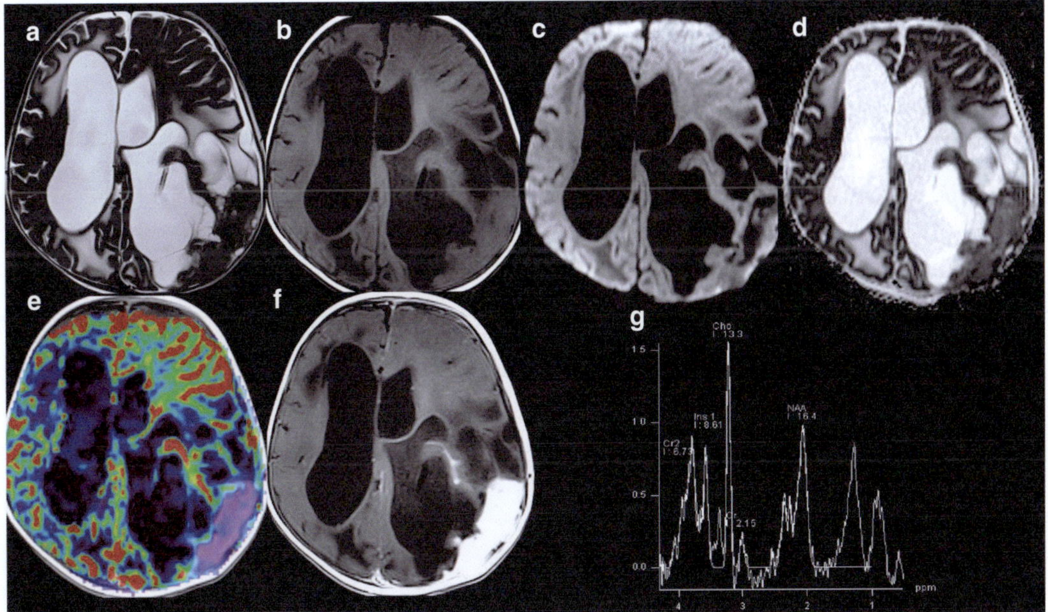

Fig. 4.6 Desmoplastic infantile astrocytoma in a 6-month-old girl. MRI T2WI (**a**), T1WI (**b**), DWI (**c**), ADC (**d**), CBV (**e**), post-contrast T1WI (**f**), spectroscopy (**g**). DIA is quite similar to DIG with the same huge superficial hemispheric cystic lesion (in this case with a shunt) and a large cortical enhancing nodule. CBV was slightly increased and spectroscopy shows a slight increase of Cho/NAA ratio and the presence of a lipid-lactate peak (Courtesy Dr. S. Colafati, Rome)

The enhancement is usually strong.

Diffusion is not restricted. Image features of DIG/DIA are summarized in Table 4.3.

4.1.4　Dysembryoplastic Neuroepithelial Tumor

WHO definition. Dysembrioplastic neuroepithelial tumor (DNT) is a benign glioneuronal slow growing tumor located in the cerebral cortex characterized by the occurrence of the pathognomonic glioneuronal element that may be associated with glial nodules and activating mutations of *FGFR1*.

It is a WHO grade 1 tumor.

Epidemiology. DNT is usually reported in epilepsy surgery series in 5–10%, the operated patients are mainly under 20 years of age.

Location. There is a predilection for temporal lobes, in particular mesial structure, but they can originate in any part of the cerbral cortex.

Clinical features. DNT is typically associated with drug-resistent seizures.

Prognosis. DNT prognosis is usually good being a stable tumor with a low rate of recurrence after surgery.

Imaging. DNT is an almost pure cortical lesion that rarely extends into subcortical areas. It can bulge over the cortical surface causing sometimes a progressive erosion of the internal calvarium (Fig. 4.7). Calcifications can be seen on CT usually in the most inner part of the tumor.

Table 4.3　DIG/DIA imaging features

Mass effect		Edema	Inhomogeneity		Cysts		Necrosis		Hemorrhage		Calcifications
+/+++		0/+	+/++		+/+++		0		0		0

CT	T1	T2	FLAIR	DWI	ADC	T1 Gd	CBV	Spec
⬤	⬤	⬤	◯	◯	⬤	+/+++	◯	↑Cho/NAA ↑lipid-lactate

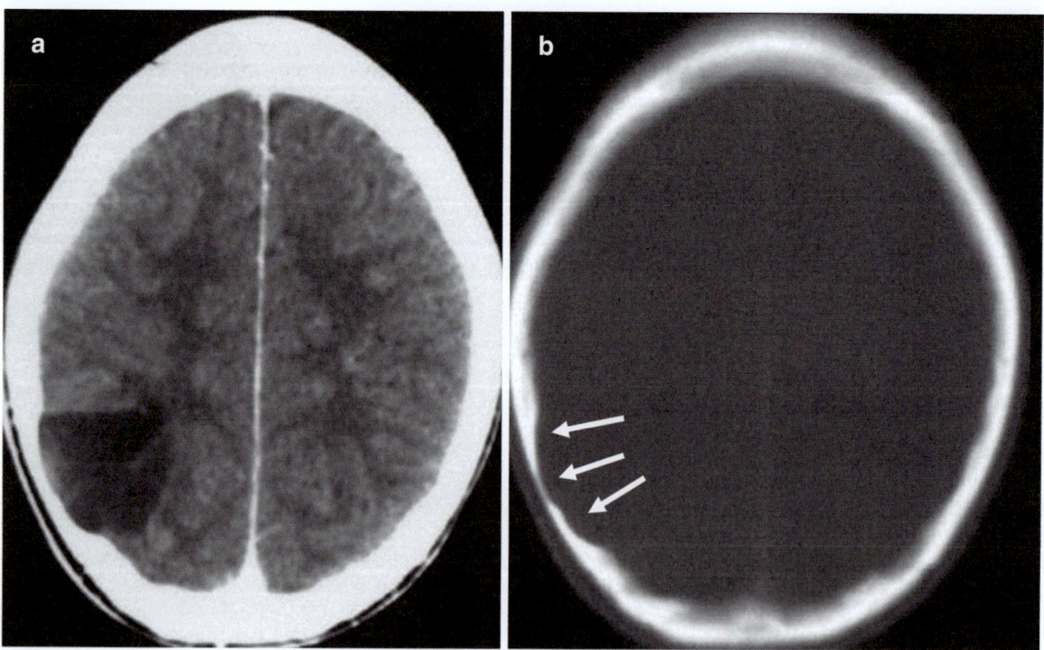

Fig. 4.7　DNT. CT parenchymal window (**a**), bone window (**b**). The neoplasm is extremely hypodense and superficial with a slight bulging over the cortex and a scalloping of the internal calvarium (arrows **b**)

The most typical feature of neuroimaging is the presence of a well demarcated lesion with a clear hypodensity on CT and a marked hyperintensity on T2WI/FLAIR sequences and hypointensity on T1WI, resembling an extremely water-rich lesion (Figs. 4.8, 4.9 and 4.10). Sometimes it appears as a cystic or multicystic lesion (Figs. 4.9 and 4.10).

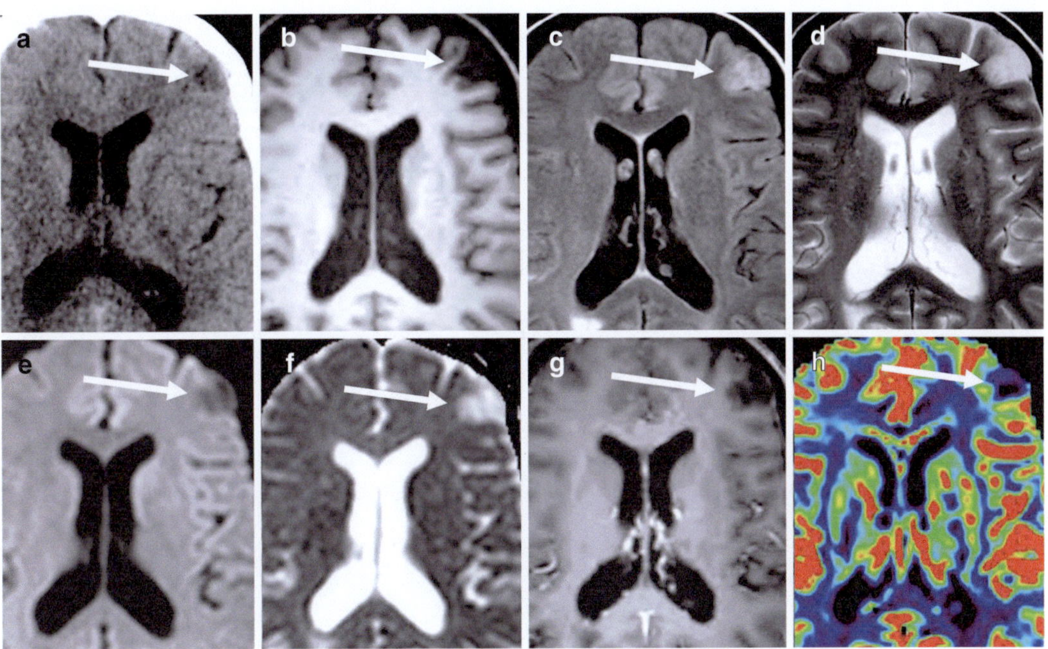

Fig. 4.8 DNT. CT (**a**), T1WI (**b**), FLAIR (**c**), T2WI (**d**), DWI (**e**), ADC (**f**), post-contrast T1WI (**g**), CBV (**h**). Left cortical frontal lesion (arrows) with a slight bulging of the most superficial part. No contrast enhancement, decreased CBV

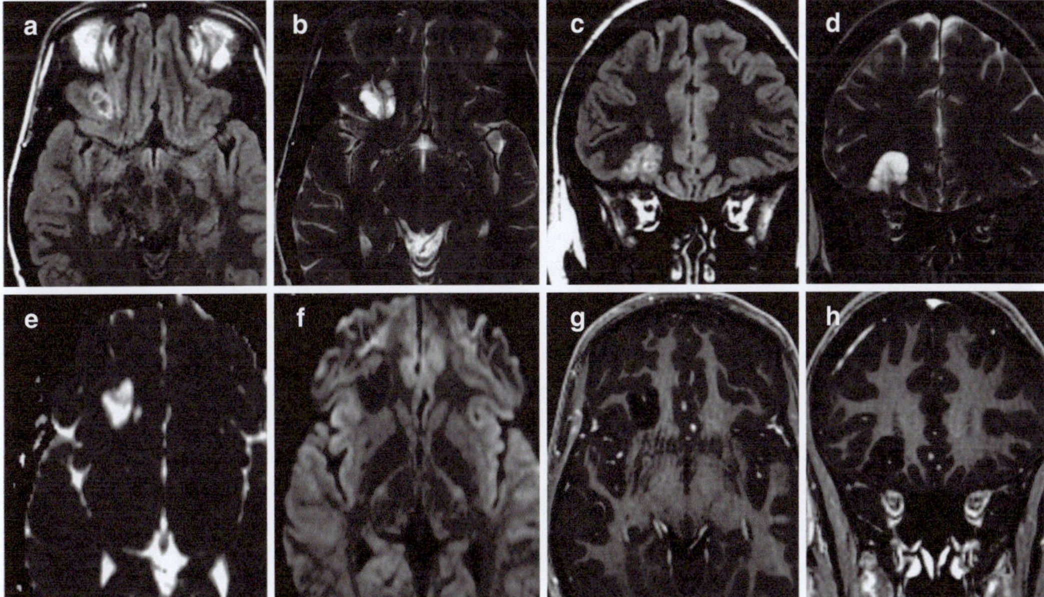

Fig. 4.9 DNT. FLAIR (**a, c**), T2WI (**b, d**), ADCI (**e**), DWI (**f**), post-contrast T1WI (**g, h**). Right cortical fronto-basal lesion with marked T1-hypointense and T2-hyperintense aspect. No contrast enhancement

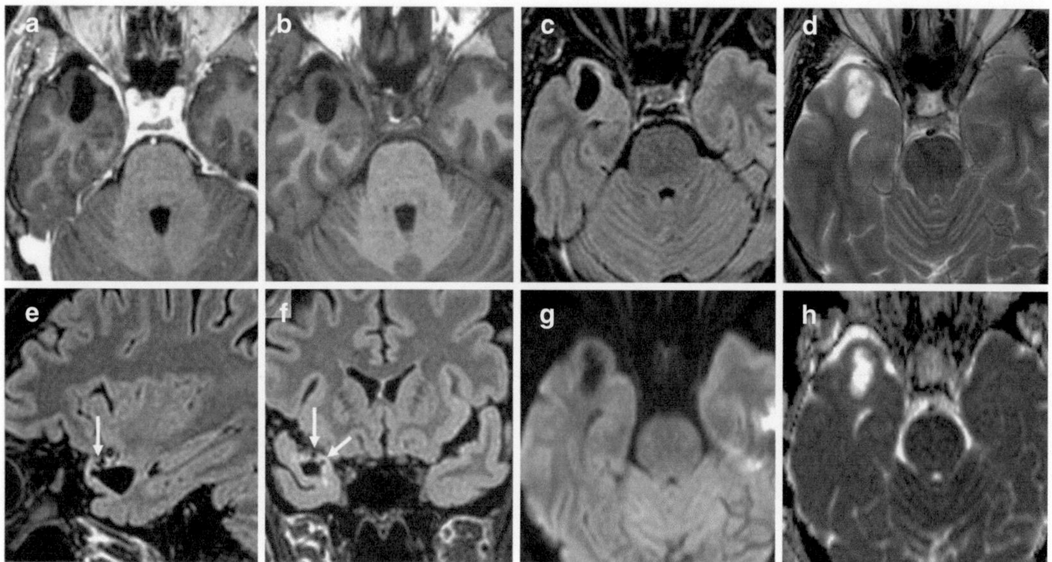

Fig. 4.10 DNT. MRI post-contrast T1WI (**a**, **b**), FLAIR (**c**, **e**, **f**), T2WI (**d**), DWI (**g**), ADC (**h**). An apparently cystic lesion is detectable on cortico-subcortical right temporo-polar region. Further very small cysts near the greater one are visible in sagittal and coronal FLAIR images (arrows **e**, **f**)

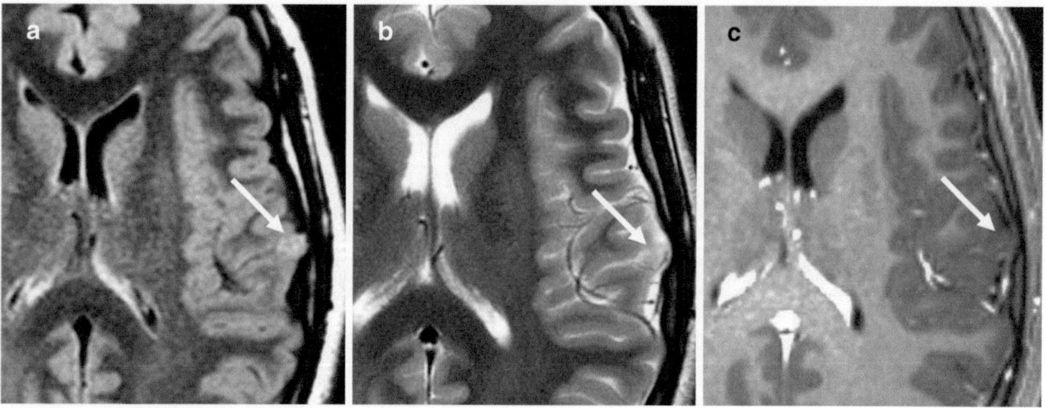

Fig. 4.11 DNT. MRI FLAIR (**a**), T2WI (**b**), post-contrast T1WI (**c**). An extremely small pure cortical lesion (arrow) is barely visible in the upper part of the left temporal region. After contrast the lesion is not clearly separable from the normal cortex

Post-contrast enhancement can be present although rare.

Diffusion is usually increased, CBV is reduced (Fig. 4.8), and a slight increase in Cho/NAA and mI/Cr was reported in spectroscopy [1].

DNT is very frequently associated with drug-resistant epilepsy: it is mandatory to carefully scrutinize in particular the region with focal spikes on EEG because the lesions can be extremely small as shown in Fig. 4.11, Image features of DNT are summarized in Table 4.4.

Table 4.4 DNT imaging summary

Mass effect	Edema	Inhomogeneity	Cysts	Necrosis	Hemorrhage	Calcifications
0/+	0	0/+	0	0	0/+	0/+

CT	T1	T2	FLAIR	DWI	ADC	T1 Gd	CBV	Spec
●	●	○	◐	●	○	0/+	●	↑Cho/NAA ↑mI/Cr

4.1.5 Diffuse Glioneuronal Tumor with Oligodendroglioma-Like Features and Nuclear Clusters

WHO definition. Diffuse glioneuronal tumor with oligodendroglioma-like features and nuclear clusters (DGONC) is a *provisional tumor type* proposed as a neuroepithelial tumor characterized by variably differentiated cells frequently showing perinuclear haloes, scattered multinucleated cells, and nuclear clusters, with a distinct DNA methylation profile and frequent monosomy of chromosome 14.

Epidemiology. Most reported cases occurred in childhood.

Location. All reported cases are located supratentorially.

Clinical features. No specific symptoms and signs.

Prognosis. The few cases reported show a survival rate at 5 years around 80%.

Imaging. Very few reports are available describing the imaging features of this rare tumor. According to these authors [2] this tumor had no appreciable perilesional edema, was hyperintense on T2WI/FLAIR images and enhanced poorly with contrast if at all. They also demonstrated internal matrix calcification, with centrally low ADC values on diffusion-weighted images (Fig. 4.12). Imaging features of DGONC are summarized in Table 4.5.

4.1.6 Papillary Glioneuronal Tumor

WHO definition. Papillary glioneuronal tumor (PGNT) is a glioneuronal tumor exhibiting a biphasic pattern with variable representation of pseudopapillary glial structures and interpapillary neuronal components and with *PRKCA* gene fusion.

It is a WHO grade 1 tumor.

Epidemiology. It is a rare tumor mainly found in young adults.

Location. It is located in the cerebral hemispheres predominantly in the temporal lobes or near lateral ventricles.

Clinical features. Headache and/or seizures.

Prognosis. If completely resected, the prognosis is good.

Imaging. It is usually composed by a cystic and a solid component with absent or scarce perilesional. Solid component of the tumor is hypodense or isodense on CT, hyperintense on T2WI/FLAIR, and mainly hypointense on T1WI and shows a heterogeneous enhancement after contrast administration (Fig. 4.13). Hemorrhage is frequently reported. Calcifications are reported in many cases.

Diffusion is usually normal even though sporadic areas of diffusion restriction in solid component have been reported.

Spectroscopy may show a Cho/NAA ratio increase and a possible lactate peak.

Data on perfusion are scarce it seems either normal or slightly increased [3]. Imaging features of PGNT are summarized in Table 4.6.

4.1.7 Rosette-Forming Glioneuronal Tumor

WHO definition. Rosette-forming glioneuronal tumor (RGNT) it is a glioneuronal tumor histologically composed by two components: neurocytes forming rosettes and/or pseudorosettes and glial elements resembling pilocytic astrocytoma.

This tumor is characterized by FGFR1 mutation and corresponds to WHO grade 1.

Epidemiology. RGNT is a rare tumor affecting mainly young adults or children.

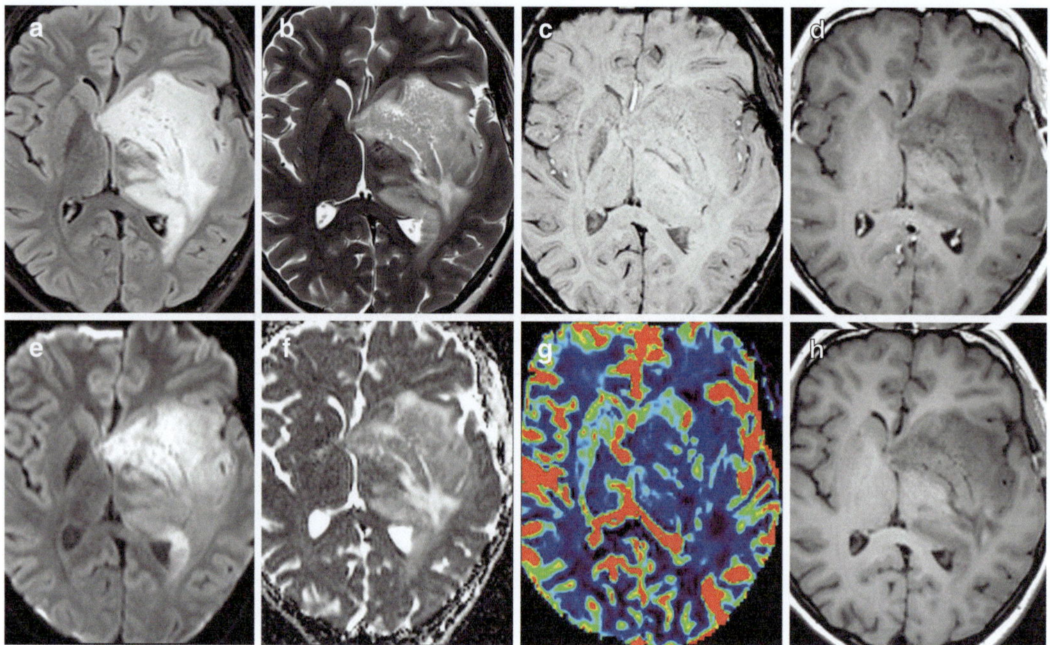

Fig. 4.12 DGONC in a 13-year-old girl. MRI FLAIR (**a**), T2WI (**b**), SWI (**c**), T1WI (**d**), DWI (**e**), ADC (**f**), CBV (**g**), post-contrast T1WI (**h**). A partly inhomogeneous lesion predominantly hyperintense on FLAIR and hypointense on T1WI is present in the deep brain structures of the left hemisphere, diffusion is slightly reduced in some parts and CBV seems to be predominantly reduced. (Courtesy Dr. S. Colafati, Rome)

Table 4.5 DGONC imaging summary

Mass effect	Edema	Inhomogeneity	Cysts	Necrosis	Hemorrhage	Calcifications
+/++	0/+	+/++	0	0	0/+	0/+

CT	T1	T2	FLAIR	DWI	ADC	T1 Gd	CBV	Spec
○	○	○	○	○	○	0/+	○	NA[a]

[a]NA (not available) = incomplete or sporadic reports

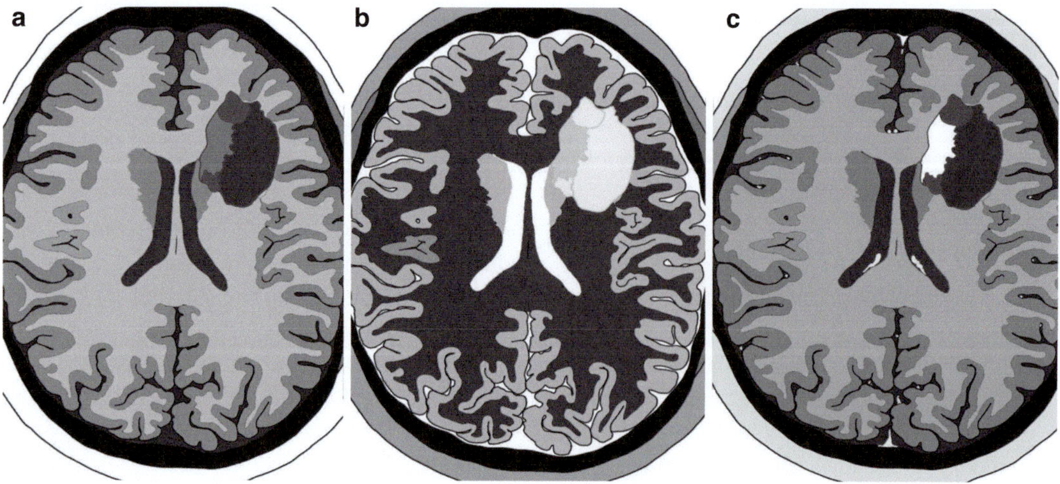

Fig. 4.13 PGNT. Schematic drawing of MRI features: T1WI (**a**), T2WI (**b**), post-contrast T1WI (**c**). Periventricular location is relatively typical

Location. Usually arise in midline structures of posterior fossa involving the fourth ventricle, the aqueduct, the cerebellar vermis, the quadrigeminal plate, and sometime the brainstem.

Clinical features. It is frequently related to intracranial hypertension due to involvement of fourth ventricle and aqueduct.

Prognosis. It is related to the possibility of a complete resection, a ventricular dissemination of the tumor is possible.

Imaging. RGNT appears as a T1WI hypointense and T2WI/FLAIR hyperintense lesion with a multinodular/cystic appearance and possible enhancement after contrast. Calcification and frequent intratumoral hemorrhage are described (Fig. 4.14).

When enhancement after contrast is present, it may be focal, multifocal, or around the cysts.

A possible slight increase in Cho/Cr ratio and presence of lipid-lactate peak have been reported [4]. Imaging features of RGNT are summarized in Table 4.7.

Table 4.6 PGNT imaging features

Mass effect	Edema	Inhomogeneity	Cysts	Necrosis	Hemorrhage	Calcifications
+/++	0/+	+/++	+/+++	0	0/++	0/++

CT	T1	T2	FLAIR	DWI	ADC	T1 Gd	CBV	Spec
○	○	○	○	○	○	+/++	○	↑Cho/NAA

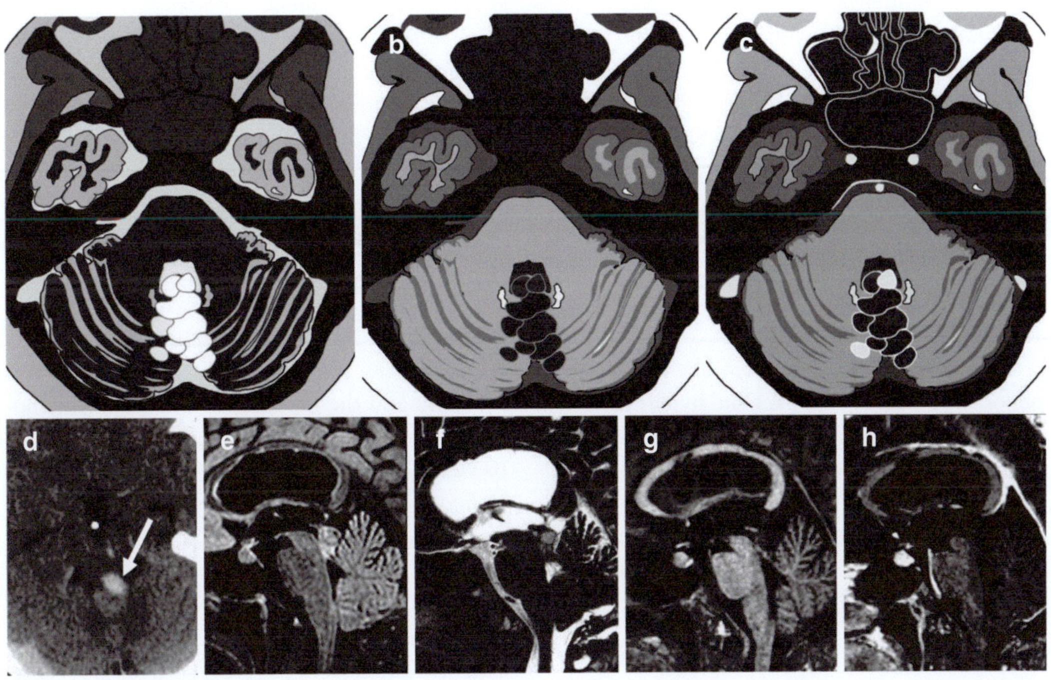

Fig. 4.14 Upper row, schematic drawing of RGNT. MRI T2WI (**a**), T1WI (**b**), post-contrast T1WI (**c**). Lower row, patients with RGNT of the quadrigeminal plate and aqueductal stenosis CT (**d**), MRI FLAIR (**e**), T2WI (**f**), T1WI (**g**), post-contrast T1WI (**h**). ON CT a small hemorrhage is visible (arrow **d**)

Table 4.7 RGNT imaging features

Mass effect	Edema	Inhomogeneity	Cysts	Necrosis	Hemorrhage	Calcifications
0/++	0	+/++	+/+++	0	+/++	0/+

CT	T1	T2	FLAIR	DWI	ADC	T1 Gd	CBV	Spec
○ (light gray)	○ (gray)	○ (light gray)	○ (white)	● (dark gray)	○ (light gray)	0/++	NA[a]	↑Cho/Cr

[a]NA (not available) = incomplete or sporadic reports

Table 4.8 Myxoid glioneural tumor imaging features

Mass effect	Edema	Inhomogeneity	Cysts	Necrosis	Hemorrhage	Calcifications
0/++	0	+/++	0/+	0	0/+	0/+

CT	T1	T2	FLAIR	DWI	ADC	T1 Gd	CBV	Spec
○ (light gray)	○ (gray)	○ (light gray)	○ (white)	● (dark gray)	○ (light gray)	0	NA[a]	NA[a]

[a]NA (not available) = incomplete or sporadic reports

4.1.8 Myxoid Glioneuronal Tumor

WGO definition. Myxoid glioneuronal tumor is a low-grade glioneuronal tumor characterized by a proliferation of oligodendrocyte-like cells embedded in a prominent myxoid stroma. There is a recurrent mutation in *PDGFRA* gene.

Epidemiology. This tumor is rare and occurs mainly in young adults.

Location. It is typically located in the septal nuclei and in the septum pellucidum, corpus callosum or periventricular white matter.

Clinical features. Clinical symptoms and signs are variable and depend on the location of the tumor.

Prognosis. If completely resected, the prognosis is good; however, it can recur locally or disseminate throughout ventricles.

Imaging. Usually, they are well circumscribed tumor hypointense on T1WI and hyperintense on T2WI/FLAIR images, with no contrast enhancement.

No restricted diffusion was reported as well as possible hemorrhages and/or calcifications [5, 6]. Imaging features of myxoid glioneuronal tumor are summarized in Table 4.8.

4.1.9 Diffuse Leptomeningeal Glioneuronal Tumor

WHO definition. Diffuse leptomeningeal glioneuronal tumor (DLGNT) is a glioneuronal tumor that diffusely involves the leptomeninges composed of oligodendrocyte-like cells. It is molecularly characterized by chromosome arm 1p deletion and a MAPK pathway gene alteration.

Epidemiology. It is a rare tumor that mostly affects pediatric patients.

Location. This tumor involves diffusely spinal and intracranial leptomeninges. In the intracranial compartment the most frequently involved structures are the leptomeninges of the posterior fossa.

Clinical features. They are usually referred to symptoms and signs of raised intracranial pressure.

Prognosis. The tumor growth is extremely slow and can be apparently quiescent for many years, but at present no effective therapy is available and the median survival after diagnosis is variable from few years to more than 10 years.

Imaging. It is characterized by multiple diffuse cysts in the subpial surface of spinal cord and brain leptomeninges with variable enhancement and diffuse leptomeningeal thickening. These findings may be present in conjunction with or without isolated spinal cord mass [7] (Fig. 4.15). As the disease progresses, hydrocephalus becomes more frequent. For its peculiar presentation diffuse infectious diseases are the main differential diagnosis. Imaging features of DLGNT are summarized in Table 4.9.

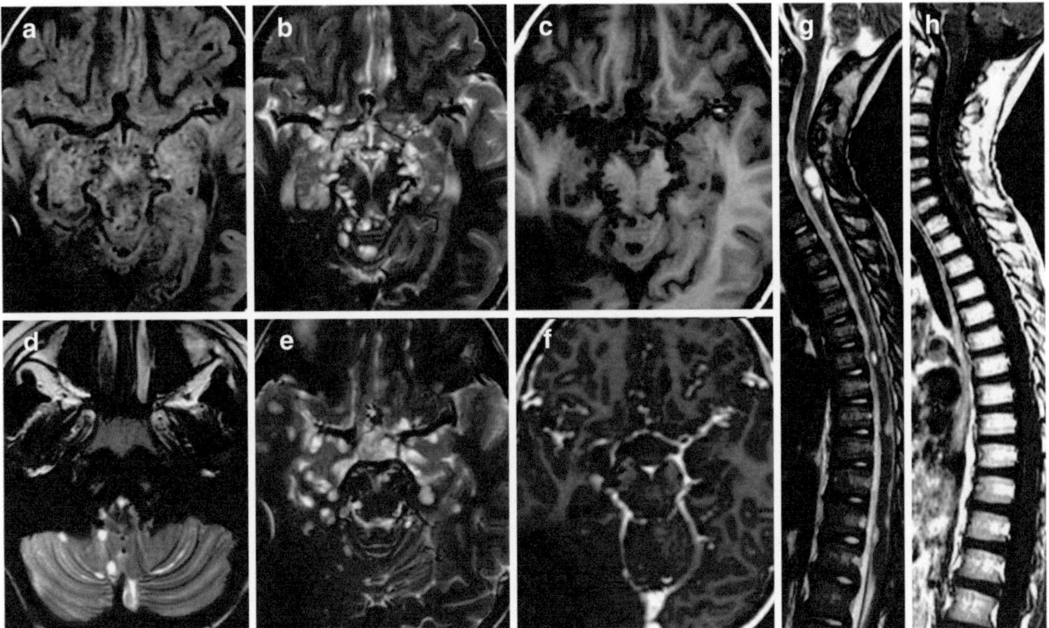

Fig. 4.15 DLGNT. MRI FLAIR (**a**), T2WI (**b, d, e, g**), T1WI (**c**), post-contrast T1WI (**f,h**). Diffuse subpial small cysts are evident both in the brain and in the spinal cord, a slight leptomeningeal enhancement is visible after contrast administration (**f, h**)

Table 4.9 DLGNT imaging features

Mass effect	Edema	Inhomogeneity	Cysts	Necrosis	Hemorrhage	Calcifications
0/++	0	+/++	+/+++	0	0/+	0/+

CT	T1	T2	FLAIR	DWI	ADC	T1 Gd	CBV	Spec
◓	◓	◯	◯	◓	◯	+/++	NA[a]	NA[a]

[a]NA (not available) = incomplete or sporadic reports

4.1.10 Multinodular Vacuolating Neuronal Tumor

WHO definition. The multinodular and vacuolating neuronal tumor (MVNT) is composed of monomorphic neuronal elements distributed in discrete and coalescent nodules, with vacuolar changes in tumor cells and their matrix.

It is a WHO grade 1 tumor.

Epidemiology. It is a rare tumor occurring mainly in adults.

Location. It is located in the deep cortical ribbon and subcortical white matter, mainly in temporal lobe.

Clinical features. It is associated with seizures.

Prognosis. It is a benign tumor that is apparently nonprogressive.

Imaging. MVNT consists of a cluster of variably sized nodular lesions located on the subcortical ribbon and superficial subcortical white matter following the gyral contour. They appear hyperintense on T2WI/FLAIR images and hypointense on T1WI and do not enhance after contrast administration (Fig. 4.16) [8]. Imaging features of MVNT are summarized in Table 4.10.

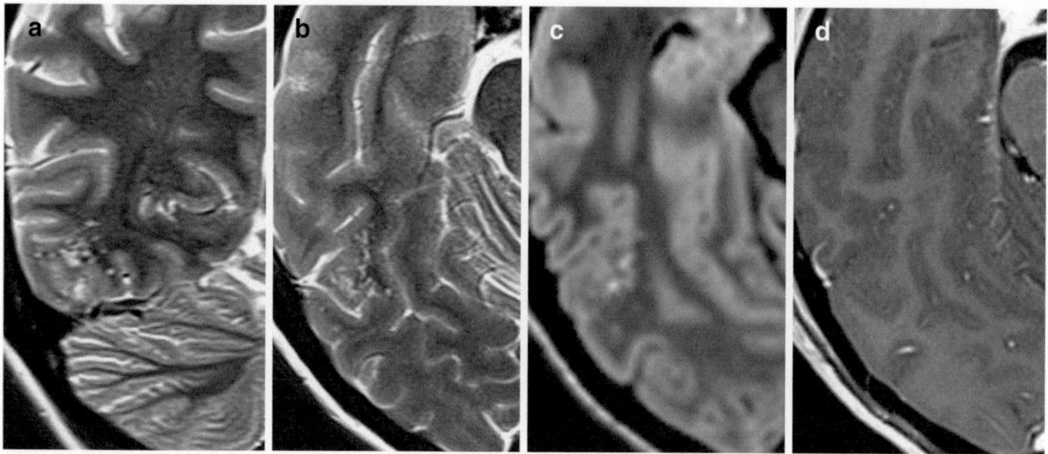

Fig. 4.16 MVNT. MRI T2WI (**a**, **b**), FLAIR (**c**), post-contrast T1WI (**d**). Small T2WI and FLAIR hyperintense subcortical nodules are visible in the right temporo-occipital lobe. No enhancement is visible (**d**). (Courtesy Dr. L. Pinelli, Brescia)

Table 4.10 MVNT imaging features

Mass effect	Edema	Inhomogeneity	Cysts	Necrosis	Hemorrhage	Calcifications
0	0	0	+	0	0	0/+

CT	T1	T2	FLAIR	DWI	ADC	T1 Gd	CBV	Spec
●	●	○	○	●	○	0	NA[a]	NA[a]

[a]NA (not available) = incomplete or sporadic reports

4.1.11 Dysplastic Cerebellar Gangliocytoma (Lhermitte-Duclos Disease)

WHO definition. Dysplastic cerebellar gangliocytoma is a rare ganglionic slow growing tumor of the cerebellum apparently maintaining the pre-existing cortical architecture. The cell of origin comes from the internal granule layer and it is not completely understood if this tumor can be considered a true neoplasm instead of an hamartomatous lesion. Usually Lhermitte-Duclos disease (LDD) is the CNS manifestation of Cowden syndrome, an autosomal dominant condition causing different hamartomas and neopalsm.

It corresponds to a WHO grade 1 tumor.

Epidemiology. This rare tumor has been described at any age of life. *PTEN* mutations have been described in adults but not in children.

Location. It is a lesion arising in one of the cerebellar hemispheres.

Clinical features. The symptoms vary from cerebellar signs to the clinical condition related to increased cranial pressure secondary to obstructive hydrocephalus, a direct mass effect of the tumor.

Prognosis. Cowden syndrome presents as a germline mutation in PTEN and for this reason it is also known as PTEN hamartomatous syndrome. Affected patients can develop a series of different neoplasms and/or hamartomas such as breast and thyroid carcinomas, gastrointestinal hamartomas, uterine leiomyomas, etc. If completely resected the prognosis for LDD is usually good, even though data on potential recurrency are scarce. In this patient the overall prognosis is mainly related to the high risk of carcinomas.

Imaging. This tumor shows a typical dysplastic macrocerebellum pattern on imaging. As shown in Fig. 4.17, a rudimental cerebellar folia

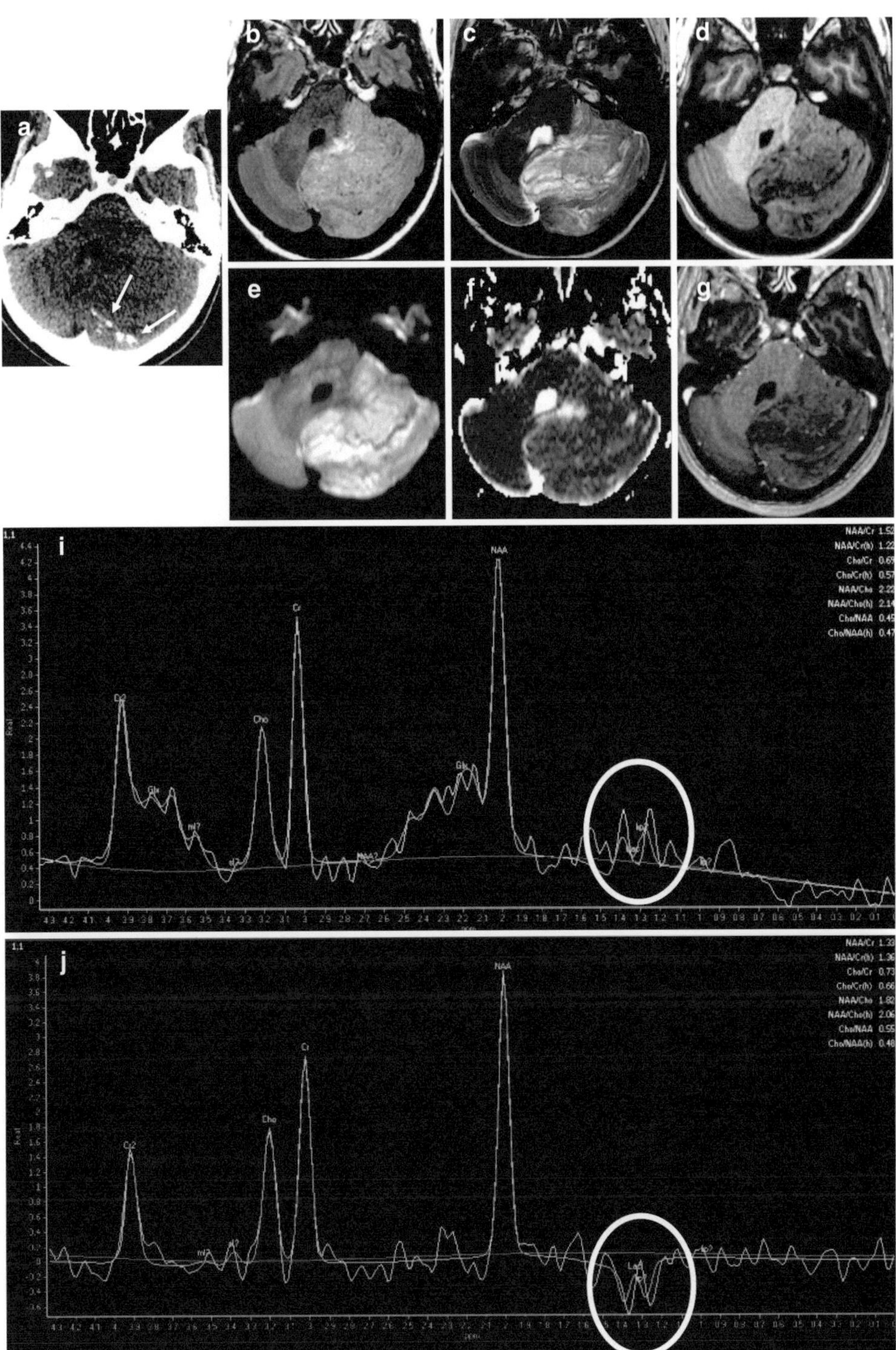

Fig. 4.17 Lhermitte-Duclos disease. Female, 48-year-old with cerebellar signs. CT (**a**), MRI FLAIR (**b**), T2WI (**c**), T1WI (**d**), DWI (**e**), ADC (**f**), post-contrast T1WI (**e**), spectroscopy, short TE (**h**), intermediate TE 144 ms (**i**). A huge neoplasm involves entirely the left cerebellar hemisphere. Enlarged dysplastic folia are visible in the most posterior part of the tumor. No tumor enhancement is detectable (**g**), whereas on CT superficial calcifications are evident. There is a slight increase of Cho/NAA and Cr/NAA peaks, whereas Cho/Cr is minimally reduced as it is not expected in a neoplasm. The doublet peak of lactate is evident in both echoes (circles **h**, **i**)

Table 4.11 LDD imaging summary

Mass effect	Edema	Inhomogeneity	Cysts	Necrosis	Hemorrhage	Calcifications
+/++	0/+	++	0	0	0	0/++

CT	T1	T2	FLAIR	DWI	ADC	T1 Gd	CBV	Spec
○	◑	○	◔	◑	●	0	NA	↑lac

[a]NA (not available) = incomplete or sporadic reports

design seems to be preserved in the superficial part of the neoplasm that is roughly homogeneous, with some aspects of T2WI/FLAIR hyperintensity at the level of the inner subcortical aspect of involved cerebellar folia. Calcifications can be present, but no pathological enhancement is usually detected.

On MR spectroscopy (Fig. 4.17) a minor increase of Cho/NAA ratio and of Cr/Naa ratio is reported. Lactate peak could be detected for some authors due to the increase in anaerobic metabolism [9]. Imaging features of LDD are summarized in Table 4.11.

4.1.12 Central Neurocytoma

WHO definition. Central neurocytoma is an intraventricular tumor composed by neuronal slow proliferating cells, it is a benign tumor but due to its potential recurrence after surgery it is classified as WHO grade 2.

Epidemiology. It affects mainly young adults.

Location. This tumor is typically located in a later ventricle and/or in the third ventricle. The commonest location is the anterior portion of one of the lateral ventricles.

Clinical features. Patients usually present with symptoms of increased intracranial pressure.

Prognosis. It is a benign tumor with a good prognosis if totally resected, but recurrence and craniospinal dissemination are reported.

Imaging. It is a mixed solid and cystic mass with frequent calcifications on CT. On MRI it is iso-hypointense on T1WI, isointense on T2WI, and hyperintense on FLAIR images with multiple small cysts and an irregular pattern of the enhancement [10] (Fig. 4.18).

No clear diffusion restriction is present.

On spectroscopy an inverted alanine peak and a notable glycine peak were reported [11].

Perfusion is variable but mainly increased. Imaging features of central neurocytoma are summarized in Table 4.12.

4.1.13 Extraventricular Neurocytoma

WHO definition. Extraventricular neurocytoma shares many histological fetures with central neurocytoma but is located within cerebral parenchyma more frequently in the frontal region.

As for central neurocytoma it corresponds to WHO grade 2.

Epidemiology. It can be present at any age even though it seems more frequent in young adults.

Location. It can arise in any location in the CNS without any clear contact with the ventricles.

Clinical features. Clinical manifestations vary according to the tumor location.

Prognosis. If completely resected, this tumor shows a good prognosis.

Imaging. Imaging features are variable, it is usually a solid-cystic lesion with calcifications. The solid portion is iso-hypointense on T1WI and hyperintense on T2WI/FLAIR images, diffusion can be slightly increased and contrast enhancement is heterogeneous [12].

Calcifications and sometimes hemorrhages can be present. In case of Fig. 4.19 permeability was increased. Imaging features of extraventricular nerocytoma are summarized in Table 4.13.

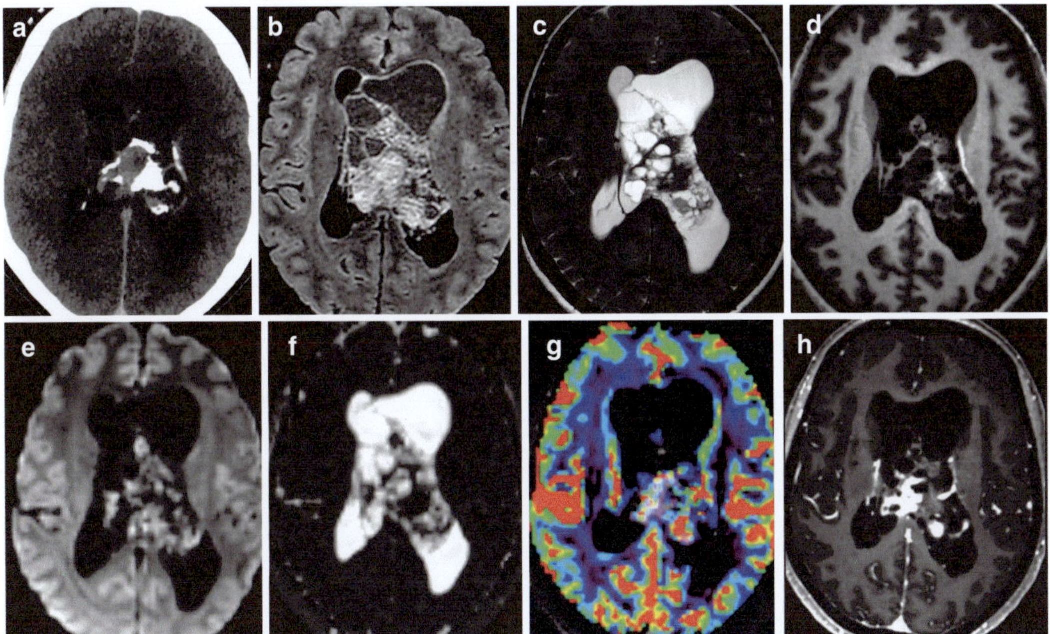

Fig. 4.18 Central neurocytoma. CT (**a**). MRI FLAIR (**b**), T2WI (**c**), T1WI (**d**), DWI (**e**), ADC (**f**), CBV (**g**), post-contrast T1WI (**h**). A large intraventricular multicystic tumor arising from the left lateral ventricle is visible. Large calcifications are present on CT (**a**), only some parts of the solid portion ehnance after contrast administration (**h**) and CBV is slightly increased

Table 4.12 Central neurocytoma imaging features

Mass effect	Edema	Inhomogeneity	Cysts	Necrosis	Hemorrhage	Calcifications
0/++	0	+/++	+/+++	0	0/+	+/+++

CT	T1	T2	FLAIR	DWI	ADC	T1 Gd	CBV	Spec
◓	◓	◓	◯	◓	◓	+/++	🟡	↑alanine, glycine

4.1.14 Cerebellar Liponeurocytoma

WHO definition. Cerebellar liponeurocytoma is a cerebellar neoplasm with advanced neuronal or neurocytic differentiation, variable glial differentiation, and focal lipoma-like changes.

It is a WHO grade 2 tumor.

Epidemiology. is a rare slow growing cerebellar tumor affecting adults.

Location. Cerebellar hemispheres.

Clinical features. Cerebellar signs or headache and other symptoms related to an increased intracranial pressure.

Prognosis. If completely resected, the prognosis is favorable.

Imaging. It can present on MRI with typical lipomatous T1WI hyperintense aspect, and fat-suppressed images can be helpful for characterizing the lesion. It must however underline that the majority of reported cases show an iso-hypointense aspect on T1WI making the differential diagnosis quite difficult. It is hyperintense on T2WI/FLAIR images, enhancement after contrast is mild [13]. Imaging features of cerebellar liponeurocytoma are summarized in Table 4.14.

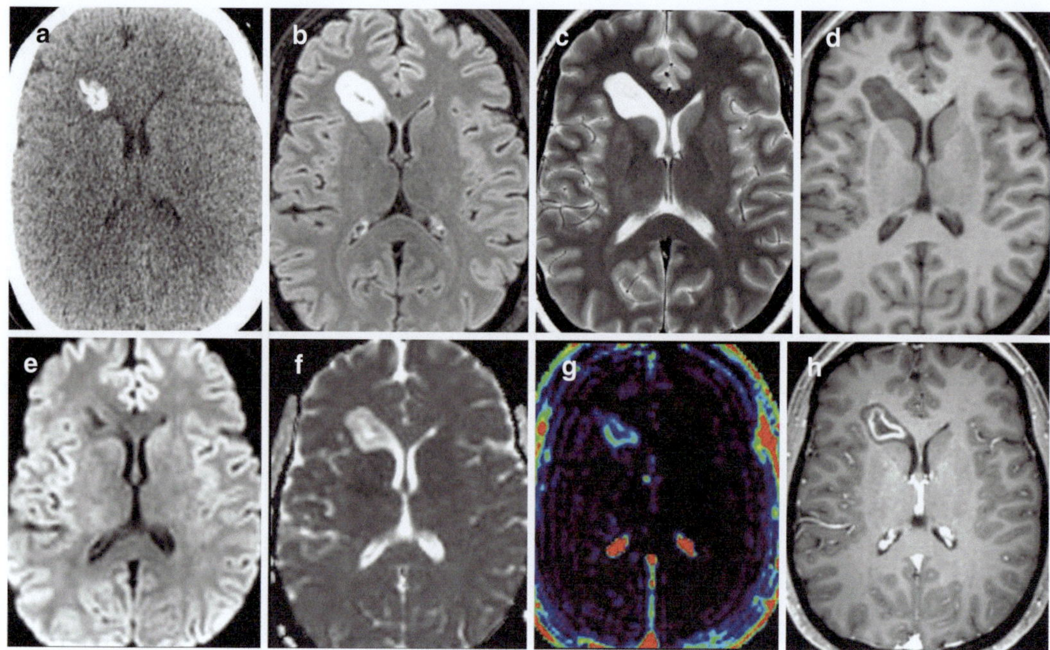

Fig. 4.19 Extraventricular neurocytoma. CT (**a**). MRI FLAIR (**b**), T2WI (**c**), T1WI (**d**), DWI (**e**), ADC (**f**), permeability, K-trans (**g**), post-contrast T1WI (**h**). The tumor was incidentally discovered in a young adult female with no sign or symptoms related to the lesion. It is a rounded well demarcated lesion with calcification and an inner shell showing enhancement (**h**) and increased permeability (**g**)

Table 4.13 Extraventricular neurocytoma imaging features

Mass effect	Edema	Inhomogeneity	Cysts	Necrosis	Hemorrhage	Calcifications
+/++	0/+	+/++	+/++	0	0/+	+/++

CT	T1	T2	FLAIR	DWI	ADC	T1 Gd	CBV	Spec
◉	◉	○	○	◉	○	+/++	◉	NA[a]

[a]NA (not available) = incomplete or sporadic reports

Table 4.14 Cerebellar liponeurocytoma imaging features

Mass effect	Edema	Inhomogeneity	Cysts	Necrosis	Hemorrhage	Calcifications
+/++	0/+	0/++	0	0	0	0

CT	T1	T2	FLAIR	DWI	ADC	T1 Gd	CBV	Spec
○◉	◉	○	○	◉	◉	+	NA	NA[a]

[a]NA (not available) = incomplete or sporadic reports

References

1. Bulakbasi N, Kocaoglu M, Sanal TH, Tayfun C. Dysembryoplastic neuroepithelial tumors: proton MR spectroscopy, diffusion and perfusion characteristics. Neuroradiology. 2007;49:805–12.
2. Pickles J, Mankad K, Aizpurua M, et al. A case series of diffuse Glioneuronal tumours with oligodendroglioma-like features and nuclear clusters (DGONC). Neuropathol Appl Neurobiol. 2021;47:464–7.
3. Yadava N, Raob S, Sainia J, Prasada C, Mahadevanb A, Sadashiva N. Papillary glioneuronal tumors: a radiopathologic correlation. Eur J Radiol. 2017;97:44–52.
4. Medhi G, Prasad C, Saini J, et al. Imaging features of rosette-forming glioneuronal tumours (RGNTs): a series of seven cases. Eur Radiol. 2016;26:262–70.

5. Lucas CHG, Villanueva-Meyer JE, Whipple N, et al. Myxoid glioneuronal tumor, PDGFRA p.K385-mutant: clinical, radiologic, and histopathologic features. Brain Pathol. 2020;30:479–94.

6. Vaz A, Cavalcanti MS, da Silva Junior EB, Ramina R, de Almeida Teixeira BC. Uncommon Glioneuronal tumors: a radiologic and pathologic synopsis. AJNR Am J Neuroradiol. 2022;43:1080–9.

7. Lakhani DA, Mankad K, Chhabda S, Feizi P, Patel R, Sarma A, Pruthi S. Diffuse leptomeningeal glioneuronal tumor of childhood. AJNR Am J Neuroradiol. 2020;41:2155–9.

8. Nunes RH, Hsu CC, da Rocha AJ, et al. Multinodular and vacuolating neuronal tumor of the cerebrum: a new "Leave Me Alone" lesion with a characteristic imaging pattern. AJNR Am J Neuroradiol. 2017;38:1899–904.

9. Klisch J, Juengling F, Spreer J, et al. Lhermitte-Duclos disease: assessment with MR imaging, positron emission tomography, single-photon emission CT, and MR spectroscopy. AJNR Am J Neuroradiol. 2001;22:824–30.

10. Chen L, Shen CC, Wang J, et al. Central neurocytoma: a clinical, radiological and pathological study of nine cases. Clin Neurol Neurosurg 2008;110:129–136.

11. Majós C, Aguilera C, Cos M, wtal. In vivo proton magnetic resonance spectroscopy of intraventricular tumours of the brain. Eur Radiol. 2009;19:2049–59.

12. Liu K, Wen G, Lv XF, et al. MR imaging of cerebral extraventricular Neurocytoma: a report of 9 cases. AJNR Am J Neuroradiol. 2013;34:541–6.

13. Wang K, Ni M, Wang, et al. Cerebellar liponeurocytoma: a case report and review of the literature. Oncol Lett. 2016;11:1061–4.

Gliomas, Glioneuronal Tumors and Neuronal Tumors: Ependymal Tumors. Choroid Plexus Tumors

5.1 Ependymal Tumors

WHO definition. The new WHO classification identifies two molecularly defined types of supratentorial ependymoma, with *ZFTA* or *YAP1* fusion, two molecularly defined types of posterior fossa ependymoma, PFA or PFB, and a spinal tumor defined by the presence of *MYCN*-amplification (Table 5.1).

In approximately 2/3 of cases these neoplasms arise in the posterior fossa within the fourth ventricle and typically in childhood.

Ependymomas account for 30% of all brain tumors in children less than 3 years old, and their incidence rate rapidly decreases with age.

Classical and anaplastic ependymomas are traditionally considered to correspond histologically to WHO grade II and III. However no association between grade and biological behavior or survival has been definitely established.

5.1.1 Supratentorial Ependymoma, NOS. Supratentorial Ependymoma, ZFTA Fusion Positive. Supratentorial Ependymoma, YAP-1 Fusion Positive

WHO definition. Supratentorial ependymoma is a circumscribed supratentorial glioma that demonstrates pseudorosettes or ependymal rosettes and comprises uniform small cells with round nuclei embedded in a fibrillary matrix.

The diagnosis should be made by a combination of histopathological and molecular features and should be made either when genetic analysis has detected a fusion gene (*ZFTA*, or *YAP1*) or when such analysis is not feasible or has been unsuccessful (not otherwise specified NOS).

The cIMPACT-NOW Update 7 [1] has replaced the 2016 WHO nosology of "ependymoma, *RELA*-fusion positive" by "Supratentorial ependymoma, C11orf95 fusion positive." This modification reinforces the idea that supratentorial ependymomas exhibiting fusion that implicates the C11orf95 (now called *ZFTA*) gene with or without the *RELA* gene represents the same histomolecular entity.

Supratentorial ependymomas are WHO grade 2 or 3 tumors.

Epidemiology. Supratentorial ependymomas affect both children and adults and account for approximately 1/3 of all intracranial ependymomas. The percentage of supratentorial ependymomas decreases with age, replaced in young adults and adults by spinal ependymomas.

Location. Supratentorial ependymomas are found in the cerebral hemispheres with or without a connection with the ventricular system, the fronto-parietal location is more frequent than the temporo-occipital one, in particular in *ZFTA* fusion positive ependymomas.

Clinical features. They comprise all the symptoms and signs typically caused by a hemispheric

Table 5.1 WHO 2021 molecular classification of EPNs

Location	Group	Genetic	Pathology	Age	Outcome
Supratentorial (30%)	ST-EPN-ZFTA	*ZFTA* fusion gene	Classic/anaplastic	Infancy/adult	Poor
	ST-EPN-YAP1	*YAP1* fusion gene	Classic/anaplastic	Infant/children	Good
	ST-SE	Balanced genome	Subependymoma	Adulthood	Good
Posterior fossa (60%)	PF-EPN-A	Balanced genome	Classic/anaplastic	Infancy	Poor
	PF-EBN-B	Genome wide polyploidy	Classic/anaplastic	Children/adult	Good
	PF-SE	Balanced genome	Subependymoma	Adulthood	Good
Spinal (10%)	SP-EPN	NF2 mutation	Classic/anaplastic	Children/adult	Good
	SP-MPE	Genome wide polyploidy	Myxopapillary	Adulthood	Good
	SP-SE	6q deletion	Subependymoma	Adulthood	Good

growing mass, from focal neurologic deficits, to seizure or signs and symptoms of raised intracranial pressure.

Prognosis. Most data are related to retrospective analysis performed before molecular classification, for which currently known the supratentorial ependymomas *ZFTA* fusion positive have the poorest outcome, whereas in case of *YAP1* fusion positive the prognosis is more favorable. Local recurrence is however frequent and radiotherapy after surgery is now considered the standard of cure.

Imaging. Supratentorial ependymomas are quite nonspecific in neuroimaging studies. They usually present as a relatively well circumscribed heterogeneous mass with cystic or microcystic component, frequent hemorrhages, and possible calcifications. Perilesional edema is variable (Figs. 5.1 and 5.2) The MRI signal is heterogeneous in most of the cases and intratumoral hemorrhage is frequent.

The solid component shows a rough isointensity with brain parenchyma on T1WI and T2WI/FLAIR images and the enhancement is irregular [2].

Diffusion. The diffusion parameters are similar to brain parenchyma or slightly reduced.

Spectroscopy. The spectroscopy profile is nonspecific and is usually similar to the typical profile of an aggressive neoplasm with clear increase in Cho/NAA ratio and possible increases in lactate.

Perfusion. Perfusion and permeability are variable, but usually increased (Fig. 5.2).

The imaging features of *YAP1*-fusion positive ependymomas are quite similar to those of *ZFTA*-fusion positive ependymomas and a differential diagnosis results are not possible [3].

Imaging deatures of supratentorial ependymomas are summarized in Table 5.2.

5.1.2 Posterior Fossa Ependymoma, NOS. Posterior Fossa Group A (PFA) Ependymoma. Posterior Fossa Group B (PFB) Ependymoma

WHO definition. Posterior fossa ependymoma is a circumscribed infratentorial glioma that demonstrates pseudorosettes or ependymal rosettes and comprises uniform small cells with round nuclei embedded in a fibrillary matrix.

The diagnosis should be established based on a combination of histopathological and molecular features. This determination should occur either when genetic analysis either can assign a molecular group or when such analysis is not feasible or has been unsuccessful (not otherwise specified NOS).

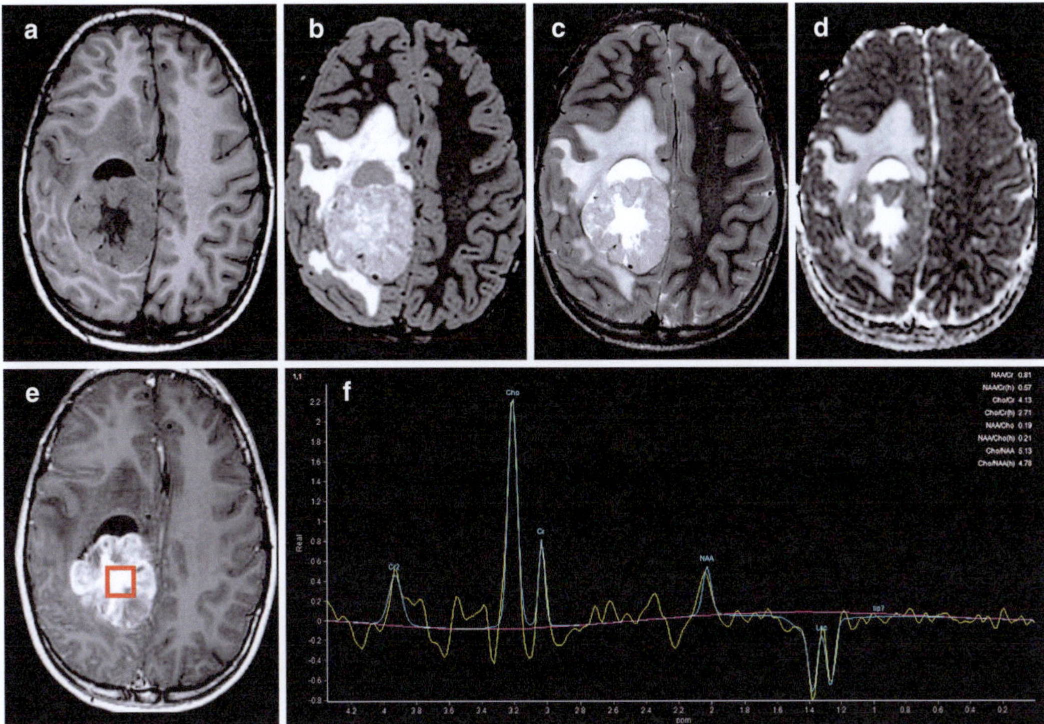

Fig. 5.1 Supratentorial RELA-fusion positive (now ZFTA fusion positive) ependymoma in a 15-year-old boy. MRI T1WI (**a**), FLAIR (**b**), T2WI (**c**), ADC (**d**), post-contrast T1WI (**e**), MR spectroscopy (**f**). An inhomogeneous well circumscribed mass with diffuse perilesional edema is visible in right peri-rolandic region. Some areas of slight diffusion restriction are present and the post-contrast enhancement is clearly evident. MR spectroscopy shows a NAA peak reduction and a relative increase of Cho peak, the lactate doublet is visible as well. (Courtesy Dr. L. Chiapparini, Pavia)

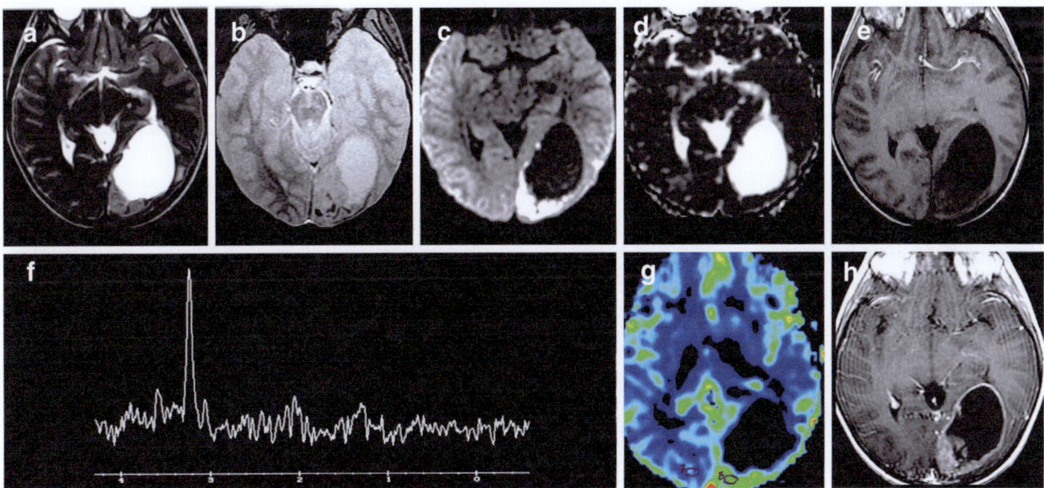

Fig. 5.2 Supratentorial ZFT fusion positive ependymoma in an 8-year-old boy. MRI T2WI (**a**), T2*WI (**b**), DWI (**c**), ADC (**d**), T1WI (**e**), MR spectroscopy (**f**), CBV (**g**), post-contrast T1WI (**h**). This lesion shows a large cyst and some possible tiny calcifications in the solid portion (**b**), diffusion is reduced (**c**, **d**). Perilesional edema is scarce and the enhancement is irregular (**h**). MR spectroscopy shows a NAA peak barely recognizable and a relative increase of Cho peak, CBV is slightly increased (Courtesy Prof G. Morana, Torino)

Table 5.2 Supratentorial ependymoma imaging features

Mass effect	Edema	Inhomogeneity	Cysts	Necrosis	Hemorrhage	Calcifications
+/+++	+/++	+/+++	+/+++	0/+	0/++	0/+

CT	T1	T2	FLAIR	DWI	ADC	T1 Gd	CBV	Spec
●	●	●	◐	○	●	+/++	●	↑Cho/NAA, ↑lac

An ependymoma can be classified as PFA identifying a loss of H3 p.K23me3 expression or by DNA methlyation profile.

An ependymoma can be classified as PFB by DNA methlyation profile.

Posterior fossa ependymomas are WHO grade 2 or 3 tumors.

Epidemiology. Posterior fossa ependymomas can occur at any age but are more frequent in children with a median age of 6 years. They represent roughly 8% of all neuroepithelial tumor in children.

A clear difference in age is present between PFA and PFB ependymomas. Under 5 years of age PFB ependymomas are virtually absent, whereas PFA subtype is exceedingly rare over 18 years of age.

Location. Posterior fossa ependymomas arise in any region of fourth ventricle including the lateral aspect, they can occur also in the cerebellopontine angle. PFA ependymomas more frequently originate from the roof and lateral aspect of the fourth ventricle, whereas PFB ependymomas seem to originate preferably from the floor of the fourth ventricle.

Clinical features. The most common clinical presentation is characterized by signs and symptoms of raised intracranial hydrocephalus due to the obstruction of the fourth ventricle.

Prognosis. The prognosis is strictly related to the radicality of the surgical intervention, recurrency is relatively frequent, and PFA ependymomas exhibit worst prognosis in comparison to PFB and more in general with other posterior fossa ependymomas.

Imaging. Posterior fossa ependymoma is usually a well circumscribed tumor occupying and enlarging the fourth ventricle with a desmoplastic growth through the Luschka and Magendie foramina (Fig. 5.3 and 5.5). It is mainly heterogeneous with a predominant T1 hypointensity and T2 mixed signal. On FLAIR it is mainly hyperintense. Even the post-contrast enhancement is quite variable from irregular and heterogenous (Figs. 5.3 and 5.4) to scarce or quite absent (Fig. 5.5).

Diffusion. Diffusion is variable from a slight increase to a slight restriction being in between from pilocytic astrocytoma and medulloblastoma.

Apart from the age difference, the only difference reported between PFA and PFB (Fig. 5.6) is given by a relatively greater enhancement after contrast from PFB. A large study in children with PFA sought to identify any differences between the two molecular subtypes of PFA, PFA-1 and PFA-2 and the 6 subgroups of PFA-1 and the three subgroups of PFA-2. In fact, there are no significant differences that allow the various subgroups to be differentiated through imaging [4].

Spectroscopy. MR spectroscopy shows usually a nonspecific redution of NAA peak and a relative increase of Cho peak. However a possible flow chart for the differential diagnosis between pilocytic astrocytoma, medulloblastoma, and ependymoma has been recently proposed. In case of Naa/Cr > 2.22 and mL/Naa < 0.65 a pilocytic astrocytoma can be considered, if not, look at the ratio mL/Cho. If the ratio is <0.85 consider a medulloblastoma, otherwise an ependymoma [5]. Imagine features od posterior fossa ependymoma are summarized in Table 5.3.

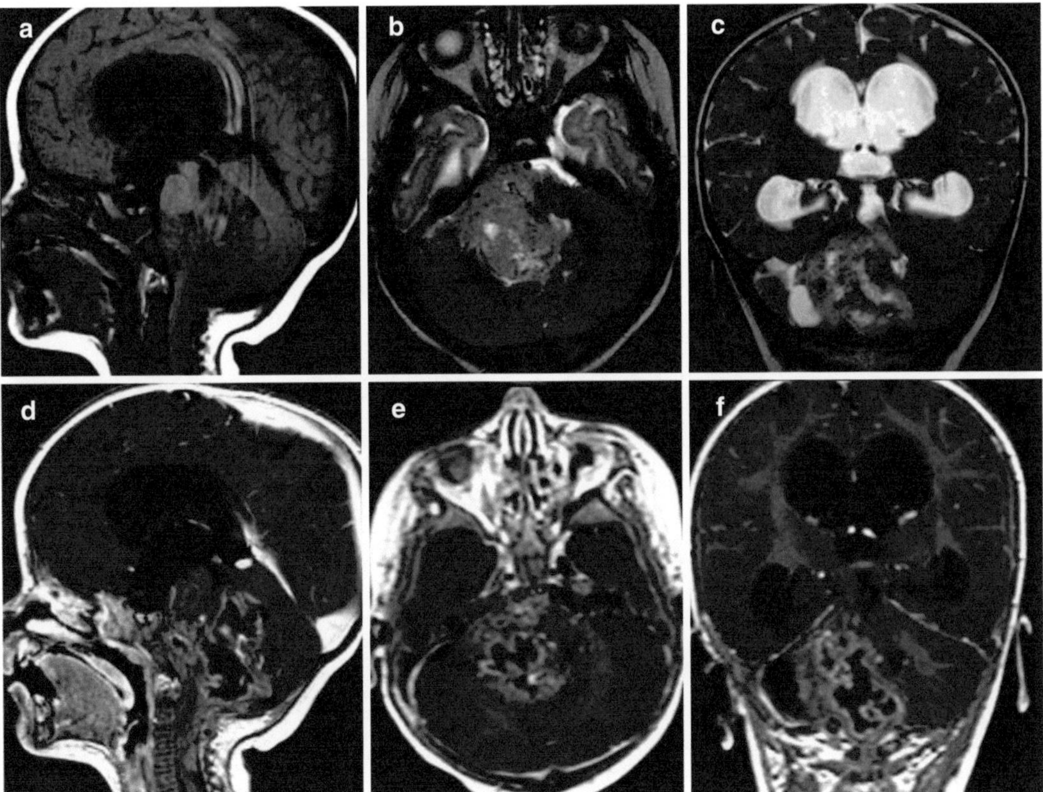

Fig. 5.3 Posterior fossa anaplastic ependymoma (PFA) in an 8-month-old girl. MRI T1WI (**a**), T2WI (**b, c**), post-contrast T1WI (**d–f**). The tumor appears as a heterogeneous lesion fully occupying the fourth ventricle with a downward diffusion through the right Lusckha foramen. A supratentorial hydrocephalus is clearly visible. The post-contrast enhancement is irregular and heterogeneous (**d–f**)

5.1.3 Spinal Ependymoma NOS. Spinal Ependymona, *MYCN*-Amplified

WHO definition. Spinal ependymoma is a circumscribed spinal glioma that demonstrates pseudorosettes or ependymal rosettes and comprises uniform small cells with round nuclei embedded in a fibrillary matrix. Classic spinal ependymoma with absent *MYCN*-amplification shows typically a low mitotic activity, and it can be find more frequently in patients with NF2. Spinal ependymomas with *MYCN*-amplification display on the contrary microvascular proliferation, necrosis and a high mitotic count.

Epidemiology. It occurs primarily in young adults and shows its peak incidence between 25 and 45 years; however, it can be present also in childhood where it represents 20% of all primary spinal tumor. Something between 20 and 50% of all patients with NF2 develop a spinal ependymoma.

Spinal ependymoma with *MYCN*-amplification is exceedingly rare and very few cases are at present reported in the literature.

Location. It is an intramedullary tumor mainly located in the cervical or cervicothoracic spinal cord.

Clinical features. Clinical signs and symptoms are nonspecific. Back pain and myelopathy can be present.

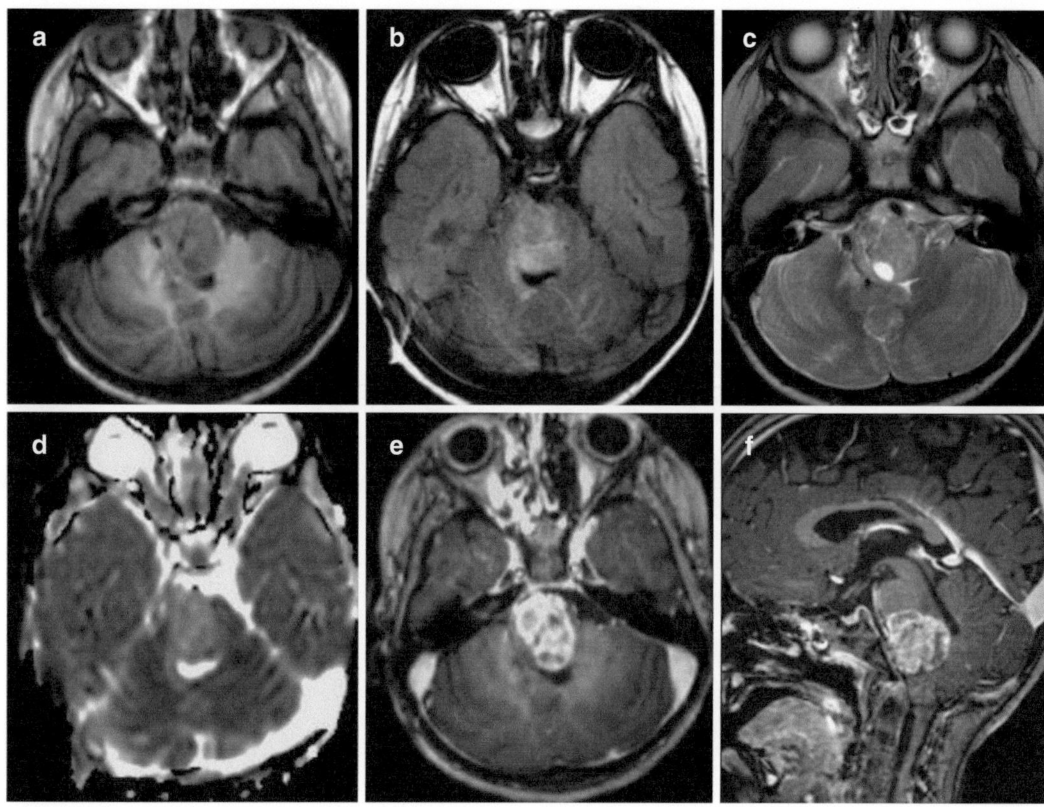

Fig. 5.4 Same case of Fig. 5.3, follow-up at 4 years of age with tumor recurrence. MRI T1WI (**a**), FLAIR (**b**), T2WI (**c**) ADC (**d**), post-contrast T1WI (**e, f**). A large still heterogeneous residual tumor shows a progressive growth through the medulla oblongata

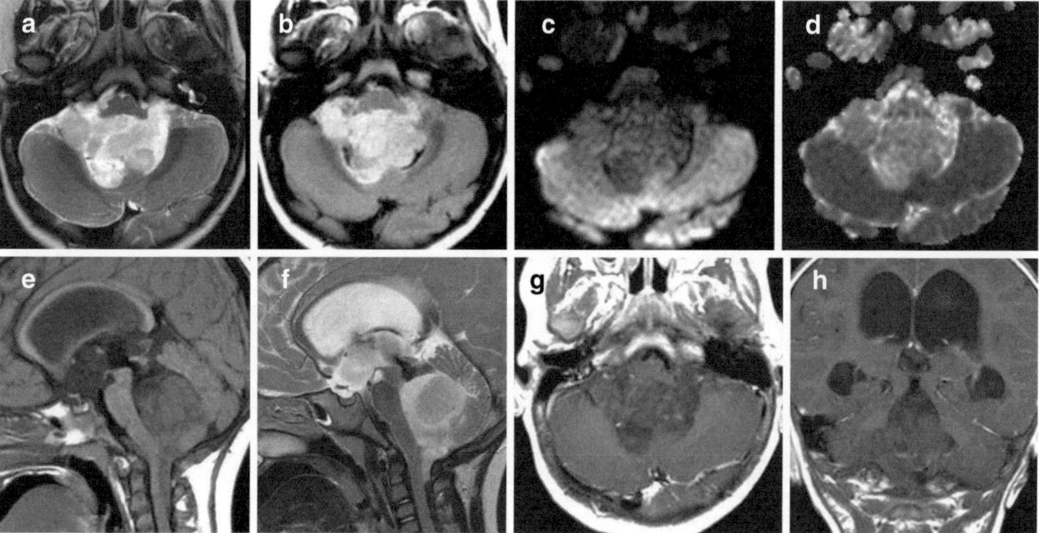

Fig. 5.5 Posterior fossa anaplastic ependymoma (PFA) in a 20-month-old girl. MRI T2WI (**a, f**), FLAIR (**b**), DWI (**c**), ADC (**d**), T1WI (**e**), post-contrast T1WI (**g, h**). A relatively more homogeneous ependymoma, with growth through both Luschka and Megendie foramina. On T2WI it is predominantly iso-hyperintense, it is clearly hyperintense on FLAIR and hypointense on T1WI. No diffusion restriction is visible and the contrast enhancement is extremely scarce

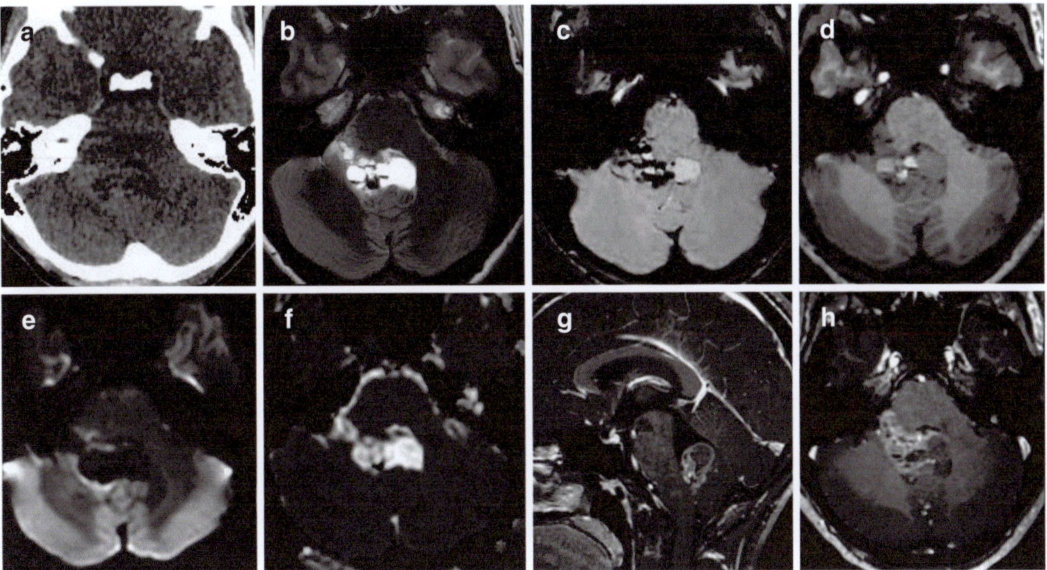

Fig. 5.6 Posterior fossa ependymoma (PFB) in a 22-year-old woman. CT (**a**). MRI T2WI (**b**), T2*WI (**c**), T1WI (**d**), DWI (**e**), ADC (**f**), post-contrast T1WI (**g, h**). A less aggressive posterior fossa ependymoma in a young woman, with a downward growth through right Lushka foramen. In this case some small cysts with hemorrhagic content (**c**) are visible and the diffusion is increased, the enhancement after contrast administration is irregular

Table 5.3 PFA and PFP ependymomas imaging features

Mass effect	Edema	Inhomogeneity	Cysts	Necrosis	Hemorrhage	Calcifications
+/+++	0/++	+/++	+	0/+	0/+	0/+

CT	T1	T2	FLAIR	DWI	ADC	T1 Gd	CBV	Spec
⬤	⬤	◯	◯	◯	⬤	+/++	🟡	↑Cho/NAA, ↑lac

Prognosis. If completely resected the prognosis is favorable, but residual tumor is not infrequent and the overall prognosis cannot be completely positive. Spinal ependymomas with *MYCN*-amplification are extremely aggressive tumor with a poor prognosis.

Imaging. Spinal ependymoma is an intramedullary tumor usually well demarcated with possible multiple small cysts and an iso-hypointense aspect on T1WI and slight hyperintense aspect on T2WI. Hemorrhages and also small calcifications can be present, as well as a cranial "cyst" due to the dilatation of the ependymal canal (Fig. 5.7) The enhancement is variable.

Diffusion can be slightly reduced (Fig. 5.7).

In the rare reported cases of spinal ependymomas with *MYCN*-amplification, there are no significant differences in imaging characteristics with traditional ependymomas. [6]. Imagin features of spinal ependymoma are summarized in Table 5.4.

5.1.4 Myxopapillary Ependymoma

WHO definition. Myxopapillary ependymoma is a glial neoplasm characterized by the radial arrangement of spindled or epitheliod tumor cells around blood vessels with perivascular myxoid change and microcystic formation.

It is a WHO grade 2 tumor.

Epidemiology. It is a rare tumor more frequent in young adults and adolescents.

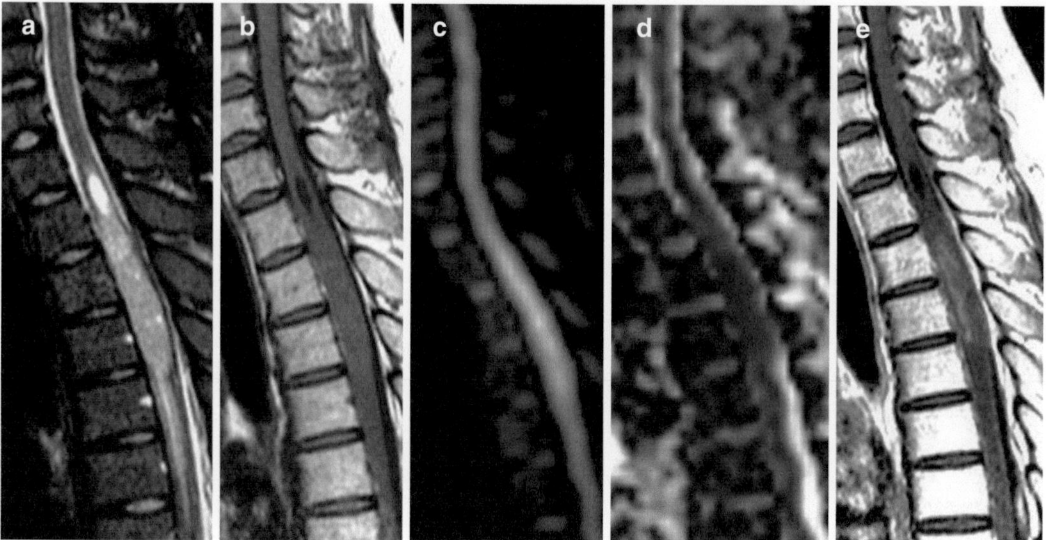

Fig. 5.7 Spinal ependymoma in a 33-year-old man. MRI T2WI (**a**), T1WI (**b**), DWI (**c**), ADC (**d**), post-contrast T1WI (**e**). A cervicothoracic intramedullary tumor is clearly demarcated with tiny cysts and a slight diffusion restriction, the post-contrast enhancement is relatively poor. The cranial cyst is due to the enlargement of the spinal canal

Table 5.4 Spinal ependymoma imaging features

Mass effect		Edema	Inhomogeneity		Cysts	Necrosis	Hemorrhage		Calcifications
+/++		0/+	+/++		++	0/+	0/+		0/+

CT	T1	T2	STIR	DWI	ADC	T1 Gd	CBV	Spec
NA[a]	◉	◉	○	○	◉	+/++	NA[a]	NA[a]

[a]NA (not available) = incomplete or sporadic reports

Location. Myxopapillary ependymoma is the most common tumor of conus medullaris and filum terminale. Rare case of extra CNS locations is reported.

Clinical features. Low back pain is the most common symptom.

Prognosis. If completely resected the prognosis is favorable.

Imaging. It is a well-defined mass in the region of conus medullaris and cauda equina characterized by a possible inhomogeneous structure with a predominantly T2WI hyperintensity and a variable T1WI appearance sometimes with spontaneous hyperintensity due to either a mucinous component of the tumor or microhemorrhages or microcalcifications [7].

Post-contrast enhancement is usually present (Fig. 5.8). Imaging features of myxopapillary ependimoma are summarize in Table 5.5.

5.1.5 Subependymoma

WHO definition. Subependymoma is a glioma characterized by the clustering of uniform tumor cell nuceli in an abundant fibrillary matrix, prone to microcystic change.

It is a WHO grade 1 tumor.

Epidemiology. It is usually found incidentally and its prevalence is not clearly known. It affects mainly adults from the fifth decade onwards.

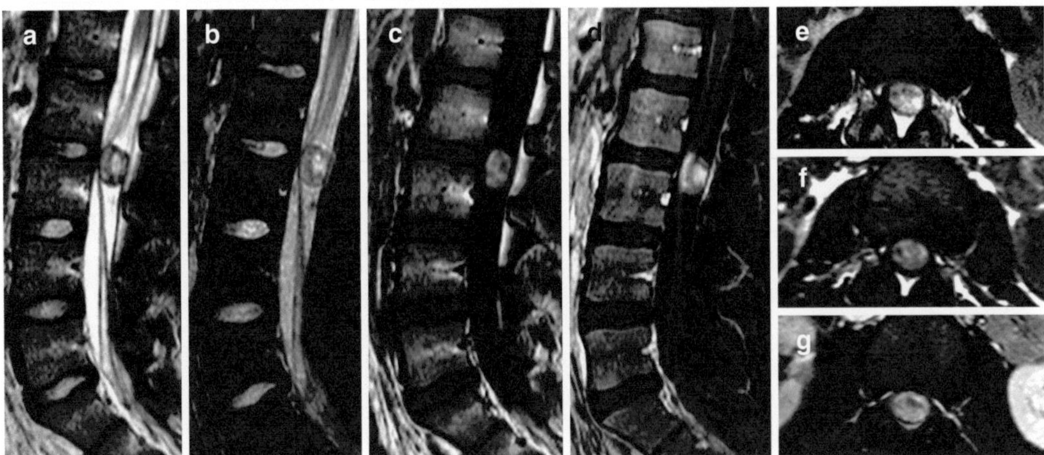

Fig. 5.8 Myxopapillary ependymoma in a 14-year-old girl. MRI T2WI (**a, e**), STIR (**b**), T1WI (**c, f**), post-contrast T1WI (**d, g**). A round intradural mass is located in the region of filum terminale at upper L3 level displac-ing anteriorly the roots of the cauda equina. Signal intensity is inhomogeneous with spontaneous hyperintensity on pre-contrast T1WI (**c, f**)

Table 5.5 Myxopapillary ependymoma imaging features

Mass effect	Edema	Inhomogeneity	Cysts	Necrosis	Hemorrhage	Calcifications
+/++	0	+/++	++	0/+	0/+	0/+

CT	T1	T2	STIR	DWI	ADC	T1 Gd	CBV	Spec
NA[a]	◉◯	◉	◯	NA[a]	NA[a]	+/++	NA[a]	NA[a]

[a]NA (not available) = incomplete or sporadic reports

Location. The fourth ventricle and the lateral ventricles are the more frequent location. It is more rare in the third ventricle and in the spinal cord.

Clinical features. Subependimomas are usually silent, clinical signs and symptoms may occur in spinal location.

Prognosis. They grow very slowly and the prognosis is good even without surgery.

Imaging. They are well defined usually small masses arising from the ependymal surface of the ventricles, mainly hypointense on T1WI and hyperintense on T2WI/FLAIR images. Cystic components or calcifications may be present and sometimes irregular contrast enhancement as well (Figs. 5.9 and 5.10).

Diffusion is increased or similar to brain parenchyma (Fig. 5.10). Imaging features of sub-ependymoma are summarized in Table 5.6.

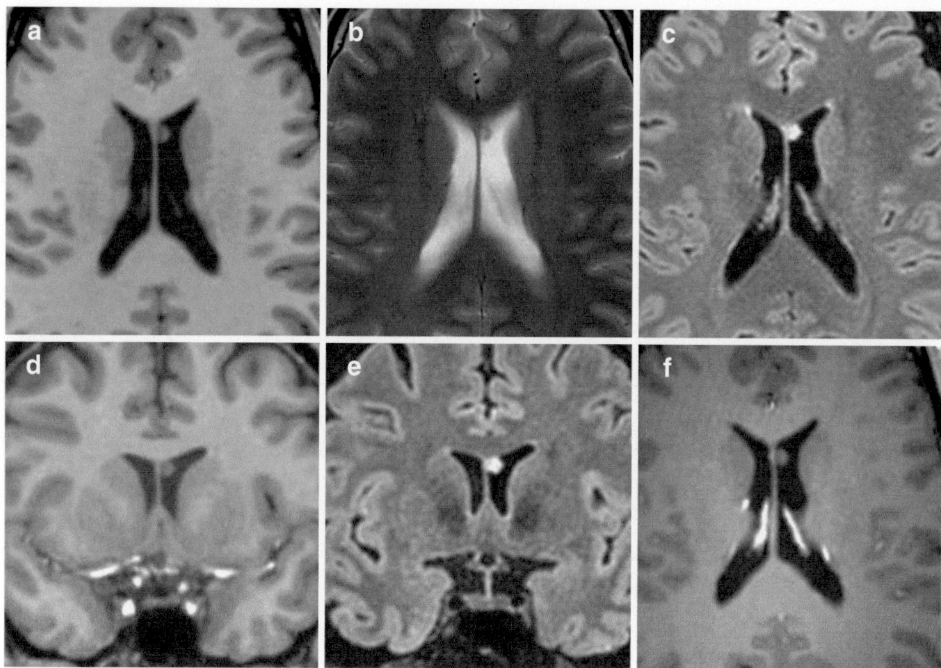

Fig. 5.9 Subependymoma. MRI T1WI (**a**, **d**), T2WI (**b**), FLAIR (**c**), post-contrast T1WI (**f**). A small nodule, hyperintense on FLAIR (**c**, **e**) and hypointense on T1WI (**a**, **d**), is visible at the angle between septum pellucidum and left frontal horn. No enhancement is visible (**f**)

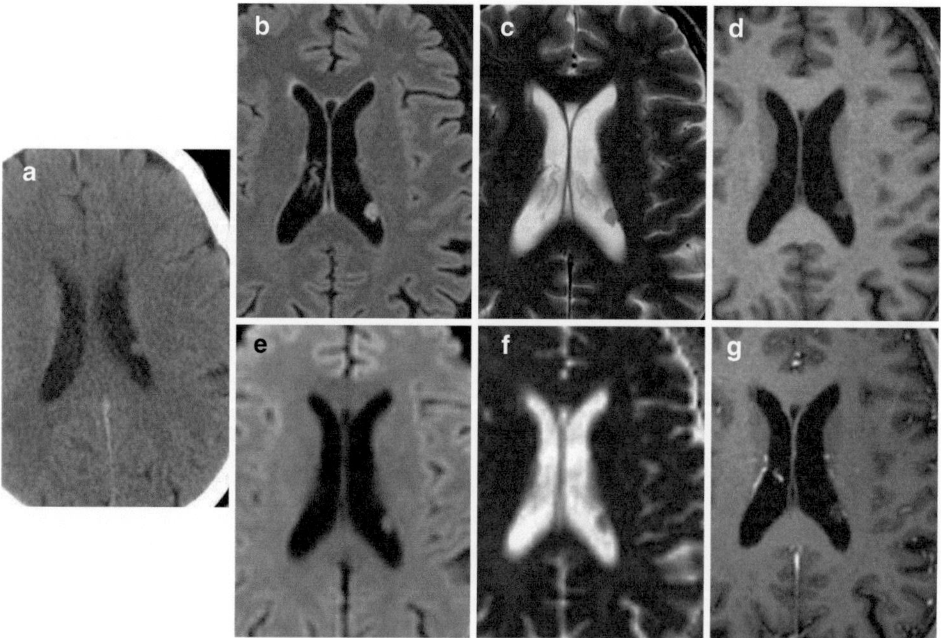

Fig. 5.10 Subependymoma. CT (**a**). MRI FLAIR (**b**), T2WI (**c**), T1WI (**d**), DWI (**e**), ADC (**f**), post-contrast T1WI (**g**). In this case the nodule is less hyperintense on FLAIR in comparison to the case of Fig. 5.9. Enhancement is absent also in this case. On diffusion the signal intensity is similar to brain parenchyma

Table 5.6 Subependymoma imaging features

Mass effect	Edema	Inhomogeneity	Cysts	Necrosis	Hemorrhage	Calcifications
0/+	0	0/+	0/+	0	0	0/+

CT	T1	T2	FLAIR	DWI	ADC	T1 Gd	CBV	Spec
●	●	◐	○	◐	●	0/+	NA[a]	NA[a]

[a]NA (not available) = incomplete or sporadic reports

5.2 Choroid Plexus Tumors

5.2.1 Choroid Plexus Papilloma. Atypical Choroid Plexus Papilloma

WHO definition. Choroid plexus papilloma is a benign intraventricular tumor arising from choroid plexus epithelium that corresponds hystologically to WHO grade 1.

Atypical choroid plexus papilloma is a choroid plexus papilloma with increased mitotic activity but does not fulfill the criteria for choroid plexus carcinoma. It is a WHO grade 2 tumor.

Epidemiology. Both choroid plexus papilloma and atypical choroid plexus papilloma occur in children but atypical variant is more frequent in young infants with a median age of less than 1 year.

Location. Choroid plexus papillomas are equally frequent in supratentorial and infratentortial region. On the contrary the atypical variant is more frequent in the lateral ventricles.

Clinical features. Clinical signs are typically related to the hydrocephalus due to the blockade of ventricular system due to the progressive tumor growth.

Prognosis. The prognosis is totally resected is favorable, recurrence is possible in the atypical variant.

Imaging. On CT and MRI both choroid plexus papilloma and atypical variant present as an irregular mass resembling sometimes a "large choroid plexus" occupying the ventricle with iso-hyperdense aspect on CT, isointense aspect on T1WI and FLAIR, and hyperintense aspect on T2WI.

A differential diagnosis between the typical and atypical variants is quite impossible; however, a very large tumor with a possible surrounding edema is most compatible with the atypical variant [8].

Diffusion. ADC values are decreased in comparison to brain parenchyma.

Perfusion. CBV is slightly increased due to the high vascularity of the neoplasm (Fig. 5.11).

Spectroscopy. On MR spectroscopy Naa and Cr peaks are usually absent and only a large peak of choline is detectable (Fig 5.11). Differently from choroid plexus carcinoma no lactate peak is usually present [9]. Imaging features of typical and atypical choroid plexus papilloma are summarized in Table 5.7.

5.2.2 Choroid Plexus Carcinoma

WHO definition. Choroid plexus carcinoma is an aggressive intraventricular tumor usually occurring within the lateral ventricles. This tumor frequently invades the surrounding brain parenchyma and metastasizes through the cerebrospinal fluid.

It is a WHO grade 3 tumor.

Epidemiology. Carcinoma of the choroid plexus is a rare occurrence, but it is relatively common during the first year of life, where it ranks as one of the most frequent intracranial malignancies.

Location. It is localized almost exclusively within and around the lateral ventricles.

Clinical features. As for papilloma, clinical signs are tipically related to the hydrocephalus.

Prognosis. The 3 year survival rate is around 60% and the 5 year survival rate is around 40%.

Imaging. Choroid plexus carcinoma presents as a huge intraventricular heterogeneous mass frequently invading the surrounding parenchyma in a way to sometimes prevent a precise localization of the tumor. It shows all the typical aspects

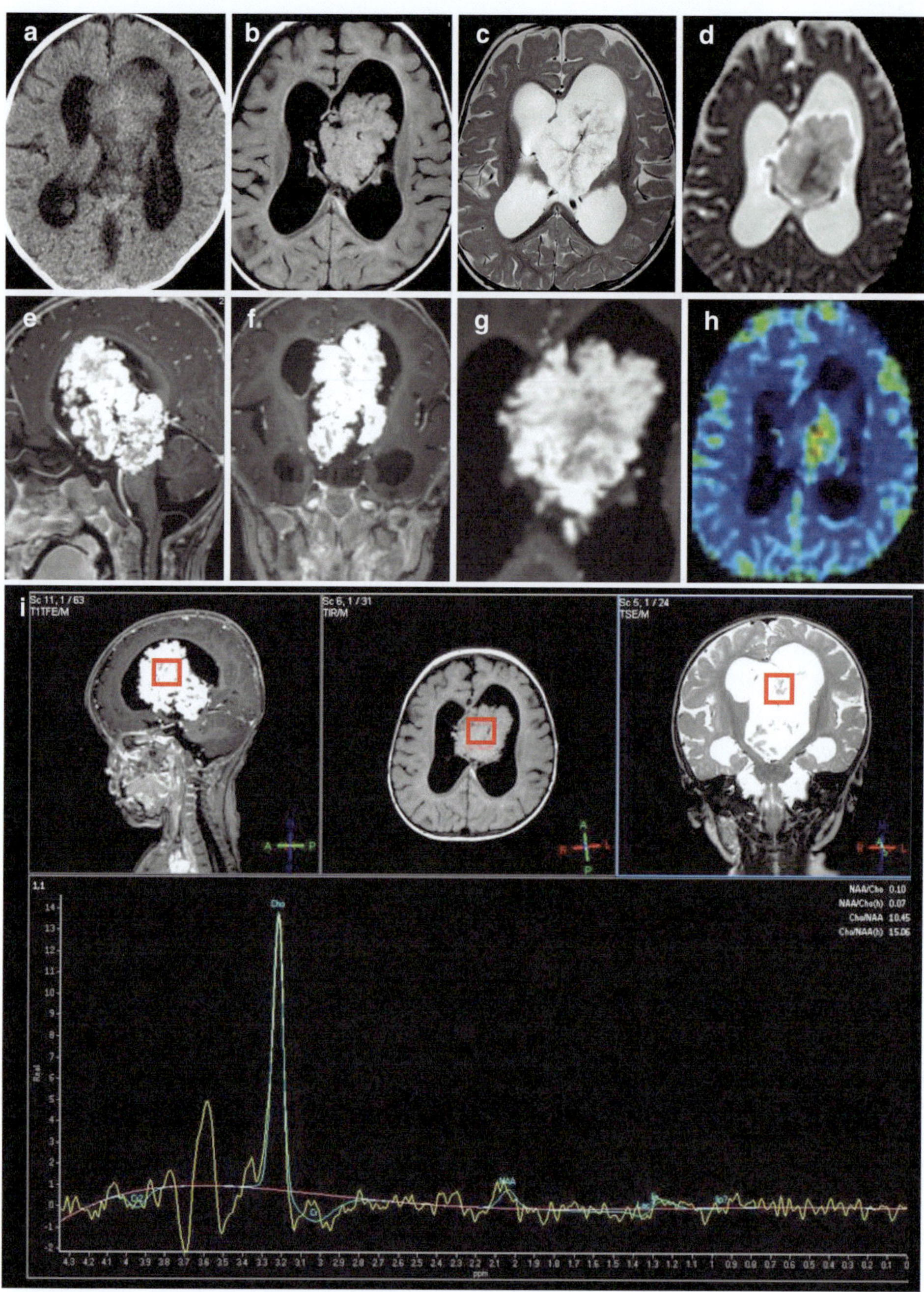

Fig. 5.11 Atypical choroid plexus papilloma in a 10-month-old boy with obstructive hydrocephalus and increased head circumference. CT (**a**). MRI FLAIR (**b**), T2WI (**c**), ADC (**d**), post-contrast T1WI (**e–g**), CBV (**h**), spectroscopy (**i**). A huge tumor with an origin most likely close to the left foramen of Monro is visible. The tumor occupies the third ventricle causing an obstructive hydrocephalus. On CT (**a**) it appears isodense such as on MRI FLAIR image (**b**), it is hyperintense on T2WI (**c**) and shows an increased ADC with respect to brain parenchyma (**d**). The typical papillary aspect of the lesion is clearly visible after contrast enhancement (**e–g**). There is a slight increase of CBV in the most vascularized areas of the tumor (**h**). MR spectroscopy (**i**) reveals a huge peak of choline, no NAA peak or Cr peak is clearly detectable

Table 5.7 Typical and atypical choroid plexus papilloma imaging features

Mass effect	Edema	Inhomogeneity	Cysts	Necrosis	Hemorrhage	Calcifications
+/++	0/+	0/++	0/++	0	0	0/+

CT	T1	T2	FLAIR	DWI	ADC	T1 Gd	CBV	Spec
○	◒	○	○	●	○	++/+++	○	Absent NAA, Cr ↑Cho

Table 5.8 Choroid plexus carcinoma imaging features

Mass effect	Edema	Inhomogeneity	Cysts	Necrosis	Hemorrhage	Calcifications
++/+++	+/++	+/+++	0/+	0/++	0/+	0/+

CT	T1	T2	FLAIR	DWI	ADC	T1 Gd	CBV	Spec
○	◒	◒	○	○	●	++/+++	●	Absent NAA, Cr ↑↑Cho, ↑lac

of an aggressive heterogeneous tumor with no specific patterns. In order to suggest a correct diagnosis the prevalent intraventricular location together with the age of occurrence (first year) has to be considered.

On MR spectroscopy the Cho peak is reported even larger than in papilloma and a lactate peak is usually reported as well [9]. Imaging features of choroid plexus carcinoma are summarized in Table 5.8.

References

1. Ellison DW, Aldape KD, Capper D, et al. cIMPACT-NOW update 7: advancing the molecular classification of ependymal tumors. Brain Pathol. 2020;20:863–86.
2. Nowak J, Jünger ST, Huflage H, et al. MRI phenotype of RELA-fused pediatric Supratentorial Ependymoma. Clin Neuroradiol. 2019;29:595–604.
3. Andreiuolo F, Varlet P, Tauziède-Espariat A, et al. Childhood supratentorial ependymomas with YAP1-MAMLD1 fusion: an entity with characteristic clinical, radiological, cytogenetic and histopathological features. Brain Pathol. 2019;29:205–16.
4. Sabin ND, Hwang SN, Klimo P Jr, et al. Anatomic neuroimaging characteristics of posterior fossa type a Ependymoma subgroups. AJNR Am J Neuroradiol. 2021;42:2245–50.
5. Manias KA, Harris LM, Davies NP, et al. Prospective multicentre evaluation and refinement of an analysis tool for magnetic resonance spectroscopy of childhood cerebellar tumours. Pediatr Radiol. 2018;48:1630–41.
6. Swanson AA, Raghunathan A, Jenkins RB, et al. Spinal cord Ependymomas with MYCN amplification show aggressive clinical behavior. J Neuropathol Exp Neurol. 2019;78:791–7.
7. Koeller KK, Scott Rosenblum R, Morrison AL. Neoplasms of the spinal cord and filum terminale: radiologic-pathologic correlation. Radiographics. 2000;20:1721–49.
8. Lin H, Leng X, Qin CH, Du YX, Wang WS, Qiu SJ. Choroid plexus tumours on MRI: similarities and distinctions in different grades. Cancer Imaging. 2019;19:17.
9. Horská A, Ulug AM, Melhem ER, Filippi CG, Burger PC, Edgar MA, Souweidane MM, Carson BS, Barker PB. Proton magnetic resonance spectroscopy of choroid plexus tumors in children. J Magn Reson Imaging. 2001;14:78–82.

6.1 Embryonal Tumors

6.1.1 Medulloblastoma Molecularly Defined

6.1.2 Introduction and WHO Definitions

In 2016 WHO brain tumors classification revision a new medulloblastoma classification according to their molecular characteritics was proposed. This classification has been considered because of growing clinical and prognostic utility. Table 6.1 summarized genetic histological and clinical characteristics of different medulloblastoma molecular subtypes as reported in the WHO 2016 and 2021 classification; however, new subgroups have been discovered in the last years through the analysis of a large number of tumors, in particular, four subgroups of SHH medulloblastoma and eight subgroups of non-WNT/non-SHH medulloblastoma are currently known, but it is very likely that other subgroups will be identified in the coming years.

Table 6.1 Molecular subtypes of medullobastomas (WHO 2016–2021)

	WNT-activated	SHH-activated		Non-WNT/non-SHH	
		TP53-wildtype	TP53-mutant	Group 3	Group 4
Age at presentation	Childhood	Infancy/adulthood	Childhood	Infancy/childhood	All age groups
Predominant histology	Classic	Desmoplastic/ nodular	Large cell/ anaplastic	Classic, large cell/ anaplastic	Classic
Genes with germlike mutation	APC	POCH1 SUFU	TP53		
Prognosis	Low risk	Standard/low risk	High risk	Standard/high risk	Standard/ high risk
Cell of origin	Low rhombic lip progenitor cells	Precursor cells of the external granule layer		Precursor cells of the external granule layer	

Generally speaking medulloblastoma is an embryonal neuroepithelial tumor typically arising in the cerebellum consisting of small rounds of undifferentiated cells with a high mitotic count.

Medulloblastoma is the second most common malignant tumor in childhood and independently from the hystological and molecular characterization it corresponds histologically to 2021 WHO grade 4.

Epidemiology, location, prognosis, and even imaging characteristics vary according to the different molecular subtypes [1, 2].

On the other hand being most frequently localized into the cerebellum clinical symptoms can often be the same for the different subtypes of medulloblastomas and are typically related to a cerebellar syndrome with ataxia and/or vertigo, even though symptoms and signs of high intracranial pressure can frequently overcome symptomatology.

6.1.2.1 Medulloblastoma, WTN-Activated

WHO definition. Medulloblastoma WNT-activated is an embryonal tumor arising from the dorsal brainstem demonstrating activation of the WNT signaling pathway.

Epidemiology. Medulloblastoma WNT subtype accounts for nearly 10% of all medulloblastomas, mostly present in children aged from 7 to 14 years.

Prognosis. Prognosis of this tumor is exceedingly good and if completely resected the survival rate is close to 100%.

Imaging

WNT-activated subtype presents all the typical aspects of the other medulloblastomas in terms of density or signal intensity: a slight hyperdensity on CT, an iso-hyperintense signal on T2WI, with slight hyperintensity on FLAIR imaging (Figs. 6.1 and 6.2).

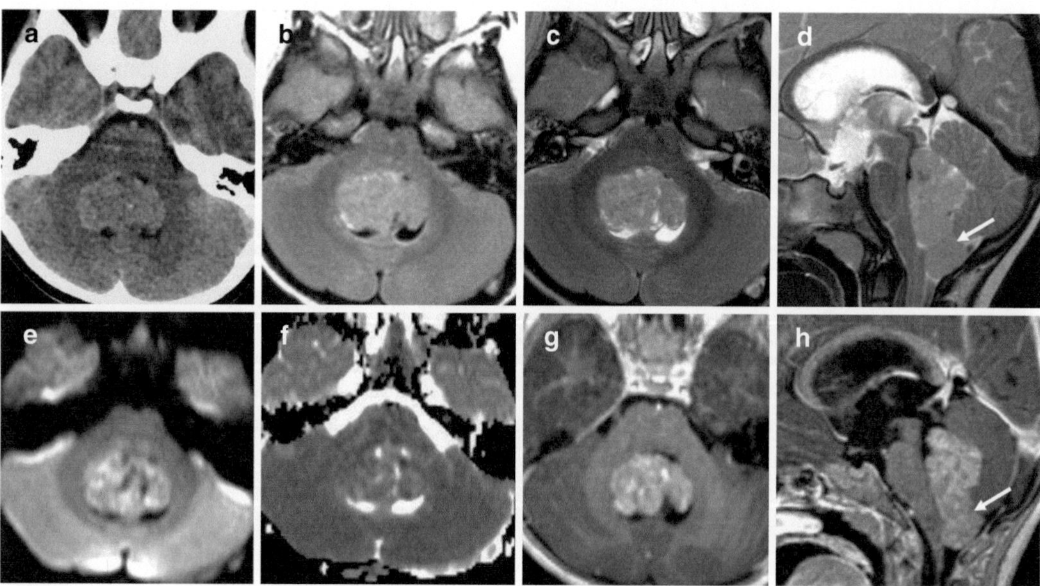

Fig. 6.1 Medulloblastoma WNT-activated in a 30-month-old girl. CT (**a**). MRI FLAIR (**b**), T2WI (**c**, **d**), DWI (**e**), ADC (**f**), post-contrast T1WI (**g**, **h**). The more typical imaging features of medulloblastomas are the slight hyperdensity on CT (**a**), the isointense pattern on T2WI and the diffusion restriction (**e**, **f**). WNT-activated medulloblastomas show usually a moderate but evident enhancement after contrast administration. The typical growing pattern is within the fourth ventricle and through the Luschka and Magendie foramina (arrow **d**, **h**)

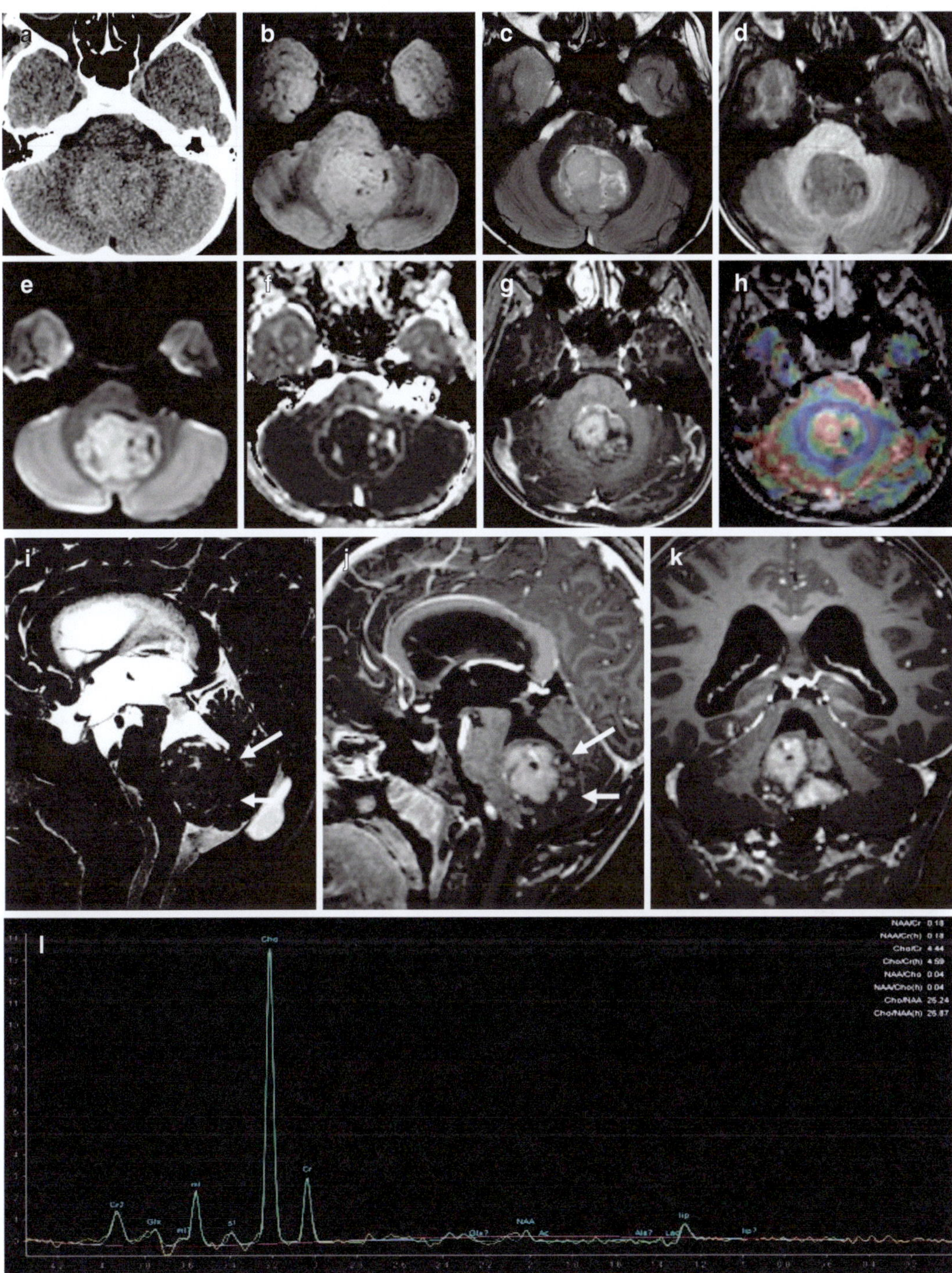

Fig. 6.2 Medulloblastoma WNT-activated in a 7-year-old boy. CT (**a**). MRI FLAIRI (**b**), T2WI (**c**), T1WI (**d**), DWI (**e**), ADC (**f**), post-contrast T1WI (**g, j, k**), CBV (**h**), bSSFP (**i**), single voxel spectroscopy (**l**). Imaging features are similar to the case of Fig. 6.1, the CBV is slightly increased. The tumor growth is through the inferior part of the fourth ventricle and the Magendie foramen (arrows **i**, **j**). The spectroscopy shows a marked increase in Cho/Cr ratio and an almost absent NAA

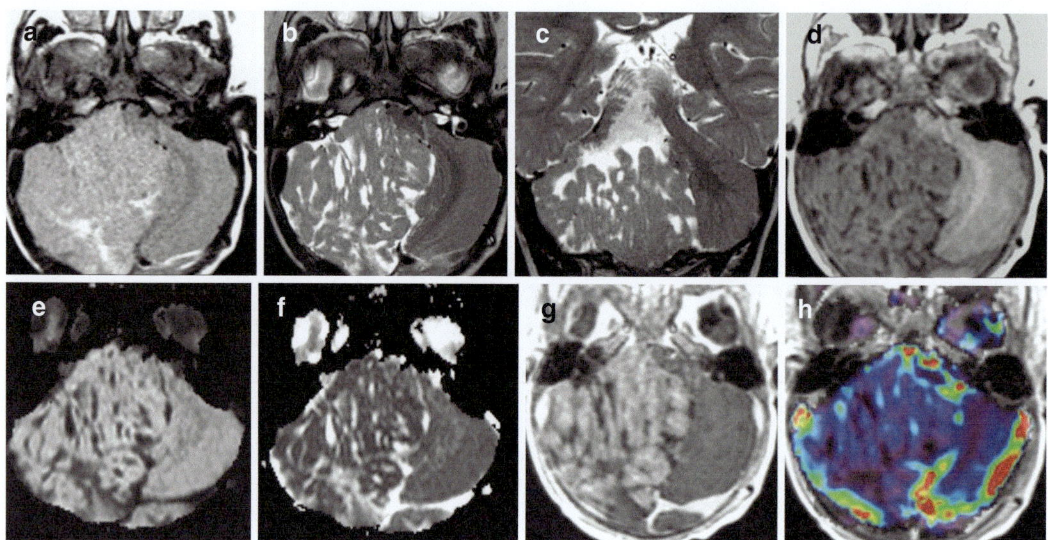

Fig. 6.3 Medulloblastoma SHH-activated in a 13-month-old boy. MRI FLAIR (**a**), T2WI (**b**, **c**), T1WI (**d**), DWI (**e**), ADC (**f**), post-contrast T1WI (**g**), CBV (**h**). The lesion occupies almost all the right cerebellar hemisphere, with a huge mass effect on fourth ventricle and brainstem, it shows a cerebriform aspect mimicking an aberrant hypertrophic cortex. Diffusion is reduced (**e**, **f**) and contrast enhancement is evident (**g**), on the contrary CBV is quite normal (**h**)

What is more typical of this medulloblastoma subtype is the growth within the fourth ventricle and through the foramina of Luschka and Magendie (Figs. 6.1 and 6.2) [3].

Presence of CSF metastases is very rare.

Diffusion. Diffusion is usually restricted.

Spectroscopy. Spectroscopy profile exhibits the typical pattern of an aggressive tumor with an increase of Cho peak and a marked decrease of Naa peak (Fig. 6.2).

6.1.2.2 Medulloblastoma, SHH-Activated and TP53-Wildtype. Medulloblastoma, SHH-Activated and TP53-Mutant

Medulloblastomas SHH-activated originate from cerebellar granule neuron precursor the proliferation of which is dependent on SHH signal activation. They account for approximately 30% of all medulloblastomas.

WHO definitions.

Medulloblastoma, SHH-activated and TP53-wildtype, is an embryonal tumor of the cerebellum demonstrating activation of the sonic hedgehog (SHH) signaling pathway in combination with a wildtype TP53 gene.

It is a WHO grade 4 tumor.

Medulloblastoma, SHH-activated and TP53-mutant, is an embryonal tumor of the cerebellum demonstrating activation of the sonic hedgehog (SHH) signaling pathway in combination with a mutant TP53 gene.

It is a WHO grade 4 tumor.

Epidemiology, prognosis.

Patients with TP53-wildtype medulloblastoma can be grouped according to age in infants with less than 4 years and in young adults. In these patients prognosis is variable but mainly good.

Medulloblastomas with the TP53 mutation are rare and found in children aged 4–17 years, their prognosis is poor.

Imaging

Medulloblastoma, SHH-activated, TP53 wildtype.

The most striking imaging feature of this tumor is the lateral localization within the cerebellar hemisphere, sometimes with a growing pattern mimicking the normal cerebellar cortex (Fig. 6.3). The lateral localization is present in roughly 2/3 of cases (Fig. 6.4), whereas in the remaining 1/3 MB SHH-activated could be present in the midline (Fig. 6.5).

This tumor typically appears as mainly isointense on T2WI and almost always exhibits diffu-

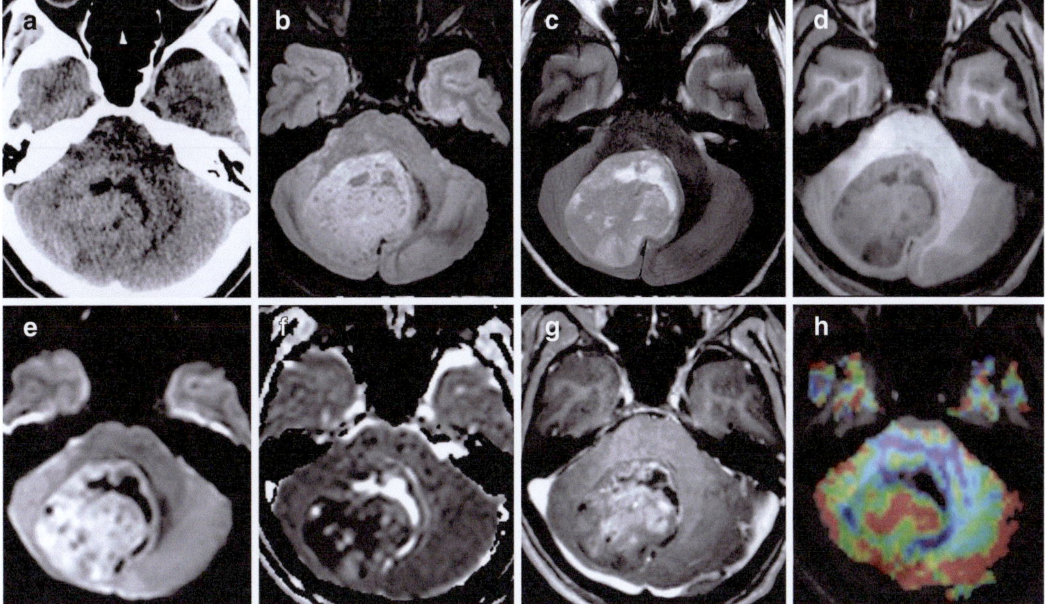

Fig. 6.4 Medulloblastoma SHH-activated in a 44-year-old woman. CT (**a**) MRI FLAIR (**b**), T2WI (**c**), T1WI (**d**), DWI (**e**), ADC (**f**), post-contrast T1WI (**g**), CBV (**h**). This kind of tumor can be found also in adults or young adult. Density and signal intensity are typical for medulloblastomas, but with a clear presence of multiple cysts. Even not so evident like in the case of Fig. 6.3, the tumor tends to localize in the right cerebellar hemisphere

sion restriction on diffusion images. Diffusion restriction is the more frequent feature on MRI in all the different medulloblastoma subtypes with a paercentage.

Calcifications are extremely unusual, such as leptomeningeal metastases, on the contrary cysts are relatively frequent.

Contrast enhancement is usually present with a moderate intensity.

Medulloblastoma, SHH-activated, TP53 mutant.

These tumors are rare and correspond histologically to anaplastic/large cell tumor. There are no specific features allowing an MR differentiation from medulloblastoma non-WNT/non-SHH.

6.1.2.3 Medulloblastoma, Non-WNT/Non-SHH

WHO definition. Medulloblastoma, non-WNT/non-SHH, is an embryonal tumor of the cerebellum without a molecular signature associated with activation of the WNT or SHH signaling pathway.

Medulloblastomas non-WNT/non-SHH are classified as group 3 or group 4 tumors and comprise eight molecular subgroup, demonstrated by DNA methylation profile.

Epidemiology. Group 3 tumors account for approximately 25% of all medulloblastoma, whereas group 4 is the largest molecular group accounting for about 40% of all cases. These two groups together represent approximately 2/3 of all medulloblastomas. Group 3 tumors are rare in adults, group 4 tumors present a peak incidence between 5 and 15 years being more rare in young infants and in adults.

Prognosis. The prognosis is variable and it is associated with the presence of metastasis at the time of diagnosis, being these two groups of tumors the most frequently associated with metastases (Table 6.2).

Imaging

From the imaging point of view group 3 and group 4 subtypes represent the most typical medulloblastomas almost always located in the

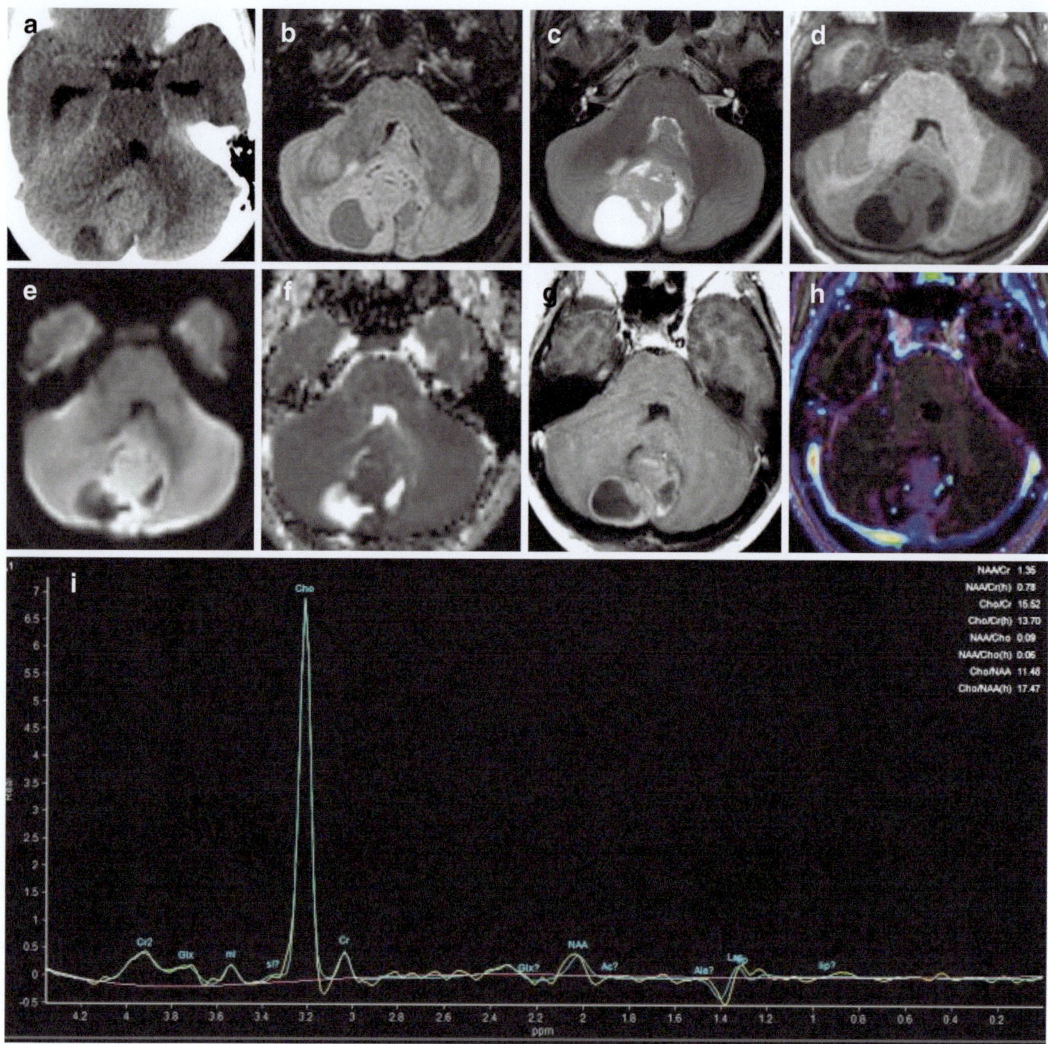

Fig. 6.5 Medulloblastoma SHH-activated in a 29-year-old woman. CT (**a**) MRI FLAIR (**b**), T2WI (**c**), T1WI (**d**), DWI (**e**), ADC (**f**), post-contrast T1WI (**g**), k-trans (**h**), spectroscopy (**i**). Another case of this tumor in a young adult. It is quite similar to the case of Fig. 6.4, but more centered on the midline with more cysts. Spectroscopy is nonspecific in medulloblastoma, in this case a large peak of choline is clearly predominant with barely visible peaks of creatine and NAA

Table 6.2 Imaging features of different molecular subtypes of medulloblastoma

MRI features	WNT	SHH	Group 3	Group 4
Location *midline*	Frequent	Rare	Almost all	All
Location *lateral*	Rare	Frequent	Almost never	Never
Contrast enhancement	Quite intense	Moderate	Moderate	Scarce
T2WI	Hypo-isointense	Isointense	Isointense	Variable
Diffusion	Restricted	Restricted	Restricted	Restricted
Peritumoral edema	Mild	Moderate	Scarce	Scarce
Calcifications	Possible	Rare	Possible	Possible
Number of (micro)cysts	Many	Many	Few	Many
Leptomeningeal metastases	Rare	Rare	Possible	Possible

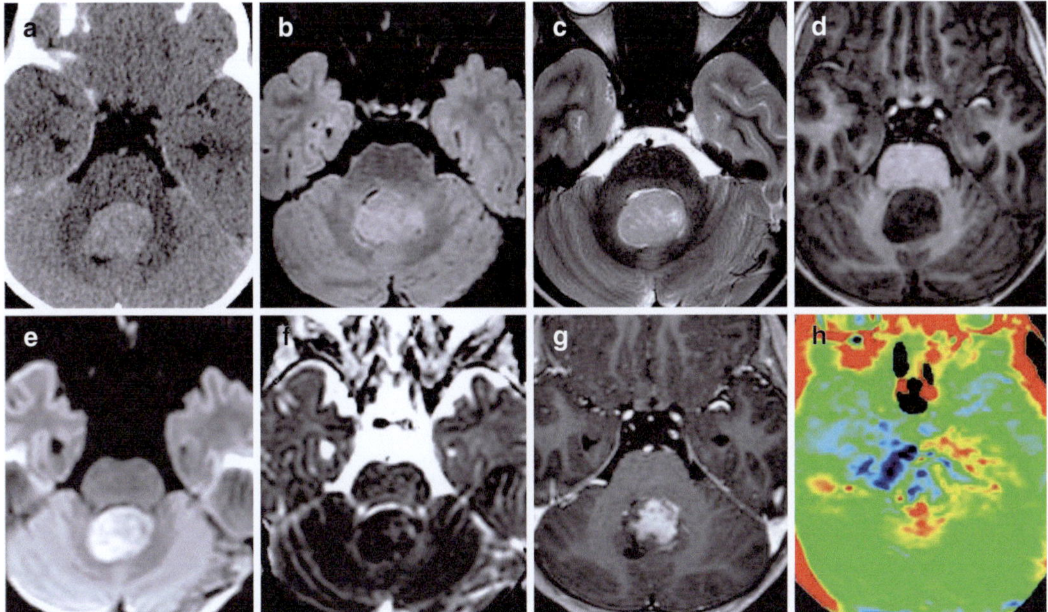

Fig. 6.6 Medulloblastoma non-WNT/non-SHH in a 7-year-old boy. CT (**a**). MRI T1WI (**b**), FLAIR (**b**), T2WI (**c**), T1WI (**d**), DWI (**e**), ADC (**f**), post-contrast T1WI (**g**), APT map (**h**). The location is in the middle portion of cerebellar vermis and the CT/MR features are quite typical with a silghtly hyperdensity on CT and a clear diffusion restriction. The amide proton transfer (APT) map shows a high amide concentration in the tumor compatible with a high-grade neoplasm

middle or inferior portion of the cerebellar midline (Figs. 6.6 and 6.7).

On CT and conventional MRI sequences the imaging features are comparable with other medulloblastoma subtypes, with a slight hyperdensity on CT, an iso-hyperintense signal on T2WI, and a slight hyperintensity on FLAIR imaging. On T1WI the tumor is mainly slightly hypointense (Fig. 6.6).

According to [2] the only difference between group 3 and group 4 medulloblastomas could be related to a possible less enhancement of group 4 medulloblastomas and to a more frequent T2 isointensity of group 3 subtype with respect to group 4 subtype. According to other authors, for patients with non-WNT/SHH tumors, the presence of an extensive gadolinium enhancement pattern predicted a worse prognosis [4].

Calcifications have been reported in roughly 1/3 of cases in both groups.

Diffusion is restricted as in the other medulloblastomas subtypes and in these two groups leptomeningeal metastases could be present at diagnosis in a higher percentage with respect to the other groups (Fig. 6.7).

MR spectroscopy in medulloblastomas. MR spectroscopy in medulloblastomas is not specific and usually shows the typical peak behavior of an aggressive tumor with a choline increase, a creatine decrease, and a marked NAA decrease (Fig. 6.5). Some statistical differences are reported between the molecular subgroups, but these data cannot be used for a single patient.

Moreover it was reported higher levels of total choline and lower levels of mobile lipids in patients with metastatic disease but also these data have a limited value in a single patient [5].

Brainstem medulloblastoma.

Medulloblastoma location is almost exclusively cerebellar; however, in one of the largest review recently published from a total of 2749 cases, 210 (7,6%) cases arose from the brainstem. In this review the cerebellar location represents approximately 85% of cases and other

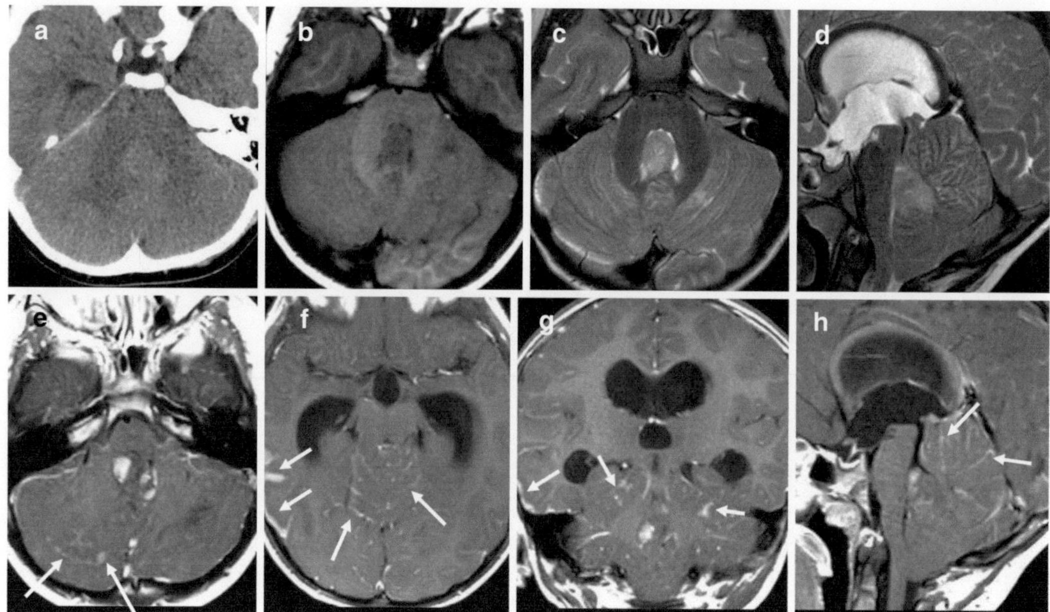

Fig. 6.7 Medulloblastoma non-WNT/non-SHH in a 4-year-old boy. CT (**a**). MRI T1WI (**b**), T2WI (**c, d**), post-contrast T1WI (**e–h**). After contrast administration a diffuse leptomeningeal enhancement is visible in posterior fossa (arrows E-H), an initial obstructive hydrocephalus is visible as well. (Courtesy Dr. L. Chiapparini, Pavia)

location outside the posterior fossa are exceedingly rare. In this series brainstem medulloblastomas exhibited worst prognosis than classical cerebellar medulloblastomas even though no data on molecular or histological classification was reported [6].

In Fig. 6.8 a rare brainstem medulloblastoma in a child of 3 years old was reported, it was a non-WNT/non-SHH type tumor. Imaging features of medullosblastoma are summarized in Table 6.3.

6.1.3 Other CNS Embryonal Tumors

From the 2016 update of the WHO classification for CNS tumors, the term primitive neuroectodermal tumor (PNET) previously used to denote a tumor belonging to a group of highly malignant, small round-cell tumors of neuroectodermal (including also medulloblastomas and atypical teratoid/rhabdoid tumors) is no longer included in the diagnostic lexicon.

6.1.3.1 Atypical Teratoid/Rhabdoid Tumor

WHO definition. Atypical teratoid/rhabdoid tumor (AT/RT) is an aggressive embryonal tumors composed by poorly differentiated cells and a variable number of rhabdoid cells with the potential to differentiate along neuroepithelial, epithelial, and mesenchymal lines. These tumors

Fig. 6.8 (**a**) Brainstem medulloblastoma. CT (**A**). MRI FLAIR (**B**), T2WI (**C**), T1WI (**D**), DWI (**E**), ADC (**F**), ASL (**G**), post-contrast T1WI (**H**). An apparently well circumscribed lesion is evident at the level of pontine-mesencephalic junction with a discrete mass effect on fourth ventricle but without perilesional edema. It appears hyperintense on FLAIR and hypointense on T1WI with diffuse microcysts and a slight diffusion restriction, perfusion is increased but no clear enhancment is evident after contrast administration. (**b**) Brainstem medulloblastoma (cont.). MRI FLAIR (**A**), post-contrast T1WI (**B, C**), spectroscopy (**E**). The location of the lesion is better appreciated in sagittal and coronal views. The absence of enhancement is confirmed in **B** and **C**. Spectroscopy exhibits the typical pattern of an aggressive lesion

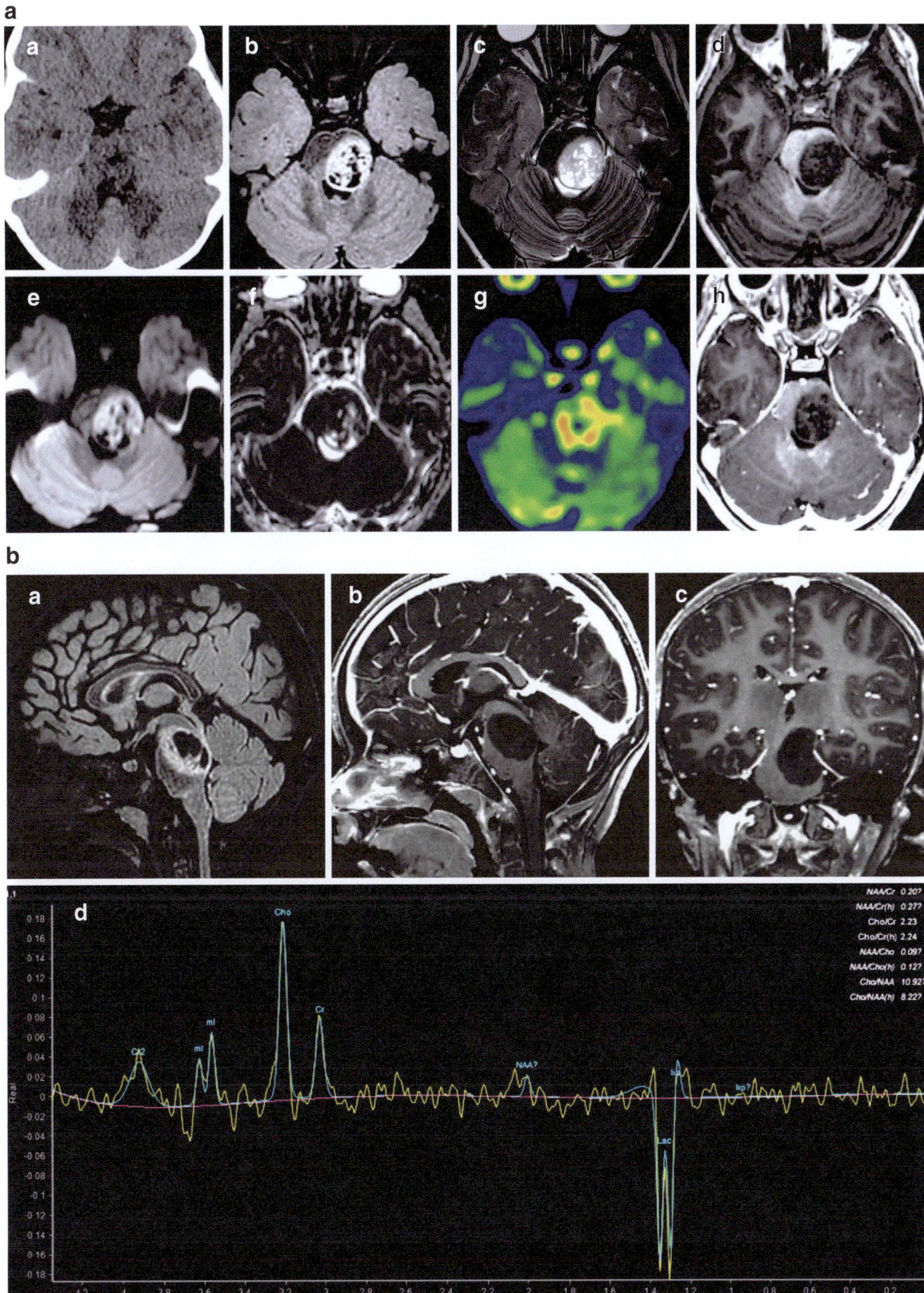

Table 6.3 Medulloblastoma general imaging features

Mass effect	Edema	Inhomogeneity	Cysts	Necrosis	Hemorrhage	Calcifications
+/+++	0/++	+/++	++	0/+	0/+	0/++

CT	T1	T2	FLAIR	DWI	ADC	T1 Gd	CBV	Spec
○	○	○	○	○	●	+/++	○	↑↑Cho/NAA

are characterized by the biallelic inactivation of *SMARCB1* or rarely *SMARCA4* genes.

AT/RT is a WHO grade 4 tumor.

Epidemiology. AT/RT is a rare tumor occurring predominantly in children under 3 years of age and rarely seen in children aged more than 6 years. About 1/3 of cases are reported under 1 year of age. A slight male predominance is reported.

Location. AT/RT can be located both infratentorially and supratentorially. When supratentorial this tumor is most frequently seen within the hemispheres, if infratentorial the most common locations are the cerebellar hemisphere or the cerebellopontine angle. The infratentorial location is more frequent under 2 years of age.

Clinical features. Most frequently the clinical onset is related to the typical signs of intracranial hypertension, but in case of infratentorial location cranial nerve palsy or head tilting can be recognized.

Prognosis. Prognosis is usually poor even though emerging data have shown some degree of variability in the 2 year overall survival rate.

6.1.3.2 Imaging

Their location on imaging can be frequently doubtful affecting both brain parenchyma and surrounding structures. AT/RT presents on CT and MR all the typical aspects of an aggressive lesion with a heterogeneous pattern with irregular enhancing solid portion and necrotic areas. Solid portions are usually slightly hyperdense on CT, iso-hyperintense on FLAIR, and iso-hypointense on T2WI and T1WI. In cases of large masses the differential diagnosis with other aggressive tumor is nearly impossible (Fig. 6.9). Perilesional edema is however usually scarce if not absent (Figs. 6.10, 6.11 and 6.12).

Diffusion, spectroscopy. Diffusion is usually restricted (Figs. 6.10, 6.11 and 6.12) and spectroscopy shows the typical profile of an aggressive lesion with very low NAA and high Cho (Figs. 6.11, 6.12) [7].

Perfusion. Perfusion is variable but usually increased. Imaging features of AT/RT are reported in Table 6.4.

6.1.3.3 Embryonal Tumor with Multilayered Rosettes

WHO definition. Embryonal tumor with multi-layered rosettes (ETMR) is an aggressive embryonal tumor conforming to one of the three morphological patterns: a. embryonal tumor with abundant neuropil and true rosettes, b. ependymoblastoma, c. medulloepithelioma. These tumors typically exhibit a C19MC a alteration or rarely a *DICER1* mutation.

ETMR is a WHO grade 4 tumor.

Epidemiology. ETMR is a rare tumor occurring usually in children under 4 years of age and in the majority of cases during the first 2 years of life.

Location. Although ETMR can occur both infra and supratentorial, the majority of cases are located in the cerebral hemisphere. Posterior fossa ETMRs occur in both cerebellum and brainstem occasionally involving the CP angle.

Clinical features. The most common clinical signs are related to increased intracranial pressure, i.e. headache, vomiting, visual disturbances.

Prognosis. ETMRs are aggressive tumors with a mean survival time reported in approximately 12 months even after therapy [8].

6.1.3.4 Imaging

ETMRs are usually large heterogeneous hemispheric tumors with an irregular enhancement on

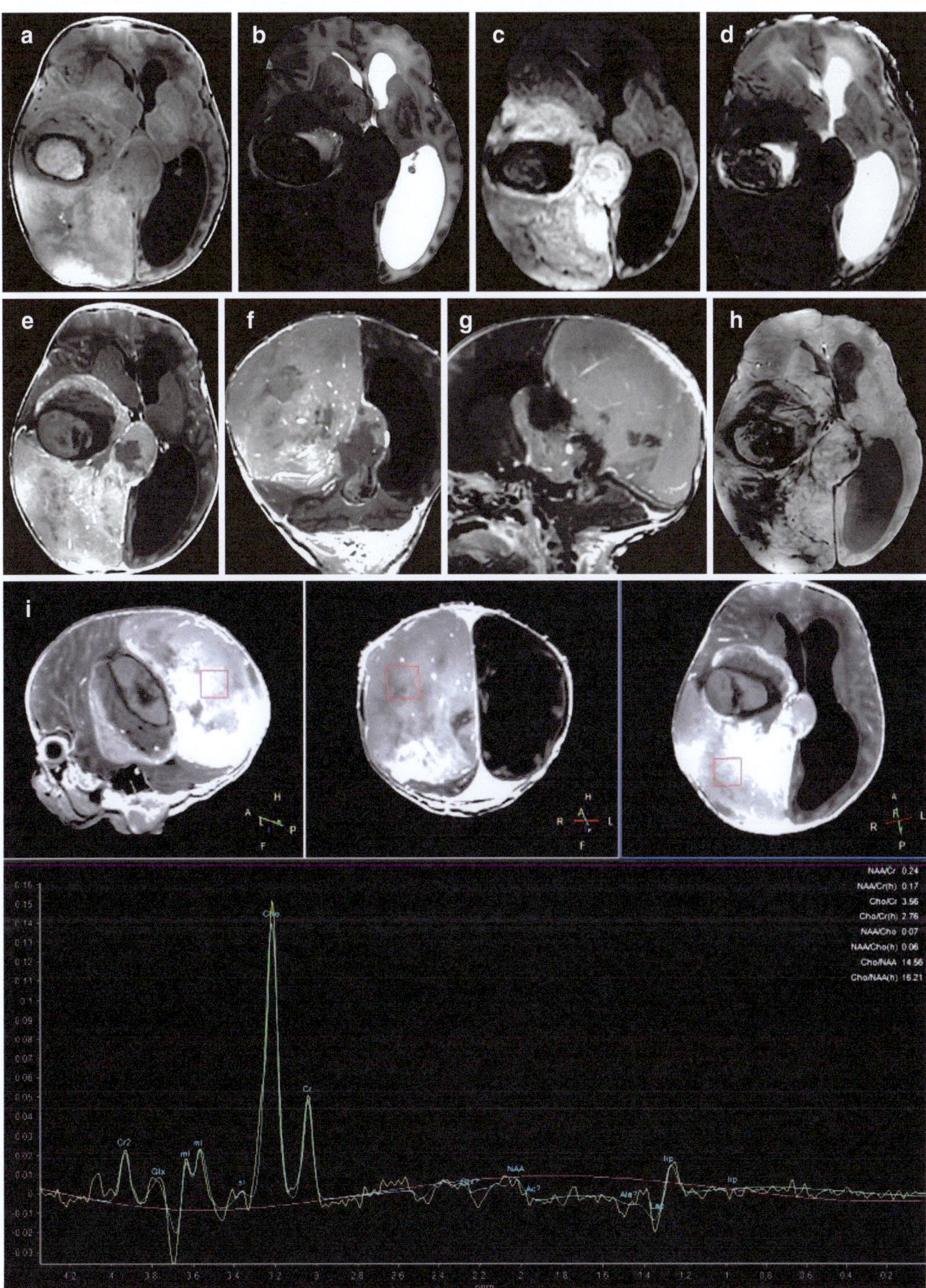

Fig. 6.9 Infat-type hemispheric glioma in a newborn, initially diagnosed as an AT/RT. MRI T1WI (**a**), T2WI (**b**), DWI (**C**), ADC (**d**), post-contrast T1WI (**e–g**), SWI (**h**), spectroscopy (**i**). A huge mass with a large hemorrhagic component is evident in the right parieto-occipital region and in the profound aspect of the right hemisphere with a dramatic mass effect. Apart from the hemorrhagic component the mass is relatively homogeneous with a diffuse T2WI hypointensity and ADC decrease. Spectroscopy profile shows the typical aspect of an aggressive tumor with an undetectable NAA

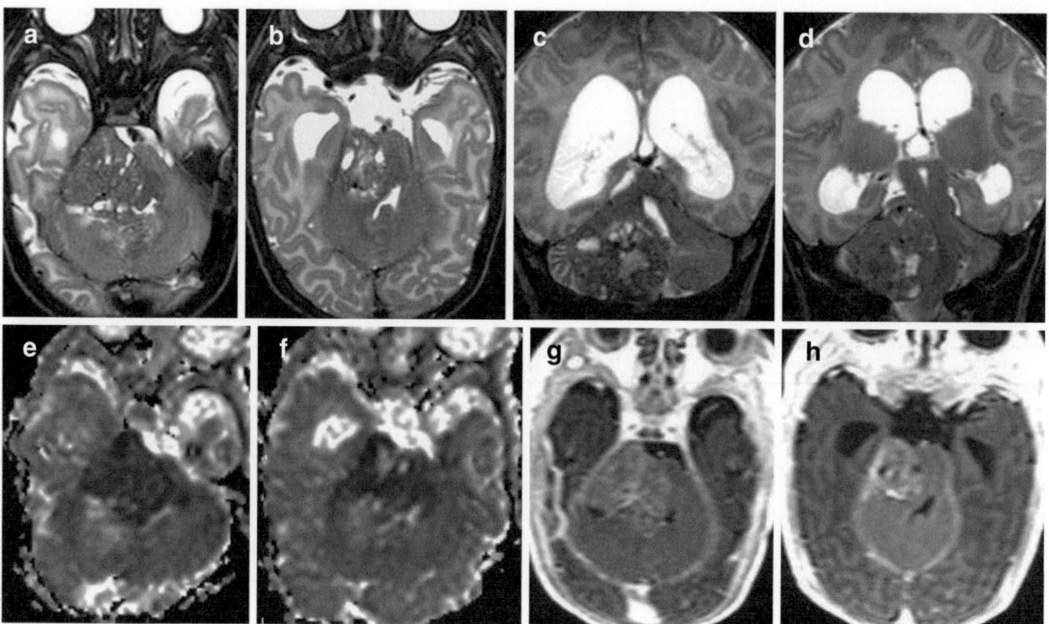

Fig. 6.10 AT/RT in a 1-month-old boy with multiple cranial nerve palsies. MRI T2WI (**a–d**), ADC (**e, f**), post-contrast T1WI (**g, h**). A heterogeneous lesion is located in the superior part of the left cerbello-pontine angle with a huge mass effect on brainstem, cerebellum and fourth ventricle causing an initial dilatation of third and lateral ventricles (**c, d**). A marked diffusion restriction is visible on ADC images (**e, f**). The lesion enhancement is scarce and irregular (**g, h**). Perilesional edema is almost absent

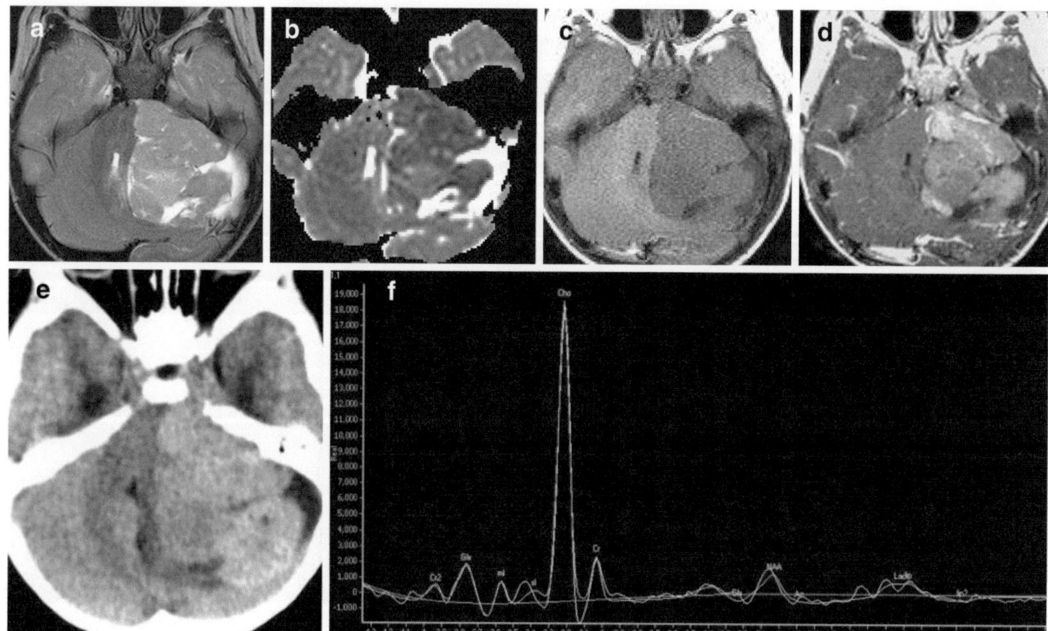

Fig. 6.11 AT/RT in a 6-month-old boy. CT (**e**). MRI T2WI (**a**), ADC (**b**), T1WI (**c**), post-contrast T1WI (**d**), spectroscopy (**f**). Also in this case the location is the CP angle with both intra- and extra-parenchymal components. The aspect of CT is slightly hyperdense. Perilesional edema is minimal

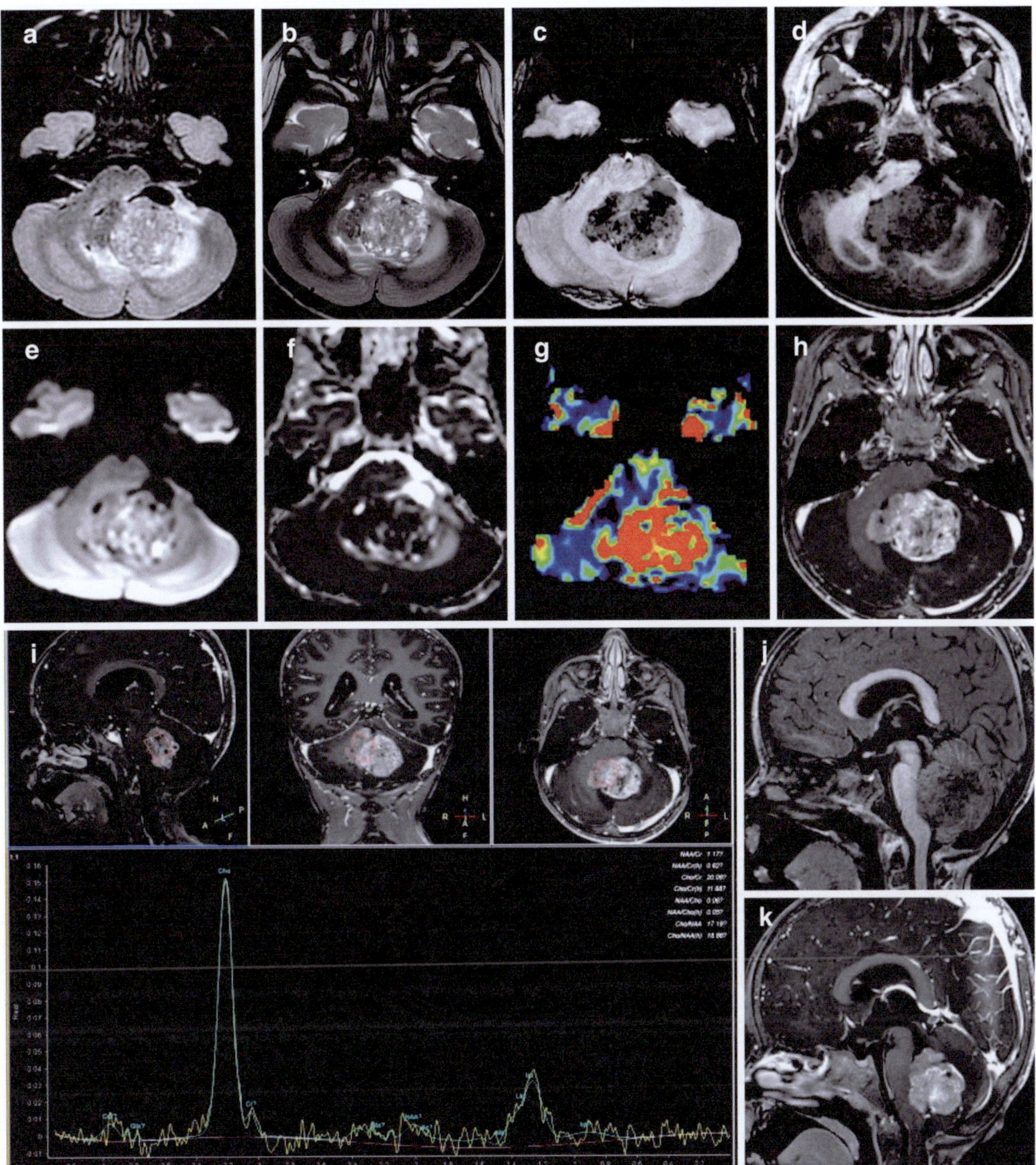

Fig. 6.12 AT/RT in a 33-month-old girl. MRI FLAIR (**a**), T2WI (**b**), SWI (**c**), T1WI (**d, j**), DWI (**e**), ADC (**f**), CBV (**g**), post-contrast T1WI (**h, k**), spectroscopy (**i**). A heterogeneous mass is located in fourth ventricle resembling a medulloblastoma or more convincingly and ependymoma with a diffusion through the left Luschka foramen. The lesions show a tiny multicystic aspect with a slight diffusion restriction, possibly microhemorrhages, irregular enhancement, and CBV increase. A differential diagnosis with the other typical pediatric lesion of the fourth ventricle is impossible. Perilesional edema is scarce. The spectroscopy profile is once again compatible with an aggressive lesion with absent NAA, high Cho peak, and some lipids. On sagittal section the location within the fourth ventricle is evident

Table 6.4 AT/RT imaging features

Mass effect	Edema	Inhomogeneity	Cysts	Necrosis	Hemorrhage	Calcifications
++/+++	0/+	+/+++	0/++	+/++	0/++	0/+

CT	T1	T2	FLAIR	DWI	ADC	T1 Gd	CBV	Spec
○	◔	◔	○	○	●	+/++	◯	↓↓ NAA ↑Cho/Cre

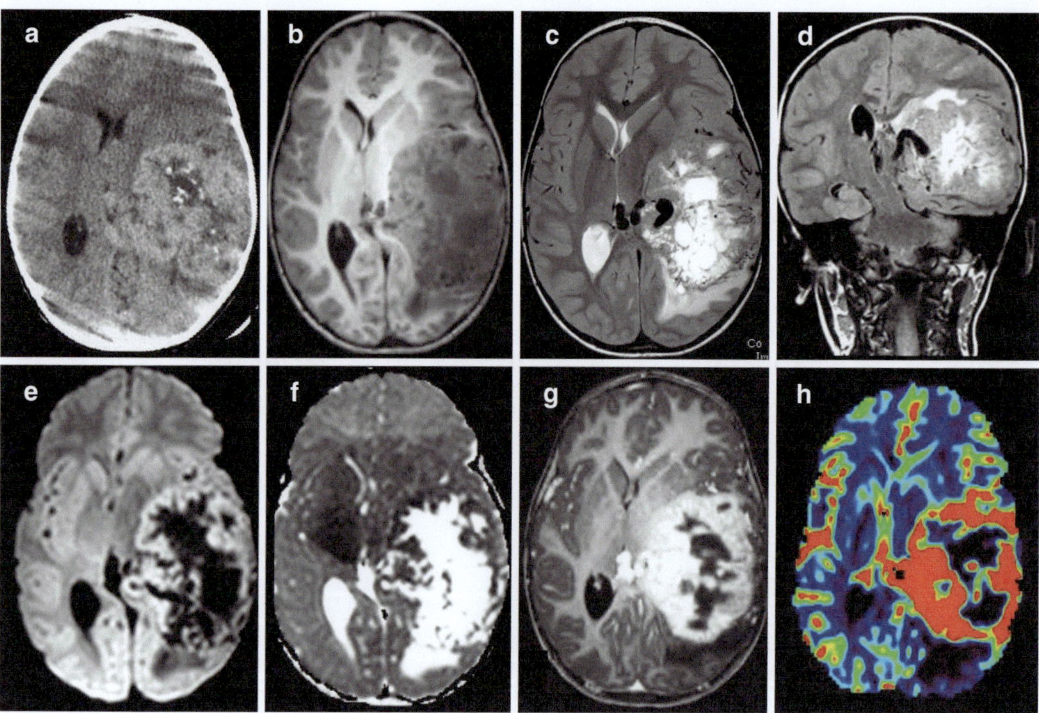

Fig. 6.13 ETMR in a 3-year-old child. CT (**a**). MRI T1WI (**b**), T2WI (**c**), FLAIR (**d**), DWI (**e**), ADC (**f**), post-contrast T1WI (**g**), CBV (**h**). A huge heterogeneous mass is visible in the left temporo-parieto-occipital region. On CT punctate calcifications are detectable in the lesion core (**a**), where large areas of necrosis are seen as well. Enhancing areas (**g**) show diffusion restriction (**e, f**), slight hyperdensity on CT (**a**) and increased CBV (**h**)

both CT and MRI. They present all the typical signs of an aggressive tumor with a slight hyperdensity on CT, an extremely heterogeneous pattern on conventional MR images with possible hemorrhages, necrosis, calcifications, and irregular enhancement after contrast administration.

Diffusion, spectroscopy. Diffusion is usually restricted and on spectroscopy a highly aggressive pattern is described with decreased NAA and increased Cho [9].

Perfusion. CBV is increased (Fig. 6.13). Imaging features of ETMR are summarized in Table 6.5.

6.1.4   CNS Neuroblastoma, *FOXR2*-Activated

WHO definition. CNS neuroblastoma *FOXR2*-activated is an embryonal neoplasm exhibiting varying degrees of neuroblastic and/or neuronal differentiation, characterized by activation of the transcription factor FOXR2.

It is a WHO grade 4 tumor.

Epidemiology. It is a rare tumor that occurs in childhood, recently described, and for which there are no epidemiological data available.

Table 6.5 ETMR imaging features

Mass effect	Edema	Inhomogeneity	Cysts	Necrosis	Hemorrhage	Calcifications
++/+++	+/++	++/+++	0/+	+/+++	0/++	0/++

CT	T1	T2	FLAIR	DWI	ADC	T1 Gd	CBV	Spec
○	◉ (gray)	○	○	○	●	+/+++	● (red)	↓↓ NAA ↑Cho/Cre

Table 6.6 CNS neuroblastoma *FOXR2*-activated imaging features

Mass effect	Edema	Inhomogeneity	Cysts	Necrosis	Hemorrhage	Calcifications
++/+++	0/+	+/+++	0/+	+/++	0/++	0/+

CT	T1	T2	FLAIR	DWI	ADC	T1 Gd	CBV	Spec
○	◉ (gray)	○	○	○	●	+/++	NA*	NA*

Location. It is typically located in cerebral hemispheres.

Clinical features. Clinical signs are related to the increased intracranial pressure.

Prognosis. It is an aggressive tumor but with limited data at present on the prognosis.

6.1.4.1 Imaging

It is a well demarcated hemispheric mass with frequently cystic component and a moderate enhancement of the solid portion.

In one of the largest reviews available us to now [10], regarding 25 patients with a median age of 4.5 years the tumors were often large, showed no (24%) or limited (60%) perilesional edema, demonstrated heterogeneous enhancement, were often calcified and/or hemorrhagic (52%), were always T2WI-hyperintense to GM, and commonly had cystic and/or necrotic components (96%). The mean ADC values were low. The tumors were always supratentorial. Metastases were infrequent (20%). Imaging features of CNS neurblastoma, *FOXR2*-activated are summarized in Table 6.6.

6.1.4.2 CNS Tumor with *BCOR* Internal Tandem Duplication

WHO definition. CNS tumor with BCOR internal tandem duplication (ITD) is a malignant tumor characterized by a predominant solid growth pattern, uniform oval or spindle-shaped cells with round to oval nuclei, a dense capillary network, focal pseudorosette formation, and an ITD in exon 15 of the *BCOR* gene.

It is a WHO grade 4 tumor.

Epidemiology. It is a rare tumor with few if any epidemiological data, the median age is around 3,5 years of age.

Location. It occurs typically in cerebral or cerebellar hemispheres.

Clinical features. Clinical signs depend on tumor location but are mainly related to increased intracranial pressure.

Prognosis. It is an aggressive tumor but with limited data at present on the prognosis.

Imaging

It is a well demarcated tumor with frequently a central cystic component and variable inhomogeneous enhancement of the solid portion.

They are usually large at diagnosis, and leptomeninges can be involved. Metastases are described.

On T2WI and FLAIR images are iso- to slightly hyperintense and on T1WI slightly hypointense. Typically perilesional edema is absent or extremely scarce (Fig. 6.14).

Diffusion is almost partly restricted, spectroscopy shows a marked increase of Cho/NAA ratio and the presence of lactate (Fig. 6.14).

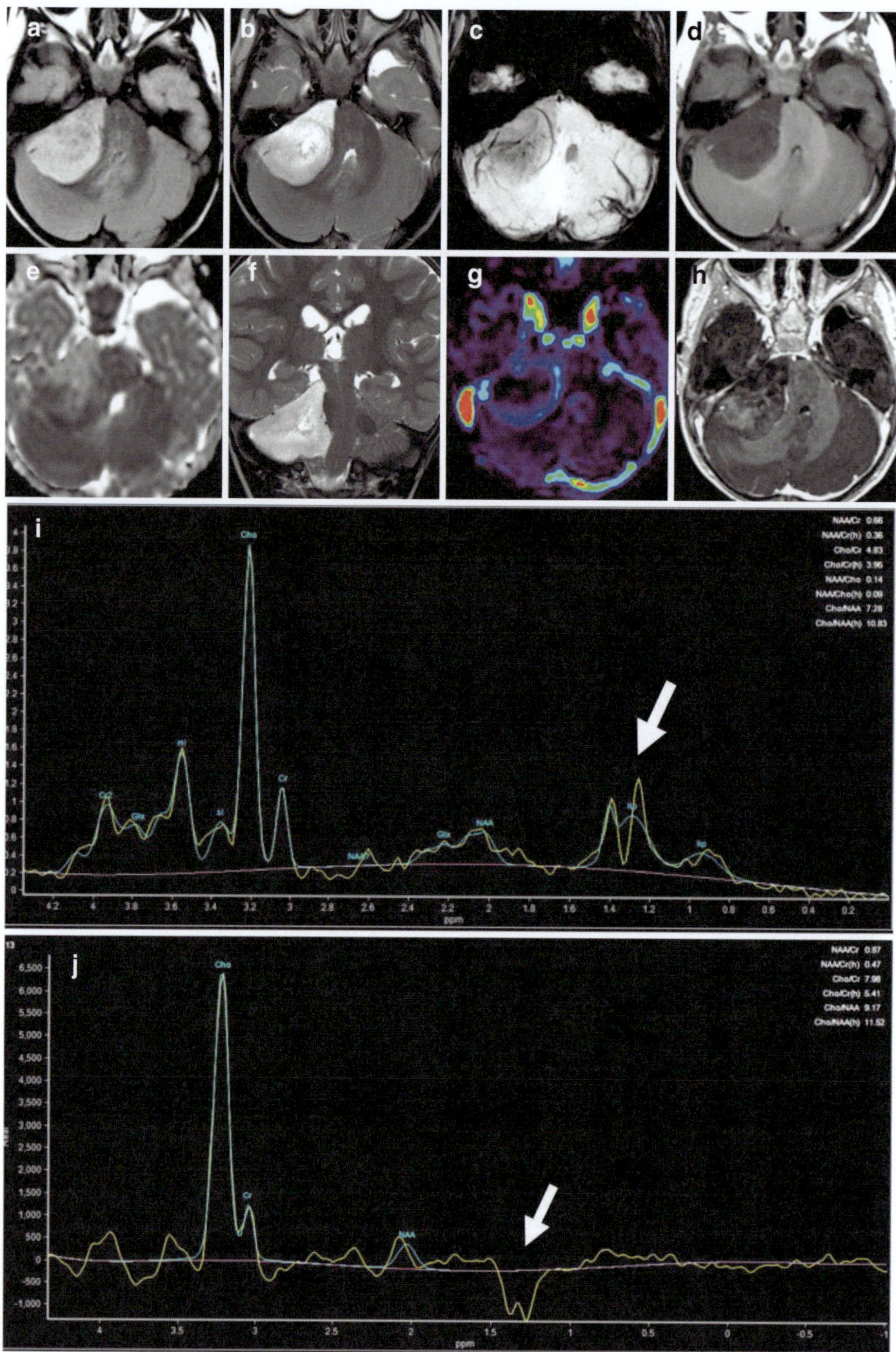

Fig. 6.14 CNS tumor with BCOR ITD in a 2-year-old girl. MRI FLAIR (**a**), T2WI (**b**, **f**), SWI (**c**), T1WI (**d**), ADC (**e**), k-trans (**g**), post-contrast T1WI (**h**), spectroscopy short TE (**i**) and intermediate TE (**j**). A large homogeneous mass is visible in the right CP angle with presumably both intra- and extraparenchymal components. A possible small cystic component is visible in the central portion of the solid homogeneous lesion, the perilesional edema is absent, the enhancement scarce and the permeability seem to be normal, whereas ADC is at least partly reduced, all these features can be suggestive of this type of embryonal tumor. NAA peak is almost absent and the lactate doublet is well evident in both echoes. (Courtesy Dr. C. Baldoli, Milan)

Table 6.7 CNS tumor with BCOR ITD imaging features

Mass effect	Edema	Inhomogeneity	Cysts	Necrosis	Hemorrhage	Calcifications
+/+++	0/+	+/++	0/+	0/++	0/+	0/+

CT	T1	T2	FLAIR	DWI	ADC	T1 Gd	CBV	Spec
○	◓	○	○	○	●	0/++	○	↑↑Cho/NAA ↑lac

Perfusion can be normal (Fig. 6.14) [11]. Imaging features of CNS tumor with BCOR ITD are summarized in Table 6.7.

6.1.4.3 CNS Embryonal Tumor NEC/ NOS

WHO definition. This is a CNS tumor with embryonal morphology and immunophenotype and: a) either lacking an alteration that would classify it as one of the molecularly defined embryonal tumor, b) or not susceptible to further analysis.

It is a WHO grade 4 tumor.

6.1.4.4 Imaging

This group of tumor encompassed all the imaging characteristics of the previous group of embryonal tumor.

6.2 Pineal Tumors

6.2.1 Pineocytoma

WHO definition. Pineocytoma is a well-differentiated pineal parenchymal neoplasm composed of uniform cells forming large pineocytomatous rosettes and/or pleomorphic cells showing gangliocytic differentiation.

It is a WHO grade 1 tumor.

Epidemiology. It represents almost 1/4 of all pineal tumors, it can be present at any age but it is more frequent in the third to fifth decade of life.

Location. It remains localized in the pineal region, compressing progressively adjacent structures.

Clinical features. Clinical signs depend on the progressive stenosis of the aqueduct with hydrocephalus and increased intracranial pressure, in case of large mass a Parinaud syndrome can occur.

Prognosis. It is a very slow growing tumor and after surgery the prognosis is favorable.

6.2.1.1 Imaging

It is a globular well defined mass of the pineal gland with calcifications, iso-hypodense appearance on CT, and hypointense aspect on T1WI. On T2/FLAIR images it can be slightly hyperintense or isointense to brain parenchyma, post-contrast enhancement is present.

Diffusion is usually similar to brain parenchyma (Figs. 6.15 and 6.16). Imaging features of pinealoma are summarized in Table 6.8.

6.2.2 Pineal Parenchymal Tumor of Intermediate Differentiation (PPTID)

Definition. Pineal parenchymal tumor of intermediate differentiation (PPTID) is a tumor with an intermediate malignancy between pineocytoma and pnealoblastoma composed by diffuse sheets of large lobules of monomorphic round cells more differentiated than those observed in pinealoblastoma.

It corresponds to a WHO grade 2 or 3.

Epidemiology. It represents 45% of pineal parenchymal tumor and occurs mainly in adults and the median patient age is 33 years.

Location. It remains localized in the pineal region.

Clinical features. Signs and symptoms are related to the mass effect on the quadrigeminal plate and aqueduct.

Prognosis PPTID is more aggressive than pineocytoma and the recurrence rate after surgery varies from 25 to 50%.

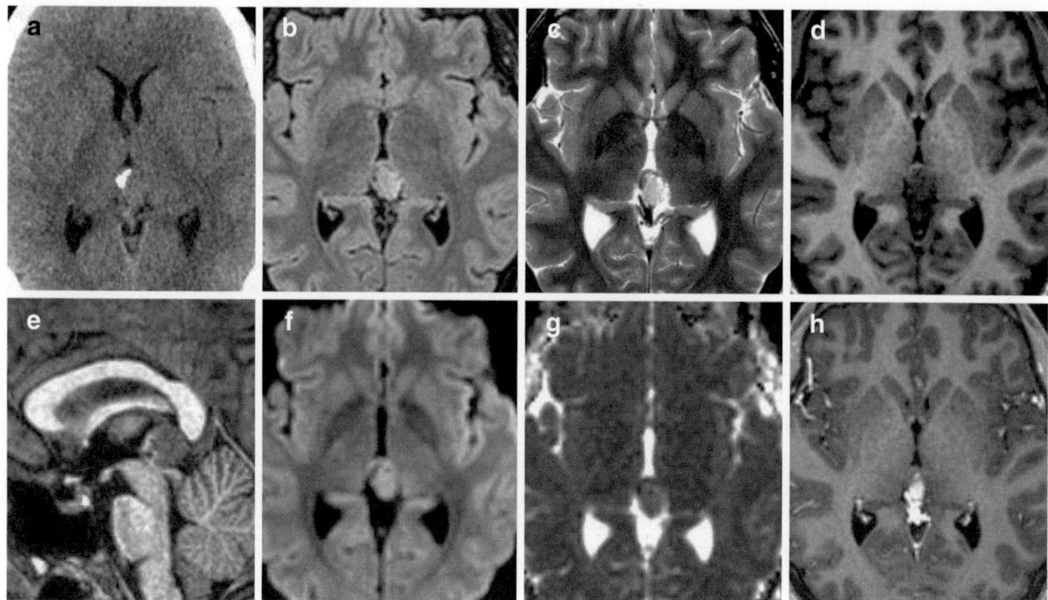

Fig. 6.15 Pineocytoma in a 24-year-old woman. CT (**a**). MRI FLAIR (**b**), T2WI (**c**), T1WI (**d, e**), DWI (**f**), ADC (**g**), post-contrast T1WI (**h**). A small pineal mass is visible with predominantly hypointense signal on T1WI and diffuse enhancement after contrast (**h**). The mass effect on the aqueduct is evident (**e**), but without supratentorial ventricular dilatation

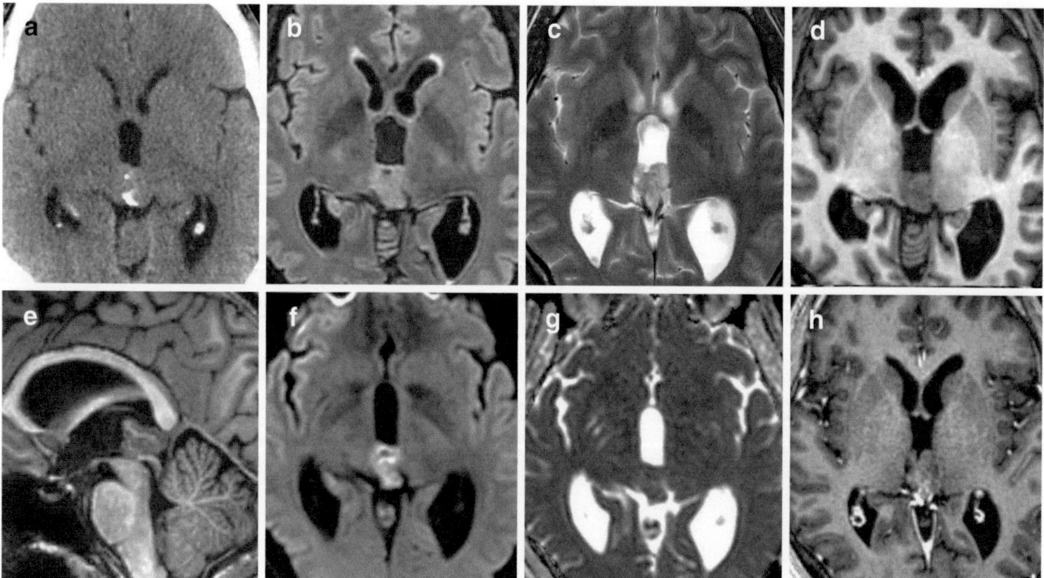

Fig. 6.16 Pineocytoma in a 37-year-old man. CT (**a**). MRI FLAIR (**b**), T2WI (**c**), T1WI (**d, e**), DWI (**f**), ADC (**g**), post-contrast T1WI (**h**). In this case the larger pineal mass causes an initial obstruction of aqueduct with a supratentorial ventricular dilatation. Small calcificazions are evident, even though the slight hyperintense signal on DWI the diffusion on ADC is similar to brain parenchyma

Table 6.8 Pineocytoma imaging features

Mass effect	Edema	Inhomogeneity	Cysts	Necrosis	Hemorrhage	Calcifications
+/+++	0	+/++	0/+	0	0	0/+

CT	T1	T2	FLAIR	DWI	ADC	T1 Gd	CBV	Spec
◯	◉	◯	◯	◯	◉	+/++	NA[a]	NA[a]

[a]NA (not available) = incomplete or sporadic reports

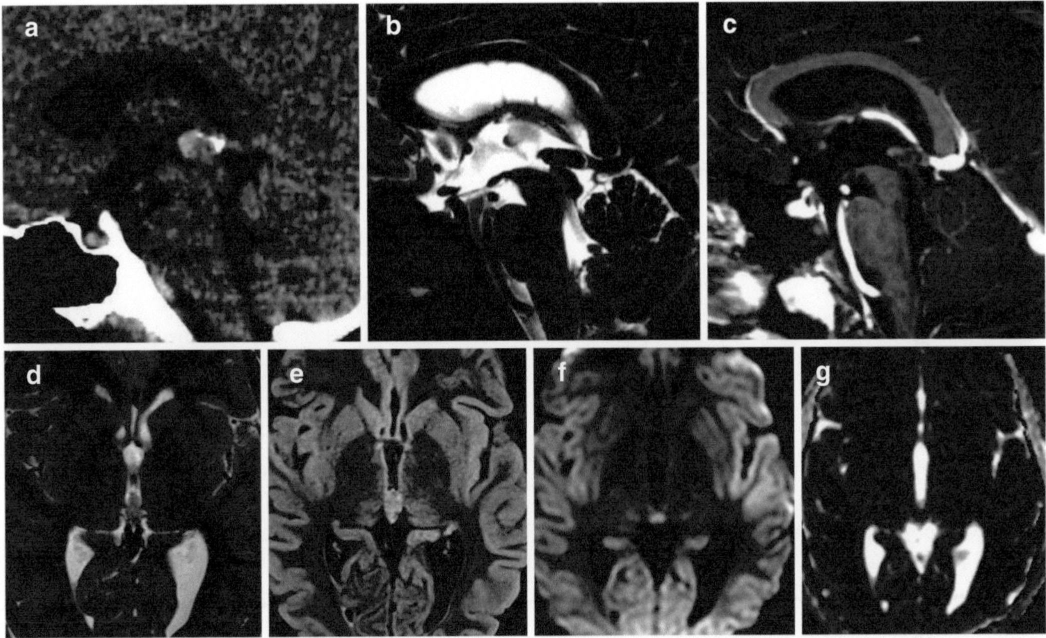

Fig. 6.17 PPTID in a 14-year-old girl. CT (**a**). MRI T2WI (**b, d**), post-contrast T1WI (**c**), DWI (**f**), FLAIR (**e**), DWI (**f**), ADC (**g**). In this case the pineal lesion slightly hyperdense on basal CT study presents a relatively small size and it is not possible to make any differential diagnosis from a pineocytoma. (Courtesy Dr. S. Colafati, Rome)

Table 6.9 PPTID imaging features

Mass effect	Edema	Inhomogeneity	Cysts	Necrosis	Hemorrhage	Calcifications
+/+++	0	+/++	0/+	0	0	+/++

CT	T1	T2	FLAIR	DWI	ADC	T1 Gd	CBV	Spec
◯	◉	◯	◯	◯	◉	+/++	NA[a]	NA[a]

[a]NA (not available) = incomplete or sporadic reports

6.2.2.1 Imaging

PPTID may usually present imaging features that may resemble pineocytoma (Fig. 6.17), the only difference is a larger size at diagnosis with a possible invasion of adjacent structures that is absent in pineocytoma [12]. Imaging features of PPTID are summarized in Table 6.9.

6.2.3   Pinealoblastoma

WHO definition. Pinealoblastoma is a poorly differentiated cellular embryonal neoplasm arising in the pineal parenchyma.

It is a WHO grade 4 tumor.

Epidemiology. It can theoretically occur at any age and according to WHO 2021 represents approximately 35% of all pineal tumors, but the vast majority of cases occurring under the age of 10 years.

There are at least four different molecular subtypes, two of those related to *DICER 1* syndrome, one to hereditary retinoblastoma with a patient median age of 2.1 years and one with *MYC* amplification and activation with a median age of 1.3 years.

Location. It is localized in the pineal region with local invasion.

Clinical features. Signs and symptoms are related to the mass effect on the quadrigeminal plate and aqueduct.

Prognosis. Diffuse craniospinal metastases are frequently discovered at diagnosis and the survival rate at 5 years varies from 10 to 80% mainly depending on the age at presentation, presence of metastases at diagnosis, and partial resection at surgery.

6.2.3.1 Imaging

It appears as a large heterogeneous mass frequently invading structures close to the pineal gland such as the quadrigeminal plate, the thalami and the splenium of the corpus callosum. On CT the lesion is iso-hyperdense with infrequent calcifications, on MRI the lesion is heterogeneous with cysts, necrosis, possible hemorrhagic components, and diffusion restriction (Fig. 6.18) [13]. Imaging features of pinealoblastoma are summarized in Table 6.10.

6.2.4   Papillary Tumor of the Pineal Region (PTPR)

WHO definition. It is a neuroepithelial tumor of intermediate malignancy characterized by combination of papillary and solid areas with epithelial-like cells and immunoreactivity for cytokeratins corresponding to WHO grade 2 or 3.

Epidemiology. It is a rare tumor with a peak incidence between 30 and 40 years.

Location. It remains localized in the pineal region.

Clinical features. Signs and symptoms are related to the mass effect on the quadrigeminal plate and aqueduct.

Prognosis. As for PPTID, even PTPR presents a high recurrence rate after surgical resection.

6.2.4.1 Imaging

It is a heterogeneous well circumscribed mass of the pineal region with a typical presence of solid portions and multiple cysts. Intrinsic T1WI hyperintensity of uncertain origin has been reported. Post-contrast enhancement is heterogeneous (Fig. 6.19) [12]. Imaging features of PTPR are summarized in Table 6.11.

6.2.4.2 Desmoplastic Myxoid Tumor of the Pineal Region, *SMARCB1-*Mutant (increase the font size)

WHO definition. DMT of the pineal region *SMRCB1*-mutant is a tumor showing desmoplasia and myxoid changes but lacks histopathological signs of malignancy.

Epidemiology. Only 7 cases are reported up to now with a median age of 40 years.

Imaging

No extensive description of these tumors with apparent no difference with pineal tumor with intermediate malignancy [14].

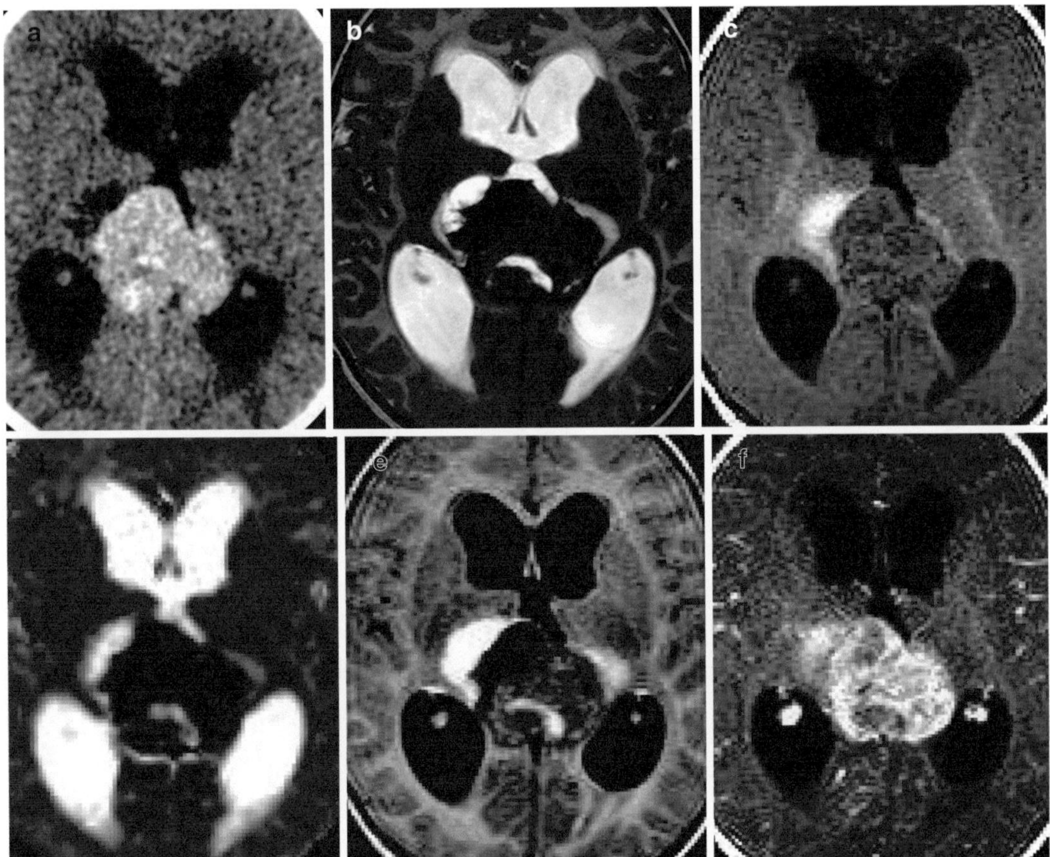

Fig. 6.18 Pinealoblastoma in a 4-month-old child with signs of intracranial hypertension. CT (**a**), MRI T2WI (**b**), T1WI (**c**), ADC (**d**), FLAIR (**e**) post-contrast T1WI (**f**). A huge pineal heterogeneous mass, with irregular enhancement T2WI hypointensity and ADC restriction due to the high cellularity is visible. On CT the tumor is diffusely hyperdense

Table 6.10 Pinealoblastoma imaging features

Mass effect	Edema	Inhomogeneity	Cysts	Necrosis	Hemorrhage	Calcifications
+/+++	+/++	+/+++	0/+	0/++	0/++	+/++

CT	T1	T2	FLAIR	DWI	ADC	T1 Gd	CBV	Spec
◯	◍	◯	◯	◯	●	+/++	NA[a]	NA[a]

[a]NA (not available) = incomplete or sporadic reports

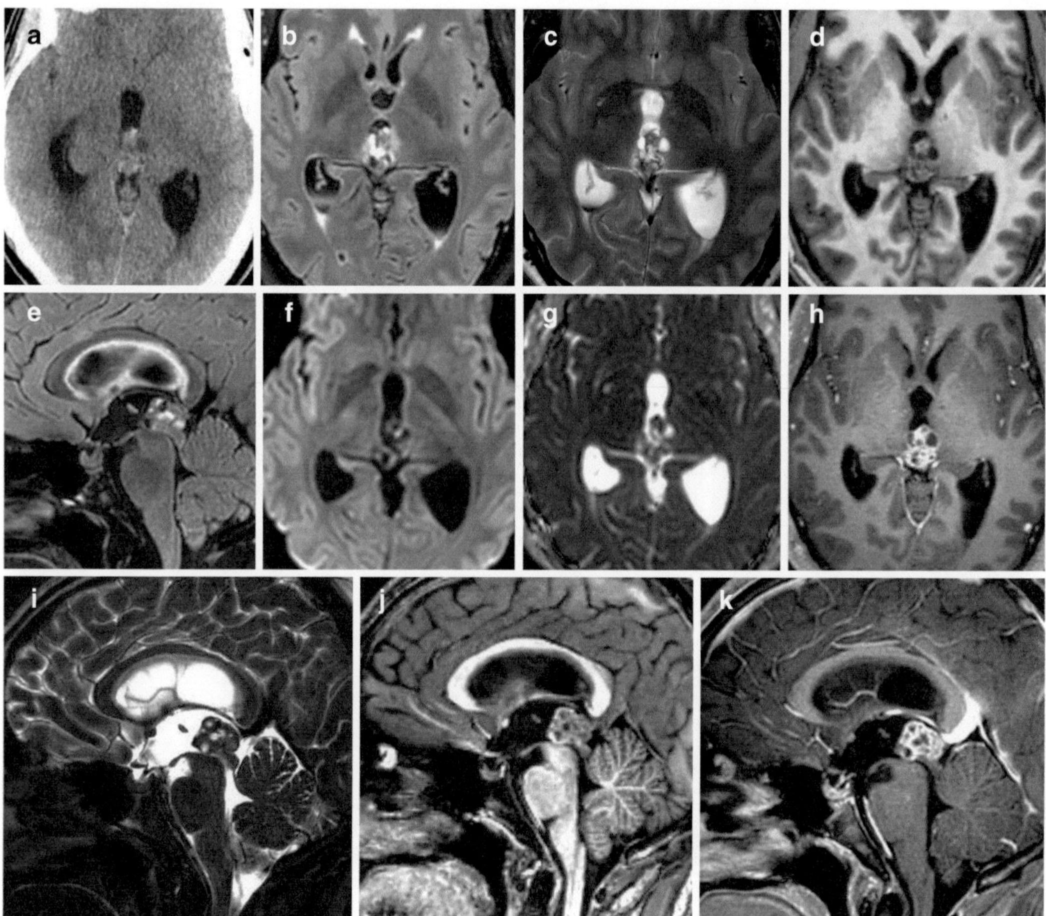

Fig. 6.19 PTPR in a 37-year-old man. CT (**a**). MRI FLAIR (**b, E**), T2WI (**C**), T1WI (**D**), DWI (**F**), ADC (**G**), post-contrast T1WI (**H**). The pineal mass exhibits its typical appearance with solid portion and multiple cysts with possible difference in signal intensity (see FLAIR images B and E). Figure 6.19 (**b**) PTPR in a 37-year-old man (cont.). MRI bSSFP (**I**), T1WI (**J**), post-contrast T1WI (**K**). The multiple cysts are well evident in the sagittal sections

Table 6.11 PTPR imaging features

Mass effect	Edema	Inhomogeneity	Cysts	Necrosis	Hemorrhage	Calcifications
+/+++	0	+/++	+/+++	0	0/+	0/+

CT	T1	T2	FLAIR	DWI	ADC	T1 Gd	CBV	Spec
◯	◓	◯	◯	◓	◓	+/++	NA[a]	NA[a]

[a]NA (not available) = incomplete or sporadic reports

References

1. Colafati GS, Voicu IP, Carducci C, et al. MRI features as a helpful tool to predict the molecular subgroups of medulloblastoma: state of the art. Ther Adv Neurol Disord. 2018;11:1–14.
2. Perreault S, Ramaswamy V, Achrol A, et al. MRI surrogates for molecular subgroups of Medulloblastoma. AJNR Am J Neuroradiol. 2014;35:1263–9.
3. Patay Z, DeSain LA, Hwang SN, Coan A, Li Y, Ellison DW. MR imaging characteristics of wingless-type-subgroup pediatric Medulloblastoma. AJNR Am J Neuroradiol. 2015;36:2386–93.
4. Łastowska M, Jurkiewicz E, Trubicka J, et al. Contrast enhancement pattern predicts poor survival for patients with non-WNT/SHH medulloblastoma tumours. J Neuro-Oncol. 2015;123:65–73.
5. Peel AC, Davies NP, Ridley L, et al. Magnetic resonance spectroscopy suggest key differences in the metastatic behavior of medulloblastoma. Eur J Cancer. 2007;46:1037–44.
6. Qin Q, Huand D, Jiang Y. Survival difference between brainstem and cerebellum medulloblastoma: the surveillance, epidemiology, and end result-based study. Medicine. 2020;99:4.
7. Jin B, Feng XY. MRI features of atypical teratoid/rhabdoid tumors in children. Pediatr Radiol. 2013;43:1001–8.
8. Korshunov A, Sturm D, Ryzhova M, et al. Embryonal tumor with abundant neuropil and true rosettes (ETANTR), ependymoblastoma, and medulloepithelioma share molecular similarity and comprise a single clinicopathological entity. Acta Neuropathol. 2014;128:279–89.
9. Wang B, Gogia B, Fuller GN, Ketonen LM. Embryonal tumor with multilayered rosettes C19MC-altered: clinical, pathological and neuroimaging findings. J Neuroimaging. 2018;28:483–9.
10. Tietze A, Mankad K, Lequin MH, et al. Imaging characteristics of CNS neuroblastoma-FOXR2: a retrospective and multi-institutional description of 25 cases AJNR. Am J Neuroradiol. 2022;43:1476–80.
11. Ferris SP, Vega JV, Aboian M, et al. High-grade neuroepithelial tumor with BCOR exon 15 internal tandem duplication—a comprehensive clinical, radiographic, pathologic, and genomic analysis. Brain Pathol. 2020;30:46–62.
12. Sadashiva N, Deora H, Arumalla K, Rao S, Saini J, Shukla D, Santosh V. Pineal parenchymal tumor of intermediate differentiation (PPTID) and papillary tumor of pineal region (PTPR): a review. Neurol India. 2021;69:1153–64.
13. Solomou AG. Magnetic resonance imaging of pineal tumors and drop metastases: a review approach. Rare Tumors. 2017;9:6715.
14. Thomas C, Wefers A, Bens S, et al. Desmoplastic myxoid tumor, SMARCB1-mutant: clinical, histopathological and molecular characterization of a pineal region tumor encountered in adolescents and adults. ·. Acta Neuropathol. 2020;139:277–86.

7.1 Cranial and Paraspinal Nerve Tumors

7.1.1 Schwannoma

WHO definition. Schwannomas are benign nerve sheath tumors composed by well-differentiated Schwann cells.

It is a WHO grade 1 tumor.

Epidemiology. They are relatively frequent intracranial neoplasms accounting for 8% of all intracranial tumors. Schwannomas can occur at any age, even though they are more frequent at middle age (40–50 yrs) and are usually sporadic. Multiple schwannomas account for 5% of all schwannomas and are usually associated with neurofibromatosis type 2 (NF2) and schwannomatosis.

Location. When located intracranially schwannomas affected the eighth cranial nerve in the vast majority of cases and represent 85% of cases of tumors of cerebellopontine angle. In the eighth cranial nerve they usually arise at the transition zone between central (oligodendrocyte) and peripheral (Schwann cell) myelination affecting usually the vestibular division and not the cochlear nerve.

Clinical features. Signs and symptoms vary according to location, being the eighth cranial nerve the typical intracranial location hearing loss, tinnitus, and vertigo can be frequently associated with intracranial schwannoma.

Prognosis. Studies in patients with NF2 demonstrated a defective production of merlin protein expressed by NF2 gene of chromosome 22. Merlin is a membrane-cytoskeleton scaffolding protein, i.e. linking actin filaments to cell membrane or membrane glycoproteins. NF2 belongs to the tumor suppressor group of genes and its abesence is an essential step in the genesis of schwannoma. Schwannomatosis is caused by a mutation in the SMARCB1 gene. This gene is located near the NF2 tumor suppressor gene.

Schwannoma is a benign tumor and if totally resected the probability of recurrence is extramely low. However surgery of large eighth cranial nerve schwannoma is complex and facial palsy is a frequent complication.

7.1.1.1 Imaging

Intracranial schwannomas are well circumscribed lesion that arises near the transitional zone from central and peripheral myelin, most frequently and typically of the vestibular nerve. In the eighth cranial nerve this area is located mainly at more than 10 mm from the origin of the nerve (approximately 11 mm), more distantly than in the other cranial nerves.

Hence the small vestibular schwannomas are found in the more external part of the internal auditory canal or just at the meatus of the canal where the transition zone is located (Figs. 7.1 and 7.2).

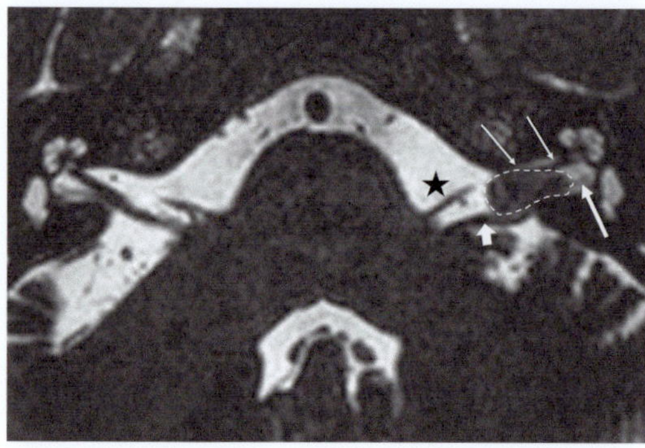

Fig. 7.1 Schwannoma of the left eighth cranial nerve. MRI 3D bSSFP high resolution sequence shows a partly intracanal left neurinoma (dotted line), with the more external part slightly protruding into the cerebellopontine angle cistern. The tumor arises from the vestibular nerve (long large arrow) compressing and anteriorly displacing the cochlear nerve (thin arrows). The common trunk of the eighth cranial nerve is indicated by the short arrow and the facial nerve from the star

From this zone schwannoma can grow within the internal canal or both within and outside the canal.

MRI is the only technique that can detect intracanalar schwannomas and the technique of choice to evaluate this tumor. On CT the evaluation of soft tissue within the internal auditory canal is obscured by the presence of beam hardening artifacts due to osseous structures. However CT can easily detect a pathological enlargement of the canal caused by the growing tumor.

Schwannomas are entirely solid when small. Larger lesions can exhibit small cystic components. On MRI they appear roughly isointense in all sequences. The enhancement is relatively intense and homogeneous when schwannoma is small but becomes irregular with the tumor growing mainly due to the presence of cysts (Figs. 7.3 and 7.4).

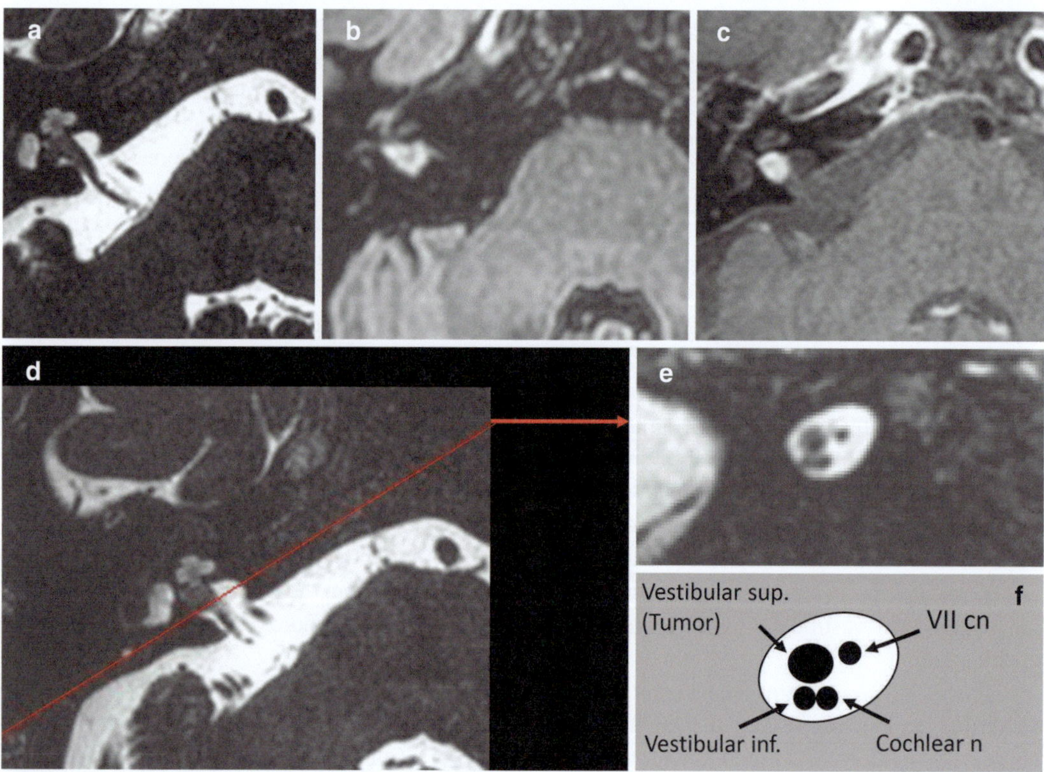

Fig. 7.2 Schwannoma of the right eighth cranial nerve. MRI bSSFP (**a**), FLAIR (**b**), post-contrast T1WI (**c**), reformatted imaging from (**a**) perpendicular to the internal auditory canal (**d**, **e**) and scheme of the position of the different nerves within the canal (**f**). In the reformatted image perpendicular to the internal auditory canal it appears clear the origin of the tumor from the superior vestibular branches of the eighth cranial nerve

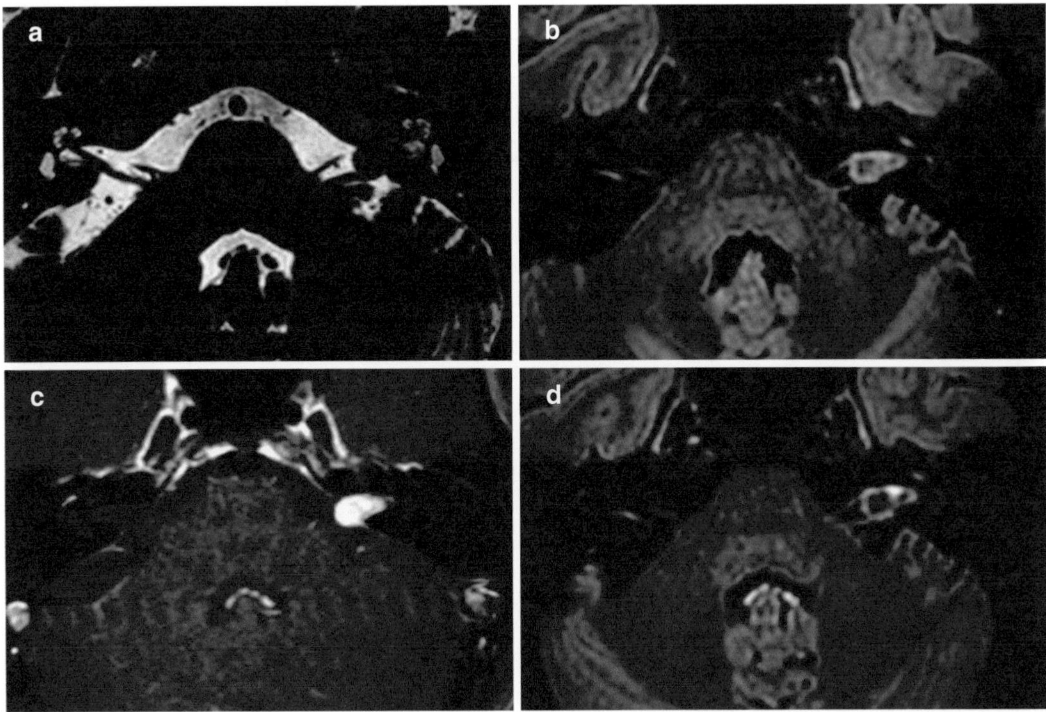

Fig. 7.3 Schwannoma of the left eighth cranial nerve. MRI bSSFP (**a**), FLAIR (**b**), post-contrast T1WI (**c**), post-contrast FLAIR (**d**). Same case of Fig. 7.1, the heteroge- neity of the lesion appears more evident on FLAIR images both before and after contrast administration

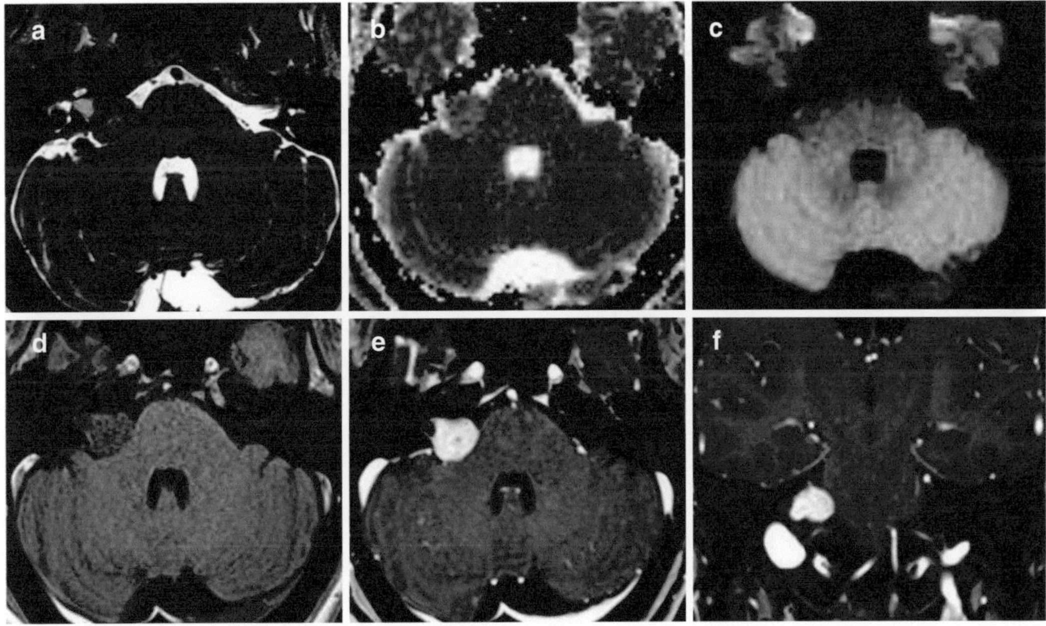

Fig. 7.4 Schwannoma of the right eighth cranial nerve. MRI bSSFP (**a**), ADC (**b**), DWI (**c**), T1WI (**d**), post- contrast T1WI (**e**, **f**). The tumor appears as roughly isoin- tense in all sequence, the component external to the auditory canal is prominent and an initial mass effect on brainstem is evident, the auditory canal is slightly enlarged

Diffusion, spectroscopy. No significant change in diffusion is usually seen and MR spectroscopy typically exhibits a large peak of lipids and the presence of lactate doublet. The presence of myoinositol peak was reported as well [1].

The presence of a peak of trimethylamine (TMA) was reported at 3.0 T in a relatively high percentage of schwannoma as well as in other peripheral nerve sheath tumors.

Perfusion. Perfusion does not usually show a significant increase.

The presence of large cysts can typically occur as a consequence of radiotherapy (gamma knife) (Fig. 7.5).

The presence of bilateral vestibular schwannoma (Fig. 7.6) is the hallmark of neurofibromatosis type 2 an autosomal dominant syndrome affecting the central nervous system with different types of tumors primarily schwannomas and meningiomas (Fig. 7.6), but also gliomas and spinal ependymoma. NF2 is caused by a mutation in NF2 gene on chromosome 22q12.

The diagnostic criteria of NF2 are reported in Table 7.1.

A diagnosis of schwannomatosis can be made in either of the following cases:

1 The person is age 30 or older and has all of the following:

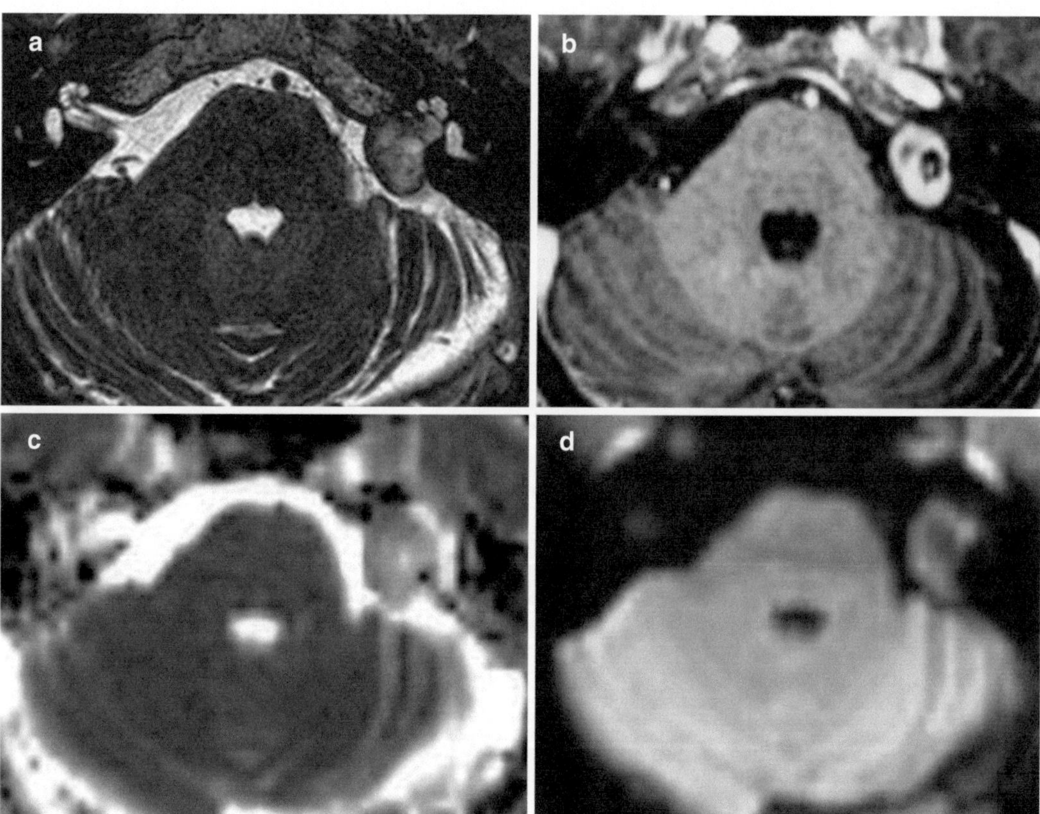

Fig. 7.5 Schwannoma of the left eighth cranial nerve. MRI bSSFP (**a**), post-contrast T1WI (**b**), ADC (**c**), DWI (**d**). This tumor was partly resected and successively treated with gamma knife. A diffuse hyperintensity of the central part is visible on T2WI image (**a**) with peripheral enhancement after contrast injection (**b**). There is an increase in diffusion (**c**, **d**) due to the large amount of water

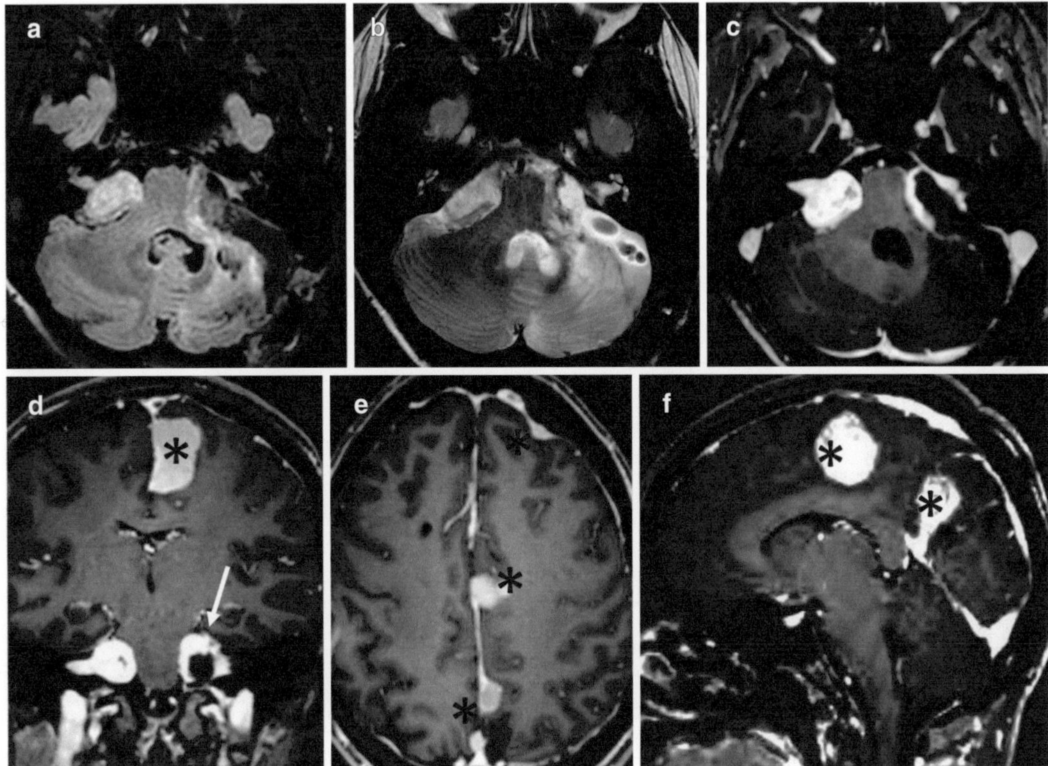

Fig. 7.6 Bilateral vestibular schwannomas in patient with NF2. MRI FLAIR (**a**), T2WI (**b**), post-contrast T1WI (**c–f**). Left vestibular schwannoma was previously oper- ated, but a residual portion is clearly visible after contrast injection (**c**, **d**). Together with bilateral schwannomas multiple meningiomas are visible as well (asteriscs **d–f**)

Table 7.1 The diagnostic criteria for NF2

The presence of one or more of the following features
(a) Bilateral vestibular schwannoma
(b) A first degree relative with NF2 AND unilateral vestibular schwannoma OR any two of: Meningioma, schwannoma, glioma, neurofibroma, posterior subcapsular lenticular opacities
(c) Unilateral vestibular schwannoma AND any two of: Meningioma, schwannoma, glioma, neurofibroma, posterior subcapsular lenticular opacities
(d) Multiple meningiomas AND unilateral vestibular schwannoma OR any of two of: Schwannoma, glioma, neurofibroma, cataract

(a) Two or more nonintradermal schwan- nomas and at least one of these tumors is con- firmed with tissue examined under a microscope

(b) No evidence of a tumor in the vestibule of the inner ear on high quality MRI scan

(c) No known physical or genetic signs of NF2

(d) No first-degree relative with NF2

2 One nonvestibular schwannoma confirmed by a pathologist, plus a first degree relative who meets the above criteria for schwannomato- sis. Imaging features of schwannoma are summa- rize in Table 7.2.

7.1.2   Neurofibroma, Plexiform Neurofibroma

WHO definition. Neurofibromas are benign nerve sheath tumors composed by well-differentiated Schwann cells mixed with non-neoplastic cells such as fibroblast and mast cells and variable myxoid or collagenous matrix.

They are WHO grade 1 tumors.

Table 7.2 Schwannoma imaging features

Mass effect	Edema	Inhomogeneity	Cysts	Necrosis	Hemorrhage	Calcifications
0/++	0/+	+/++	+/++	+	0	0

CT	T1	T2	FLAIR	DWI	ADC	T1 Gd	CBV	Spec
						++		↑↑lipids,↑lac ↓NAA. ↑TMA

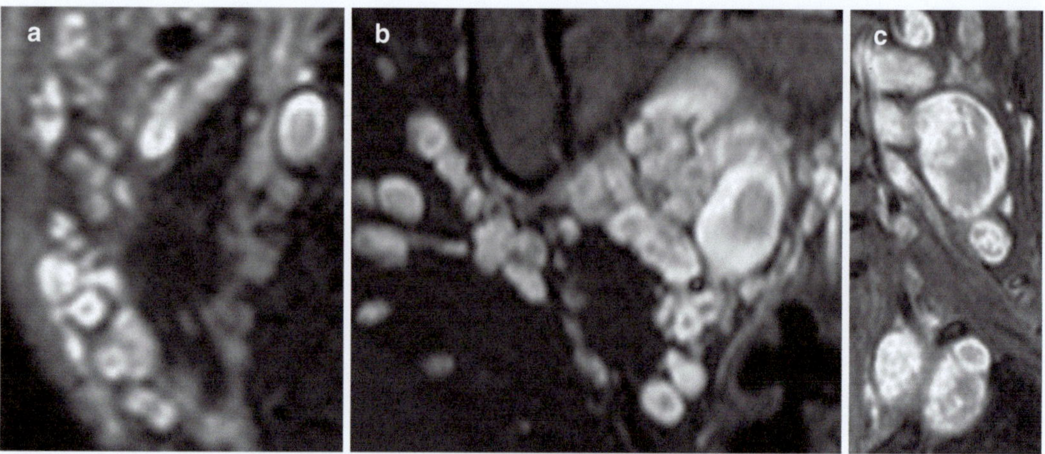

Fig. 7.7 Multiple subcutaneous and plexiform neurofibromas in NF1 patient. MRI T2WI (**a–c**), the typical "fried-egg" appearance is clearly visible in almost all the lesions

Epidemiology. Neurofibromas are the most common peripheral nerve sheath tumors and they are usually solitary sporadic lesion, less frequently they are multiple, and sometimes widely diffuse in subjects with NF1. There is no sexual predilection and the solitary lesions appear in childhood.

Location. They may be present everywhere, more commonly as cutaneous nodule, and less frequently as a circumscribed mass in a peripheral nerve or a plexiform mass in a major nerve trunk or plexus. Differently from the general population in patients with NF1 neurofibromas commonly involve spinal nerve roots bilaterally being associated with different degree of scoliosis.

Clinical features. Neurofibromas are rarely painful and their sign and symptoms are related mainly to mass effect.

Prognosis. Neurofibromas are related to the loss of function of NF1 gene. Even though benign a malignant transformation of large plexiform tumors in NF1 patients has been reported in 5–10% of cases.

7.1.2.1 Imaging

Neurofibromas are solid mass most frequently in subcutaneous location with a typical hyperintense aspect on T2WI and particularly on STIR sequence. This sequence allows the better conspicuity for this kind of lesion and has to be provided when neurofibromas are suspected. The enhancement is moderate to low and mainly peripheral. Frequently neurofibroma shows on T2 and STIR images a target or "fried-egg "sign with the more inner part of the mass relatively isointense and the more external part clearly hyperintese (Fig. 7.7) [2, 3].

Neurofibromas are one of the typical hallmarks of NF1, where they can be found in a subcutaneous location or as a plexiform mass. When located subcutaneously they can form huge aggregates of multiple lesions with variable sizes causing characteristic deformity such as in the case of Fig. 7.8.

Plexiform neurofibromas are typically found along the spinal roots where they can cause nerve compression, osseous reabsorption resulting in

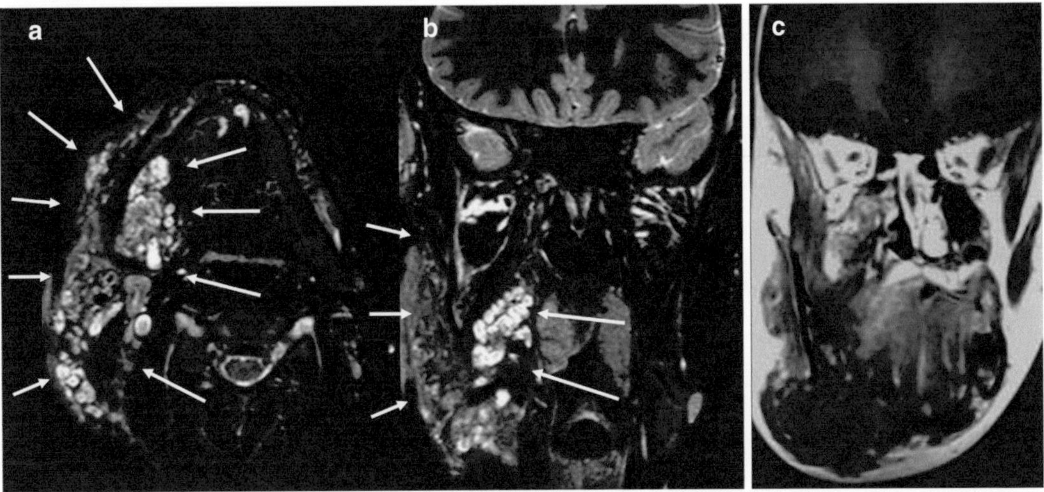

Fig. 7.8 Multiple subcutaneous and perineural neurofibromas in NF1 patient. MRI STIR (**a, b**), post-contrast T1WI (**c**). These multiple diffuse neurofibromas cause a large irregular perimandibular mass with a head and neck deformity

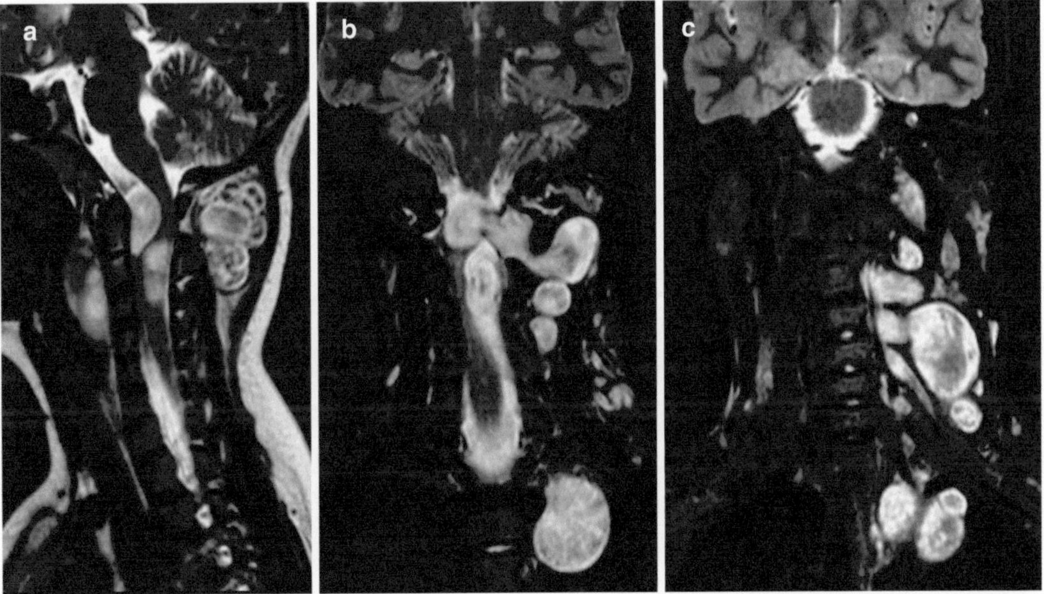

Fig. 7.9 Multiple cervical plexiform neurofibromas in NF1 patient. MRI T2WI (**a**), STIR (**b, c**). The huge plexiform neurofibromas cause enlargement of neural foramina and a compression of the upper cervical spinal cord

the enlargement of neural foramina, and eventually a possible direct mass effect on spinal cord (Figs. 7.9 and 7.10).

Spectroscopy. MR spectra show a complete different profile with respect to central nervous system tissue and the presence of trimethylamine (TMA) is quite characteristic for peripheral nerve sheath tumors. Imaging features of neurofibromas are summarized in Table 7.3.

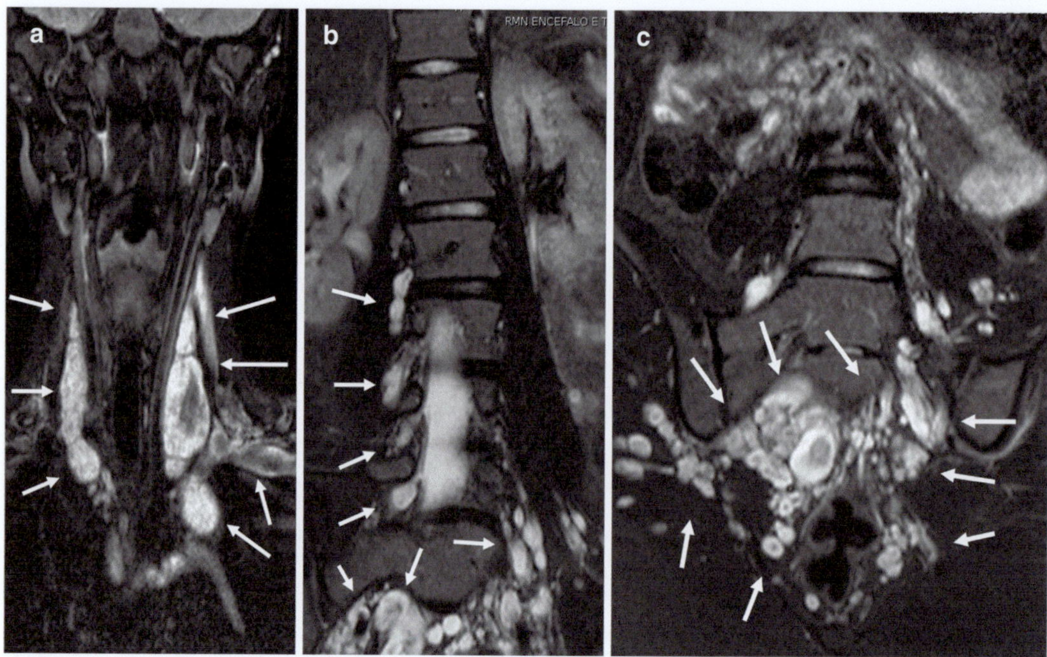

Fig. 7.10 Multiple subcutaneous and plexiform neurofibromas in NF1 patient. MRI STIR (**a–c**). Plexiform neurofibromas are evident in both cervical (**a**) and lumbo-sacral location (**b, c**)

Table 7.3 Neurofibromas imaging features

Mass effect	Edema	Inhomogeneity	Cysts	Necrosis	Hemorrhage	Calcifications
+/+++	0	+/++	0	0	0	0

CT	T1	T2/STIR	FLAIR	DWI	ADC	T1 Gd	CBV	Spec
⬤	⬤	◯	◯	⬤	◯	🟡	⬤	TMA

7.1.3 Rare Nerve Sheath Tumors

1. **Perineurioma** *Definition.* Is a benign tumor composed of neoplastic perineural cells. It is a WHO grade 1 tumor. IMAGING. Perineuriomas are fusiform enlargement of a peripheral nerve with increased T2 signal and contrast enhancement.
2. **Hybrid nerve sheath tumor** *Definition.* Hybrid nerve sheath tumors are benign peripheral nerve sheath tumors with combined features of more than one conventional type (neurofibroma, schwannoma, perineurioma). IMAGING. There are no criteria to differentiate this type of tumor from the other three benign peripheral nerve sheath tumors.
3. **Malignant melanotic nerve sheath tumor** *Definition.* Malignant melanotic nerve sheath tumor (MMNST) is composed uniformly of tumor cells with features of both Schwann cell and melanocytic differentiation and frequently shows aggressive clinical behavior. IMAGING. The only difference wuth peripheral schwannoma is the possibile presence of a T1WI hyperintensity due to the presence og melanin.

7.1.4 Malignant Peripheral Nerve Sheath Tumor

WHO definition. Malignant peripheral nerve sheath tumor (MPNST) is a malignant tumor of

Table 7.4 MPNST imaging features

Mass effect	Edema	Inhomogeneity	Cysts	Necrosis	Hemorrhage	Calcifications
+/+++	0	+/++	0	0/++	0/+	0

CT	T1	T2/STIR	FLAIR	DWI	ADC	T1 Gd	CBV	Spec
●	○	○	◐	◐	●	+	NA[a]	↑↑ TMA

[a]NA (not available) = incomplete or sporadic reports

Table 7.5 Cauda equina neuroendocrine tumor imaging features

Mass effect	Edema	Inhomogeneity	Cysts	Necrosis	Hemorrhage	Calcifications
+/+++	0	0/++	0	0	0/+	0

CT	T1	T2/STIR	FLAIR	DWI	ADC	T1 Gd	CBV	Spec
0	○	◐	◐	NA[a]	NA[a]	++/+++	◐	NA[a]

[a]NA (not available) = incomplete or sporadic reports

Schwann cells or perineural cells arising in peripheral nerve or in soft tissue. A precise grading of this tumor is lacking; however, according to WHO about 85% of these tumors are highly aggressive.

Epidemiology. They account for less than 5% of all malignant soft tissue tumor and arise usually in young or middle aged adults. In about 50% of cases MPSNT is associated with NF1 where it usually arises from a pre-existing neurofibroma.

Location. MPSNT affected predominantly large and middle sized nerves and sciatic nerve is one of the more typical location.

Clinical features. They present as a rapidly growing indolent mass of the trunk or buttocks. Radicular pain can be present in case of MPSNT arising from spinal nerves.

Prognosis. These tumors are aggressive with a high rate of recurrence and in case of truncal location and size greater than 5 cm the prognosis is usually poor. Patients with NF1 are at high risk to develop this kind of tumor.

7.1.4.1 Imaging

MR features are highly nonspecific and present similar characteristic to other soft tissue malignancies such as a sarcoma. MPNST presents as a nonhomogeneous mass with variable signal intensity and highly irregular enhancement, with frequent areas of necrosis [3].

According to some authors MR spectroscopy at 3.0 T shows the presence of TMA in higher concentration with respect to benign lesions [4]. Imaging features of MPNST are summarized in Table 7.4.

7.1.5 Cauda Equina Neuroendocrine Tumor (Previously Paraganglioma)

WHO definition. Cauda equina neuroendocrine tumor is a neuroendocrine neoplasm arising from specialized neural crest cells in the cauda equina/filum terminale region.

Epidemiology. These are very rare tumors affecting mainly adult population.

Location. Cauda equina/filum terminale.

Clinical features. Usually a common low back pain followed by paraparesis and sphincter symptoms.

Prognosis. If completely resected the prognosis is good.

7.1.5.1 Imaging

It presents as an ovalar intradural mass in the lumbar region with a hypointense signal on T1WI and a hyperintense signal on T2WI/STIR images. It is an highly vascular lesion with a strong post-contrast enhancement and an increase in CBV [5].

Hemorrhages can be present. Imaging features of cauda equina neuroendocrine tumor are summarized in Table 7.5.

7.2   Meningioma

7.2.1   Meningioma

WHO definition. Meningiomas comprise a family of neoplasms that are most likely derived from the meningothelial cells.

They are WHO grade 1 tumors, but in a small percentage also WHO grade 2 or 3 tumors.

Epidemiology. Meningiomas are the most frequent intracranial tumor in the USA accounting for more than 1/3 of all intracranial tumors (WHO 2021). Females are at greater risk to males with an incidence rate of 10.5 cases for 100.000 female population versus 4.6 cases for 100.000 male population. The lifetime risk of developing meningiomas is about 1%, the median age is around 65 years, and the risk increases with age.

Location. Meningiomas can develop wherever meningothelial cells are present and even (rarely) within the ventricles. They are located intracranially in the majority of cases, but spinal meningiomas are not infrequent, particularly in dorsal location.

Clinical features. They present as a slow growing mass and the symptomatology is related to the mass effect and to the compression of adjacent structures.

Prognosis. Prognosis is usually good for grade 1 tumors and is mainly related to the location of the tumor and consequently to its complete resectability at surgery. If completely removed, the recurrence rate is very low. Prognosis is worst in case of meningiomas grade 2 and in particular in the case of meningiomas grade 3.

From a histopathological point of view 2021 WHO CNS brain tumor classification reported 15 subtypes (Table 7.6),

The most frequent subtypes are meningothelial, fibrous, and transitional meningiomas and the majority of subtypes have a benign clinical course corresponding to grade 1. However features of a more aggressive growth can arise in any subtypes of meningiomas and the criteria of atypical or anaplastic meningiomas defining a menin-

Table 7.6 Histopathological subtypes (WHO 2021)

Meningothelial meningioma
Fibrous meningioma
Transitional meningioma
Psammomatous meningioma
Angiomatous meningioma
Microcystic meningioma
Secretory meningioma
Lymphoplasmacyte-rich meningioma
Metaplastic meningioma
Chordoid meningioma (grade 2)
Clear cell meningioma (grade 2)
Rhabdoid meningioma (grade 3)
Papillary meningioma (grade 3)
Atypical meningioma (grade 2)
Anaplastic (malignant) meningioma (grade 3)

gioma grade 2 or a meningioma grade 3, respectively, can be assigned to any meningioma subtypes.

Independently from these considerations, chordoid and clear cell meningiomas are assigned to grade 2, whereas rhabdoid and papillary meningiomas to grade 3.

7.2.1.1 Imaging

On imaging meningiomas typically present as a relatively homogeneous dural mass with a clear enhancement and frequent calcification on CT. The most typical finding on image is the so-called *dural tail sign*, a progressively thinning area of dural enhancement surrounding the meningeal mass that frequently helps in defining the origin site or the tumor (Fig. 7.11). Dural tail is however a nonspecific sign and can be encountered in other diseases [6].

On CT meningiomas appear mostly iso-hyperdense with frequent calcifications and a typical hyperostotic reaction at the level of the involved leptomeninges. Sometimes the tumor presents a growth through the meninges to the skull, invading the diploe and the cortical bone. In these cases the skull shows a diffuse sclerotic appearance and the presence of subtle spiculae at the bone surfaces (Fig. 7.12).

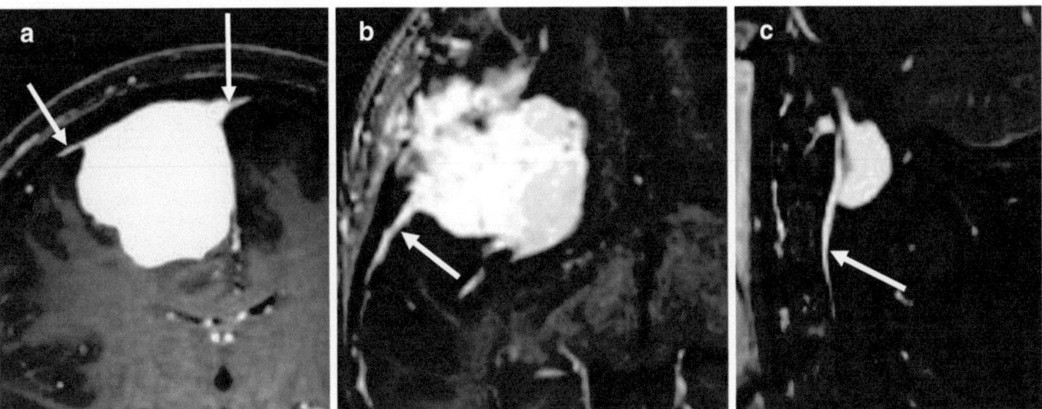

Fig. 7.11 Meningiomas. MRI post-contrast T1WI of three different meningiomas at the convexity (**a**), in the sphenoid-temporal region (**b**), and at the cervico-cranial junction (**c**). In all the cases the dural tail sign (arrow) allows to easily localize the tumor within the leptomeninges

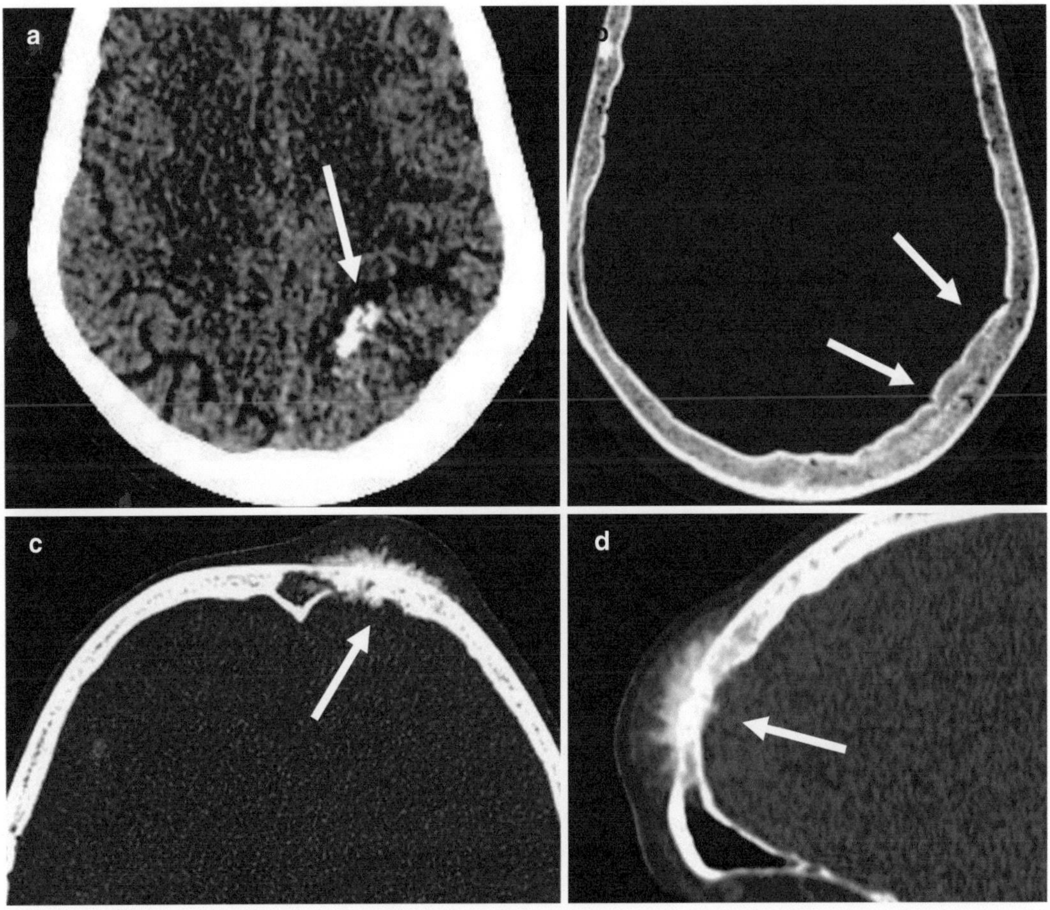

Fig. 7.12 Meningiomas. CT, two different cases: left parietal location with calcification (arrow **a**) and parietal bone sclerosis (arrows **b**), left frontal intra-osseous location with hyperostotic reaction, tiny osseous spiculae (arrow **c**, **d**), and extracranial growth

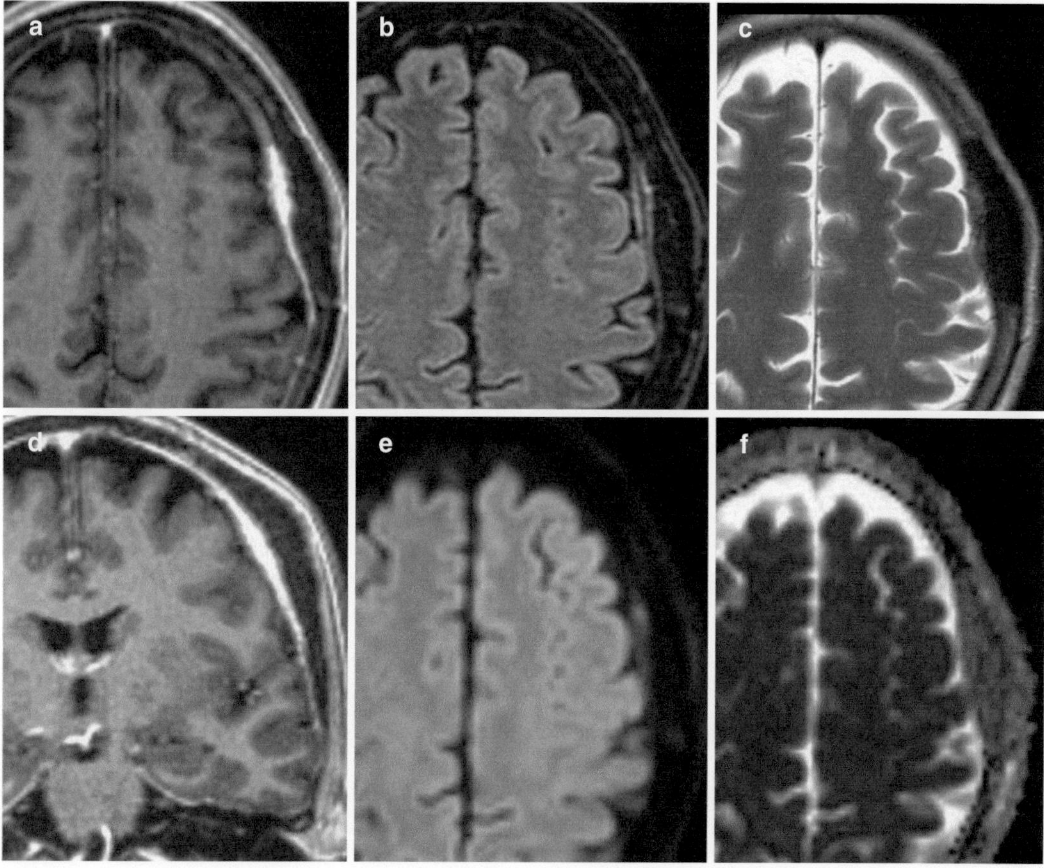

Fig. 7.13 Meningioma "en plaque." MR post-contrast T1WI (**a**, **d**) FLAIR (**b**), T2WI (**c**), DWI (**e**), ADC (**f**). The left frontal meningioma grows tangentially to the lepto-meninges, a sclerotic bone reaction is present with a thick bone directly involved by the tumor

Meningioma is defined as "en plaque" when the growth is almost only along the dural surface or "intra-osseous" when the growth is almost completely within osseous structure and eventually in the extracranial spaces (Fig. 7.13).

The hyperdensity on CT derives from both the relatively high cellularity of the tumor and to the presence of microcalcification. Microcalcification can be easily assessed on MRI by SWI sequence (Fig. 7.14).

On MRI meningioma exhibits a variable signal intensity most often isointense in all sequences, sometimes with slight hypointensity on T1WI or slight hyperintensity on FLAIR and T2WI.

The enhancement is usually strong and homogeneous, even though the presence of large calcification can cause some post-contrast heterogeneity (Figs. 7.14 and 7.15).

Perilesional edema is variable, usually scarce, but it can be extensive in case of secretory meningiomas.

Diffusion. On diffusion meningioma is quite similar to normal gray matter diffusion.

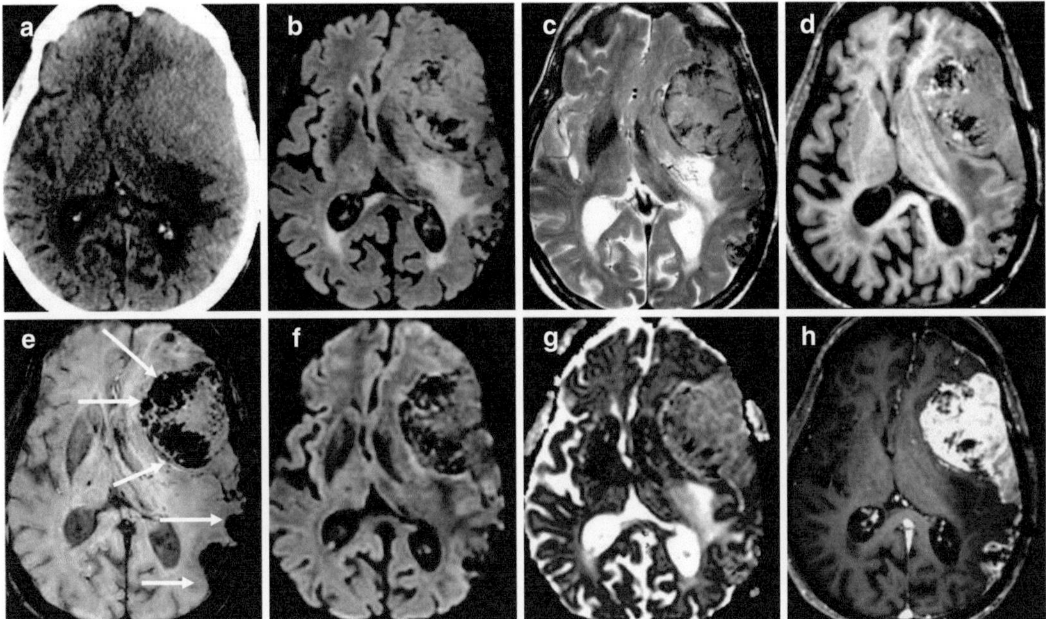

Fig. 7.14 Meningioma. CT (**a**), MRI T1WI (**b**), FLAIR (**c**), T2WI (**d**), SWI (**e**), post-contrast T1WI (**f**), DWI (**g**), ADC (**h**). A large left fronto-temporoparietal meningioma with diffuse microcalcifications easily detectable on SWI sequence (arrows **e**). Perilesional edema is visible only in the posterior part of the lesion

Spectroscopy. Spectroscopy shows the absence of NAA, low Cr, and a Cho increase with a typical lipid peak (Figs. 7.15 and 7.16).

Perfusion. MR perfusion shows an increase in both CBV and CBF (Fig. 7.16).

In the current state of knowledge, there are no valid criteria for identifying the potentially more aggressive histological meningiomas variants or in any case predicting a less favorable course in terms of tumor growth rate or its recurrence. A possible help could come from radiomics techniques even if at present we do not yet have concrete results in this regard [7, 8].

In the diagnosis of meningioma it is most important to define the exact location of the tumor being strictly related to the prognosis. The relationship with great venous sinuses should be carefully evaluated in order to rule out any possible invasion from the tumor. The superior sagittal sinus is frequently involved due to the proximity of the falx and of the dura of the cranial vault a region where meningiomas are typically located. The cavernous sinus is another typical location of intracranial meningiomas. In this case a cavernous sinus syndrome can progressively become evident with a reduction of the internal carotid artery caliber in its intracavernous course (Fig. 7.17) [9].

Cavernous sinus may be involved also by meningioma arising from the tuberculum sellae and from the dura of the sellar diaphragm. In the case of large lesion, almost partly extending into the sellar fossa, meningiomas have to be differentiated from macroadenomas. In the majority of cases the compressed pituitary gland is still differentiable from the neoplasm, but most important the dural tail sign of the meningioma is usually present (Fig. 7.18).

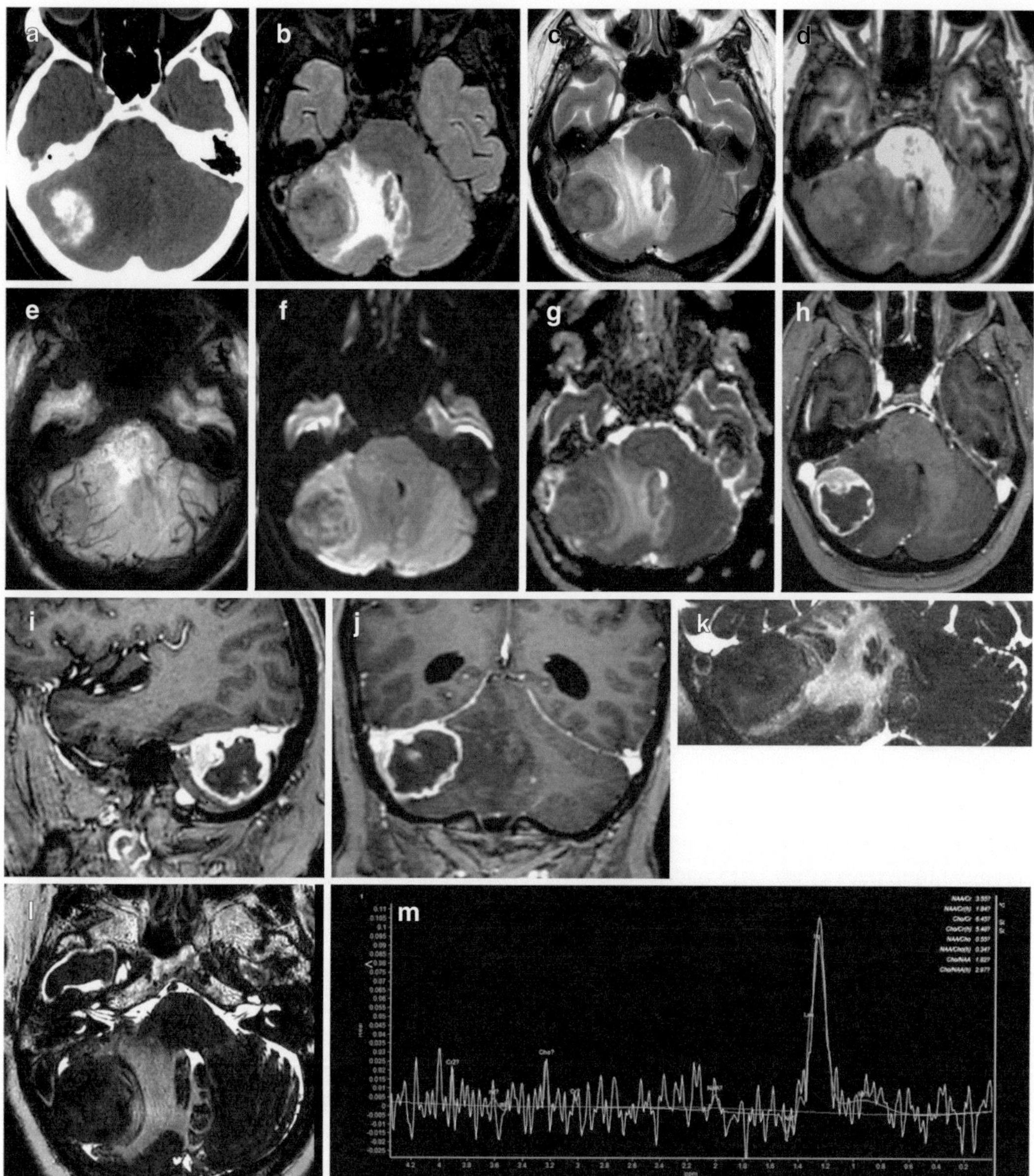

Fig. 7.15 Fibrous meningioma. CT (**a**). MRI FLAIR (**b**), T2WI (**c**), T1WI (**d**), SWI (**e**), DWI (**f**), ADC (**g**), post-contrast T1WI (**h, i, j**), bSSFP (**k, l**), spectroscopy (**m**). Posterior fossa fibrous meningioma, with extensive mass effect and perilesional edema. These aspects together with an unusual peripheral enhancement make the diagnosis challenging. Even with high resolution bSSFP images are difficult to exclude a direct cerebellar involvement of the tumor. Spectroscopy exhibits only a solitary huge lipids peak

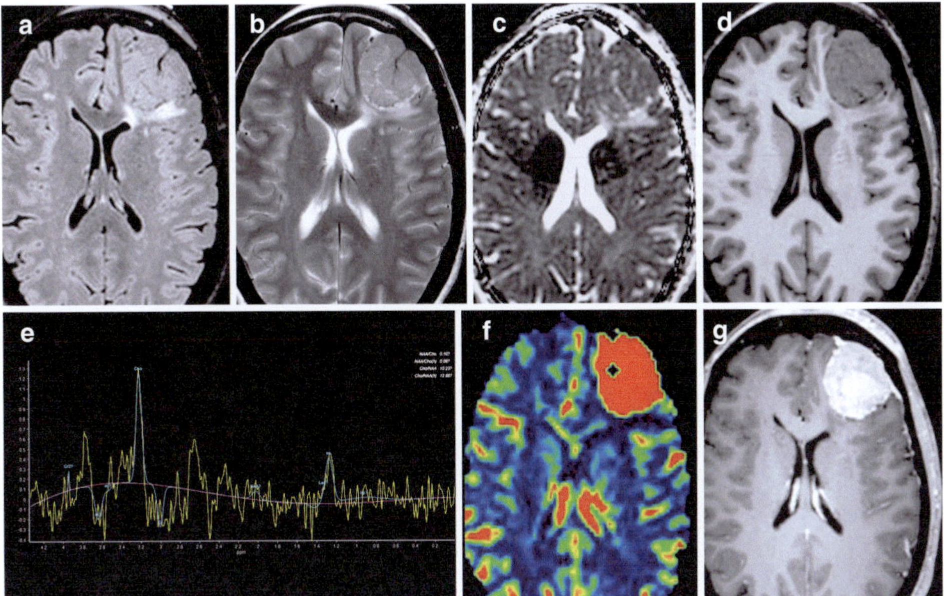

Fig. 7.16 Meningioma. MRI FLAIR (**a**), T2WI (**b**), ADC (**c**), T1WI (**d**), spectroscopy TE 144 (E), CBV (**f**), post-contrast T1WI (**g**). This left frontal meningioma shows a substantial isointensity in all pre-contrast sequences (**a–d**). A striking enhancement (**g**) and CBV (**f**) increase is evident after contrast injection. Spectroscopy reveals the absence of NAA, the relative increase of Cho, and the presence of a lipid peak

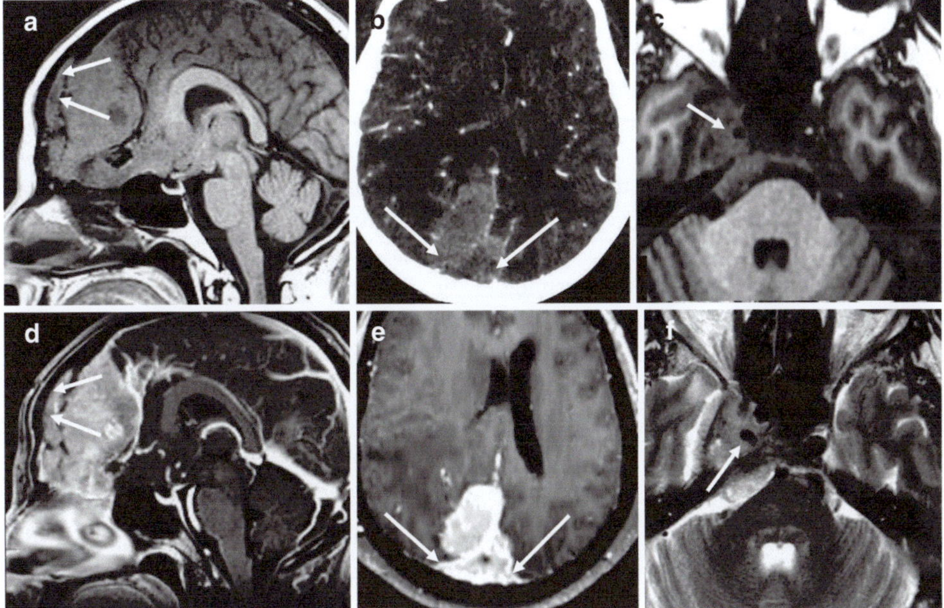

Fig. 7.17 Meningiomas, venous sinuses invasion. Case 1 (**a, d**), superior sagittal invasion, MRI T1WI (**a**), and post-contrast T1WI (**d**). A huge frontal meningioma extensively involves the anterior part of the superior sagittal sinus (arrows). Case 2 (**b, e**), superior sagittal sinus invasion, post-contrast CT (**b**), MRI post-contrast T1WI (**e**). In this case the meningioma involves the postero-inferior part of the superior sagittal sinus close to the torcular region (arrows). Case 3 (**c, f**), cavernous sinus invasion, MRI T1WI (**c**), T2WI (**f**). The meningioma occupies the right cavernous sinus, extending laterally through the middle cranial fossa and posteriorly through the petrous apex. The vessel diameter of the right internal carotid is reduced (arrows)

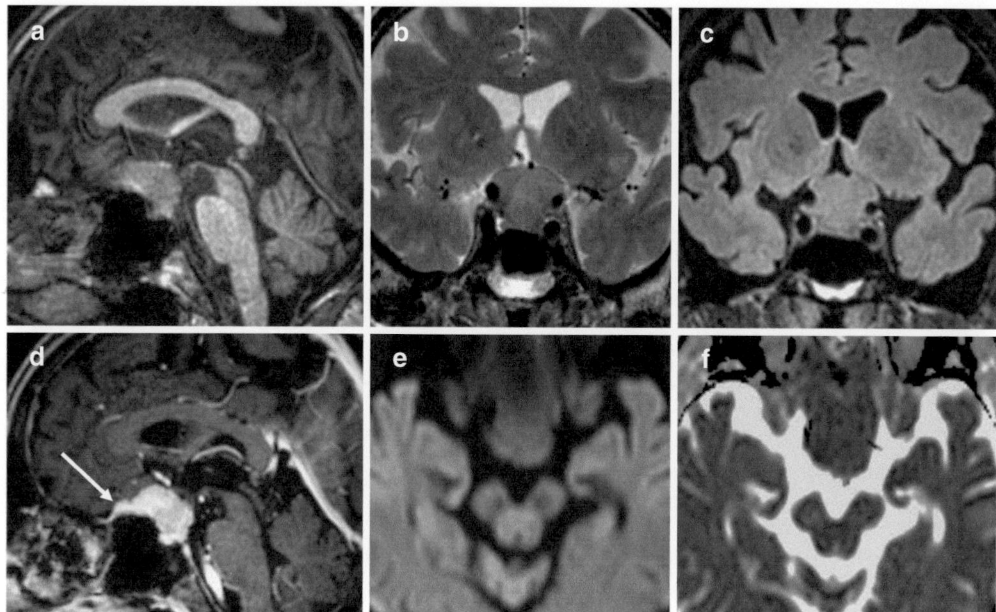

Fig. 7.18 Meningioma of the tuberculum sellae. MRI T1WI (**a**), T2WI (**b**), FLAIR (**c**), post-contrast T1WI, DWI (**e**), ADC (**f**). Meningiomas of the tuberculum sellae are most easily to evaluate in sagittal section where their relationship with dura and dural tail (arrow **d**) is clearly appreciable. On coronal (**b**, **c**) and axial (**e**, **f**) sections the differentiation with a pituitary gland macroadenoma can be more difficult even though in the coronal sections the normal pituitary gland is usually demonstrable

Cranio-cervical junction is a particularly critical region due to confounding symptomatology and to the difficulty to recognize a meningioma of this site on a routine basal CT scan of the head (Figs. 7.19 and 7.20). Lesions at this level can reach large size before to be diagnosed.

Rarely meningioma can also originate within the ventricles, most likely from meningothelial inclusion bodies located in the tela choroidea or in the choroid plexuses. The typical location is in the region of the choroid plexus of the lateral ventricles (Fig. 7.21).

Meningiomas can arise also along the optic nerve sheath, MRI axial or sagittal sections reveal a typical tram-like enhancing lesion around the involved nerve, or a concentric enhancing lesion in the coronal section. In the pre-contrast scan the lesion can be difficult to disclose (Fig. 7.22).

Spinal meningiomas are relatively rare in comparison to the intracranial compartment accounting for approximately 1.2% of all meningiomas of the central nervous system. In a review of 131 operated cases, the mean age was 69 years. Thoracic location results in the most frequent (73%) followed by cervical (16%) and cervicothoracic (5%). The dural attachment of the spinal meningioma was predominantly localized laterally or ventrolaterally (Fig. 7.23) [10]. Imagin features of meningioma are summarized in Table 7.7.

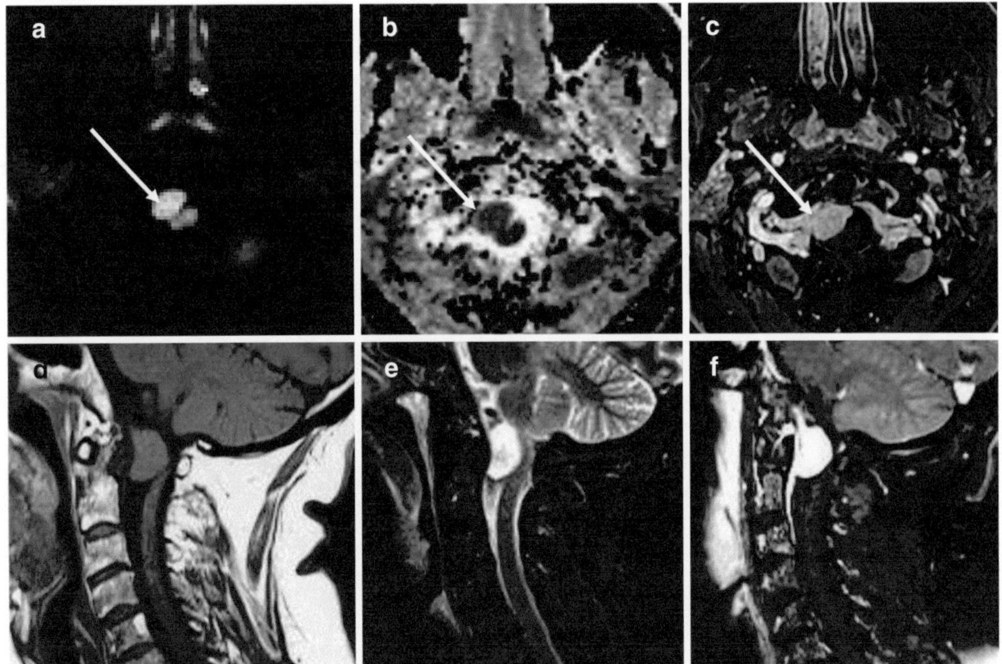

Fig. 7.19 Meningioma of the cranio-cervical junction. MRI DWI (**a**), ADC (**b**), post-contrast T1WI (**c, f**), T1WI (**d**), T2WI (**e**). The tumor arises from the dura covering the tip of the dens and tectorial membrane laterally (arrows A-C). A slight mass effect on the spinal cord is evident

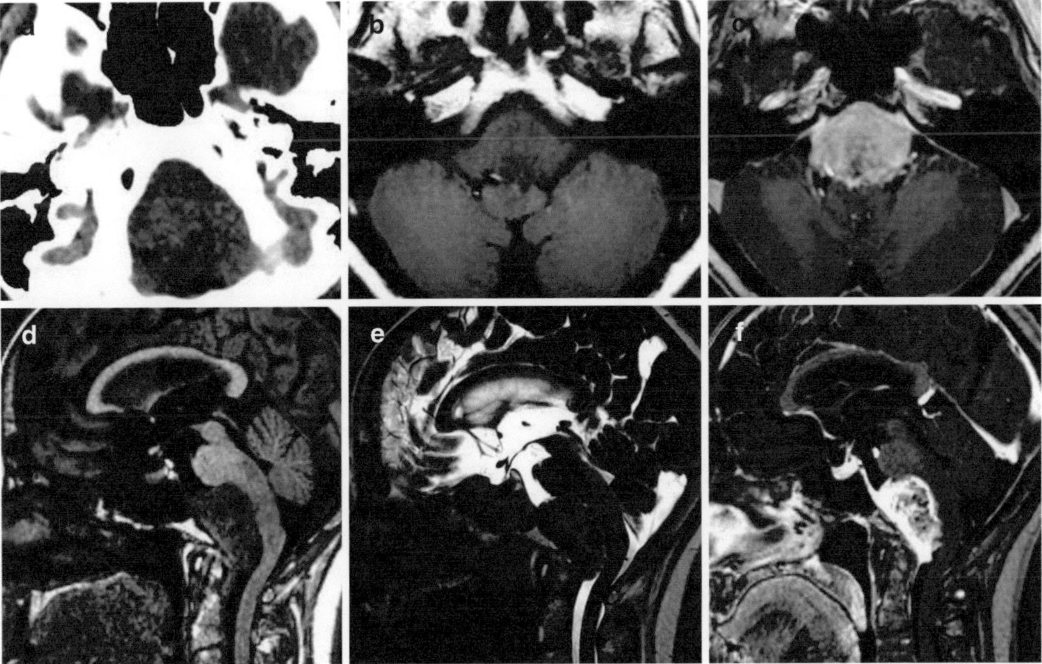

Fig. 7.20 Meningioma of the cranio-cervical junction. Basal CT (**a**), MRI T1WI (**b, d**), post-contrast T1WI (**c, f**), bSSFP (**e**). A large cranio-cervical neoplasm extending superiorly along the clivus is visible, with a huge mass effect on brainstem. On basal CT study it is difficult to differentiate the tumor from the brainstem, sagittal MR sections are mandatory in order to fully identify the tumor and its relationship with dural sheats

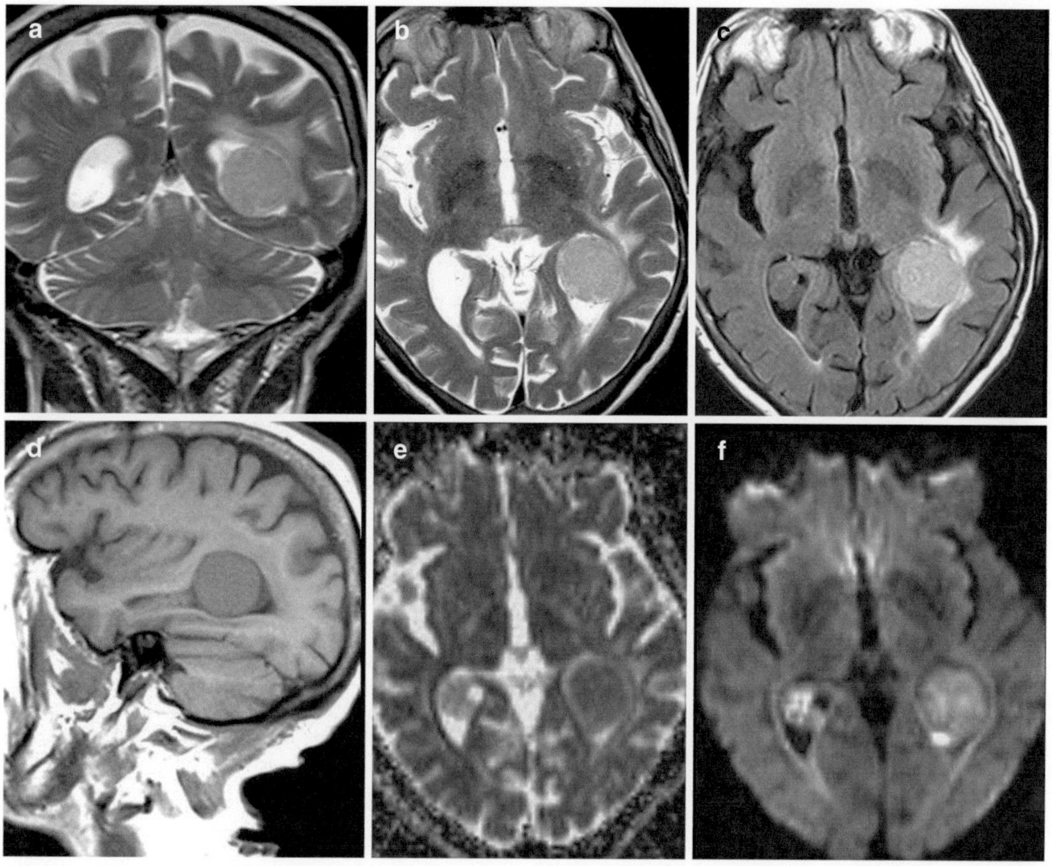

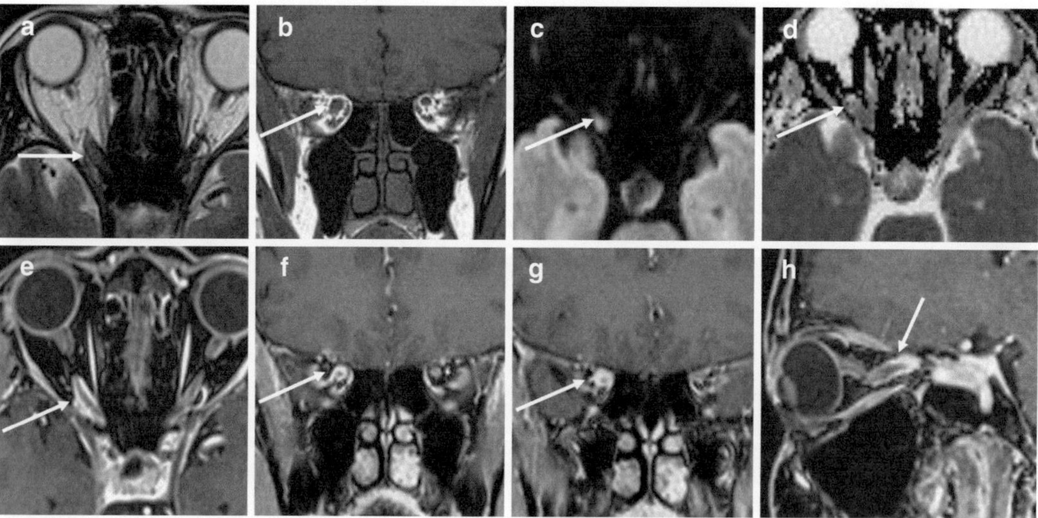

Fig. 7.21 Intraventricular meningioma. MRI T2WI (**a**, **b**), FLAIR (**c**), T1WI (**d**), ADC (**e**), DWI (F). A round large meningioma is visible within the trigonal region of the left lateral ventricle in the location of the choroid plexus. There is a slight mass effect with edema in the surrounding brain structures, however ventricular size is normal

Fig. 7.22 Meningioma of the optic nerve sheath. MRI T2WI (**a**), T1WI (**b**), DWI (**c**), ADC (D), post-contrast T1WI (**e–h**). The tumor arises from the left optic nerve sheath in the region of orbital apex (arrows). The post-contrast T1W images allow to demonstrate the location of the tumor externally to the proper optic nerve

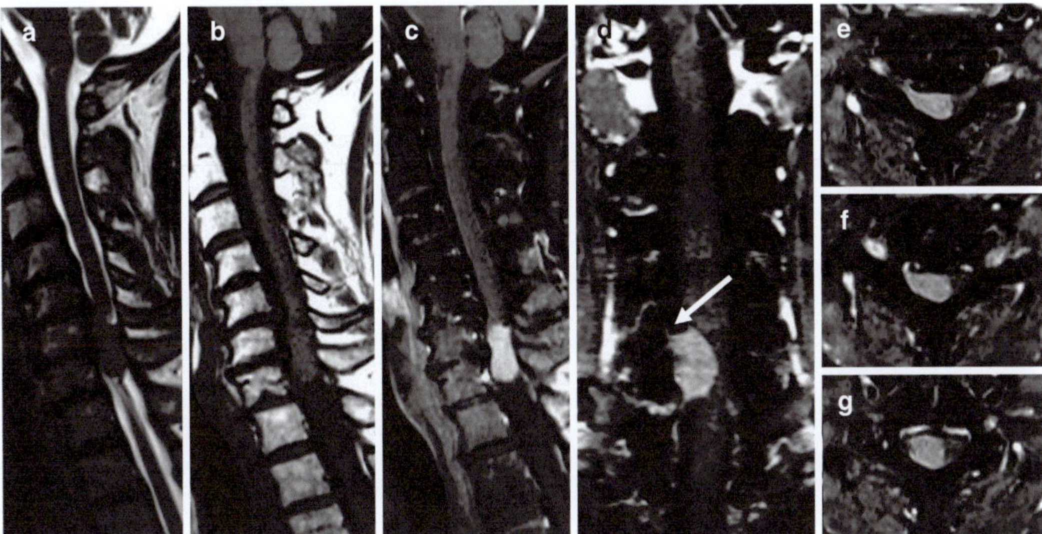

Fig. 7.23 Meningioma of the cervical spine. MRI T2WI (**a**), T1WI (**b**), post-contrast T1WI (**c–g**). The tumor arises from postero later aspect of the cervical dura with a marked mass effect on the spinal cord. The MRI features are nonspecific and the main differential diagnosis is usually with neurinoma, the presence of a dural tail, as it is visible in this case in the coronal section (arrow **d**), may help in the diagnosis

Table 7.7 Meninigioma imaging chracteristics

Mass effect	Edema	Inhomogeneity	Cysts	Necrosis	Hemorrhage	Calcifications
+/+++	0/+++	0/++	0/++	0	0	+/+++

CT	T1	T2	FLAIR	DWI	ADC	T1 Gd	CBV	Spec
⬤	◯	⬤	◯	◯	⬤	+/+++	⬤	↑↑lipids,↑Cho ↓↓Naa

References

1. Khaled M, Moghazy K, Elsaadany W, Eissa L. Additional diagnostic role of MRI spectroscopy, diffusion and susceptibility imaging in differentiation of CPA masses: our experience with emphasis on schwannomas and meningiomas. Egypt J Radiol Nucl Med. 2020;51:137.
2. Lim R, Jaramillo D, Young Poussaint T, Chang Y, Korf B. Superficial Neurofibroma: a lesion with unique MRI characteristics in patients with neurofibromatosis type 1. AJR. 2005;184:962–8.
3. Liu J, Huang JN, Wang MH, et al. Image based differentiation of benign and malignant peripheral nerve sheath tumors in neurofibromatosis type 1. Front Oncol. 2022;12:898971.
4. Fayad LM, Wang X, Blakeley JO, et al. Characterization of peripheral nerve sheath tumors with 3T proton MR spectroscopy. AJNR Am J Neuroradiol. 2014;35:1035–41.
5. Méndez JC, Carrasco R, Prieto MA, Fandiño E, Blázquez J. Paraganglioma of the cauda equina: MR and angiographic findings. Radiol Case Rep. 2019;14:1185–7.
6. Sotoudeh H, Yazdi HR. A review on dural tail sign world. J Radiol. 2010;2:188–92.
7. Gu H, Zhang X, di Russo P, Zhao XT. The current state of radiomics for meningiomas: promises and challenges. Front Oncol. 2020;10:567736.
8. Ugga L, Pinto SGL, Cuocolo R, Brunetti A. Meningioma Radiomics: at the nexus of imaging, pathology and biomolecular characterization. Cancers. 2022;14:2605.
9. Vachhrajani S, Jea A, Rutka JA, Blaser S, Cusimano M, Rutka JT. Meningioma with dural venous sinus invasion and jugular vein extension. J Neurosurg Pediatr. 2008;6:391–6.
10. Sandalcioglu IE, Hunold A, Muller O, Bassiouni H, Stolke D, Asgari S. Spinal meningiomas: critical review of 131 surgically treated patients. Eur Spine J. 2008;17:1035–41.

Mesenchymal, Nonmeningothelial Tumors Involving the CNS. Melanocytic Tumors

8.1 Mesenchymal, Nonmenigothelial Tumors Involving the CNS

The histological features of mesenchymal tumors affecting the CNS are quite similar to those of the corresponding extracranial soft tissue and bone tumors. They range from benign neoplasm corresponding to grade 1 WHO to extremely aggressive sarcomas corresponding to grade 4 WHO.

Mesenchymal nonmeningiomatous tumors are very rare accounting for no more than 0.1–0.2% of all intracranial tumors. Even rare they are quite numerous and the 2021 WHO classification subdivided them into six different categories (Table 8.1).

Table 8.1 Mesenchymal nonmeningiomatous tumors categories according to 2021 WHO classification of brain tumors

1. Fibroblastic and myofibroblastic tumors
2. Vascular tumors
3. Skeletal muscle tumors
4. Tumors of uncertain differentiation
5. Chondrogenic tumors
6. Notochordal tumors

8.2 Fibroblastic and Myofibroblastic Tumors

8.2.1 Solitary Fibrous Tumor

Definition. Solitary fibrous tumor (SFT) is a fibroblastic tumor with a genomic inversion at the 12q13 locus, leading to *NAB2* and *STAT6* gene fusion as well as STAT6 nuclear expression. This gene fusion is present in most cases regardless of the histological grading.

This tumor corresponds to the hemangiopericytoma or solitary fibrous tumor/hemangiopericytoma of the previous classifications.

The WHO grade ranges from 1 to 3.

Epidemiology. It is a rare tumor and due to the previous ambiguous nomenclature no clear epidemiological data are at present available. In the largest series this tumor occurred between the fifth and seventh decade of life without any sex prevalence.

Location. SFTs are usually located within the dura, and falcine, parasagittal. And skull base area are the most frequent locations. About 10% arises in the dura of the spine.

Clinical features. Signs and symptoms vary by location, they can reach large dimensions

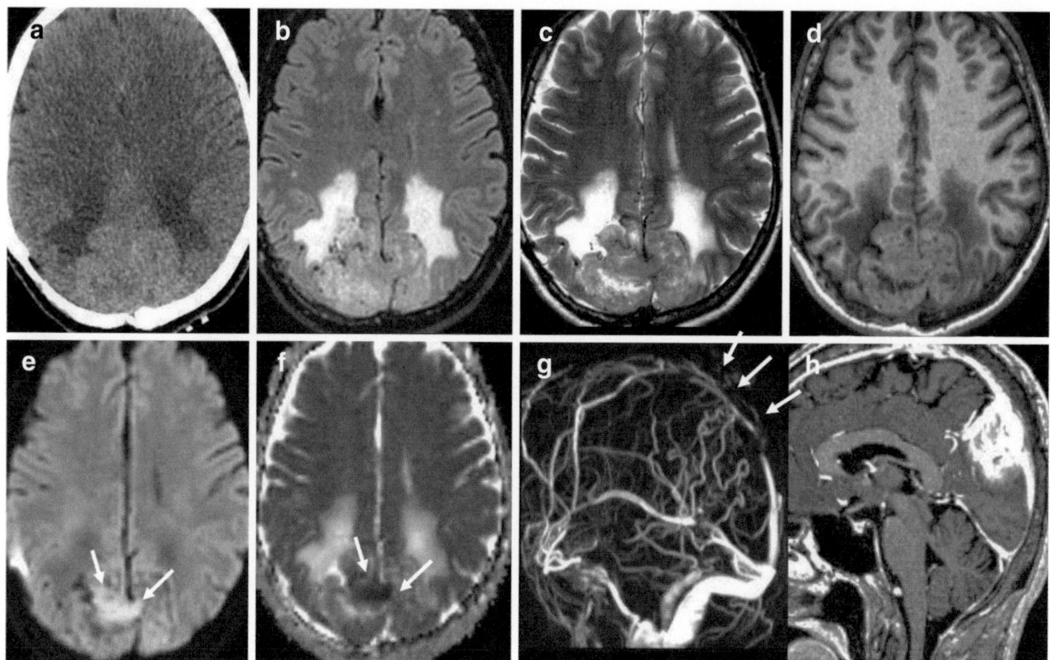

Fig. 8.1 SFT, posterior falcine recurrence in a 60-year-old man, 10 years after surgery of the first tumor. CT (**a**). MRI FLAIR (**b**), T2WI (**c**), T1WI (**d**), DWI (**e**), ADC (**f**), 3D PC angio (**g**), post-contrast T1WI (**h**). A huge heterogeneous tumor slightly hyperdense on CT (A) and with vascular flow voids on MR (**b**, **c**) is visible across the posterior falx with invasion of the superior sagittal sinus (**g**, **h** arrows). The contrast enhancement is heterogeneous and an area of decreased diffusion is visible in the central part of the tumor (arrows **e**, **f**)

without any symptoms, so that intracranial hypertension is often the first clinical evidence of the neoplasm.

Prognosis. The prognosis is primarily related on tumor grading and location. Even though apparently completed resected SFT has typically a high rate of recurrence (Fig. 8.1), and it is one of the few intracranial neoplasms associated with extracranial metastases (Fig. 8.2). The most common sites of metastases are bone, lung and pleura, liver, and vertebrae.

Higher primary tumor grade is associated with an increased risk of extracranial metastases [1].

8.2.1.1 Imaging

SFT has to be differentiated firstly from a common meningioma.

SFT is traditionally described as a well-defined, usually round like mass on CT and MRI. On MR T1WI SFTs are iso- or hypointense, whereas on T2WI and FLAIR most of the SFTs are predominantly isointense. Prominent internal vessel void can be evident.

Contrast enhancement is always present, and it can be both homogeneous and heterogeneous. A dural tail is reported in the majority of SFTs and something around ¼ of case may show peritumoral edema. As a matter of fact a differential diagnosis with a classic meningioma is frequently impossible[2, 3].

The mean of minimum ADC of SFTs has been reported as significantly higher than the mean of minimum ADC of meningiomas (Figs. 8.1 and 8.2) [4] but areas of decreased ADC can be detected also in SFTs (Fig. 8.1).

Report on spectroscopy and perfusion is scarce; however, an increase of CBV has been reported on spectroscopy and an increase of lipid, lactate, and myoinositol peaks has been reported on spectroscopy studies. Imaging features of SFT are summarized in Table 8.2.

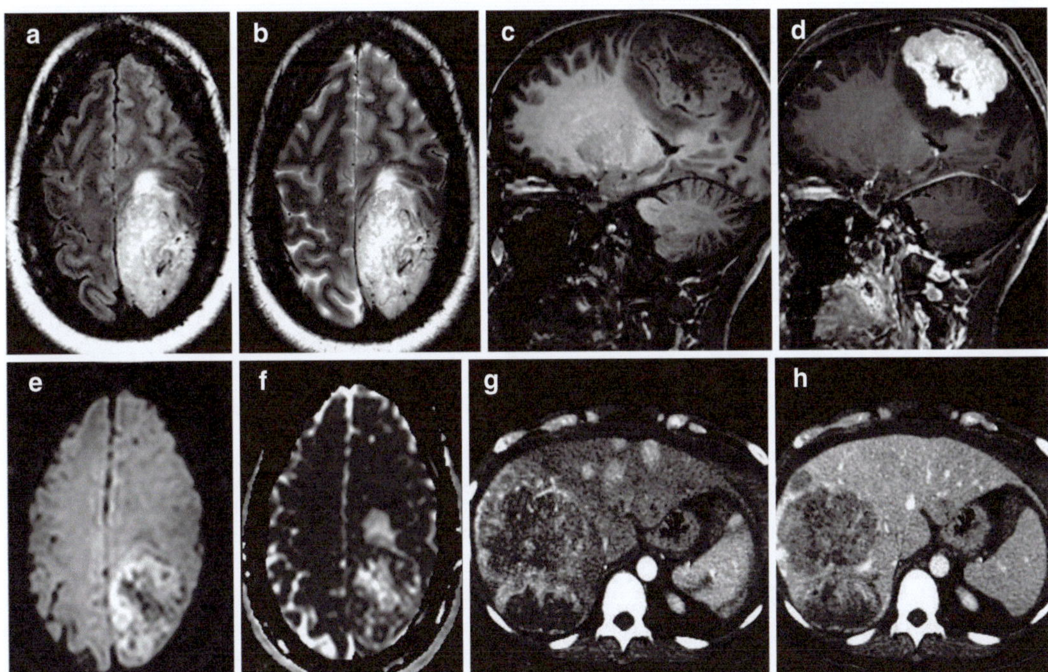

Fig. 8.2 SFT, left parasagittal parietal huge tumor in a 45-year-old female with secondary metastases on the liver. MRI FLAIR (**a**), T2WI (**b**), T1WI (**c**), post-contrast T1WI (**d**), DWI (**e**), ADC (**f**). CT of the abdomen, post-contrast arterial phase (**g**), post-contrast venous phase (**h**). SFT shows the typical heterogeneous aspect with flow voids (**a–f**). It was apparently completely resected and a diagnosis of WHO grade 3 was made, 3 years later a large liver metastases was diagnosed (**g, h**)

Table 8.2 SFT imaging features

Mass effect	Edema	Inhomogeneity	Cysts	Necrosis	Hemorrhage	Calcifications
+/+++	0/++	+/+++	0/+	0/+	0/+	0/++

CT	T1	T2	FLAIR	DWI	ADC	T1 Gd	CBV	Spec
⬤	⬤	⬤	⬤	⬤	⬤	++/+++	🟠	↑Lipids, lactate, myoinositol

8.3 Vascular Tumors

8.3.1 Hemangioma and Vascular Malformations

(a) Hemangioma is a benign neoplastic vascular lesion with multiple tightly packed capillary sized and cavernous vessels that can be isolated, multiple or part of an overgrowth syndrome.

It is extremely frequent and typically located in the spine and less frequently in the skull.

It is usually asymptomatic, but in rare case they can present a more aggressive behavior leading to vertebral fracture and/or spinal cord compression.

IMAGING. On CT it presents the typical honeycomb appearance with thickened trabeculae, on MR it is usually hyperintense on both T1 and T2 weighted images (Fig. 8.3);

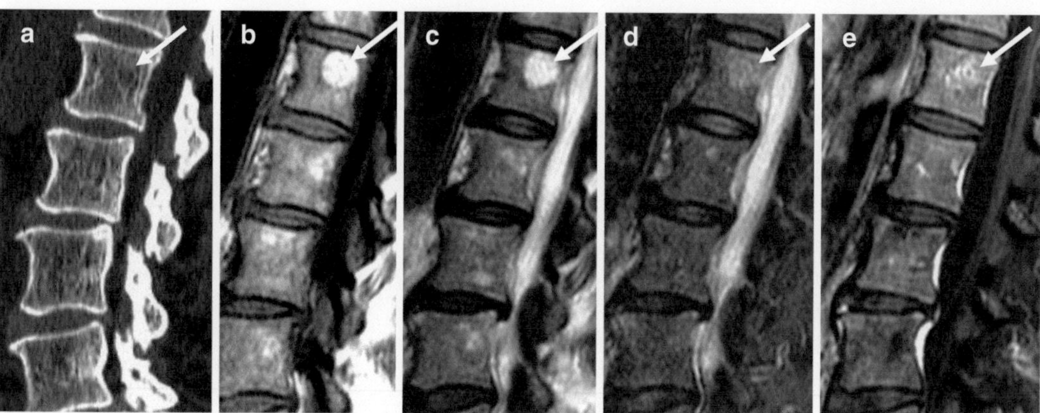

Fig. 8.3 Spinal hemangioma. CT (**a**), MRI T1WI (**b**), T2WI (**c**), STIR (**d**), post-contrast T1WI (**e**). A spinal hemangioma of L1 vertebral body is visible as hyperintense lesion on both T1WI and T2WI sequences (arrows **b** and **c**). A slight hyperintensity is visible also on STIR sequence (**d**) and mild enhancement is visible after contrast administration (**e**). A minimal trabecular appearance of hemangioma is seen on CT image (**a**)

however, some hemangiomas may be hypointense on T1WI and hyperintense on STIR with some problem in differential diagnosis with other more aggressive lesions.

(b) Cavernous malformations (CMs) are angiografically occult solitary or multifocal vascular anomalies characterized by multiple tightly packed sinusoidal vessels with fibrotic walls lacking arterial or venous features. Multiple CMs are associated usually with familial syndromes with mutations in *KRIT1* (CCM1), *CCM2*, or *PDC10* (CCM3).

They can be present everywhere within the CNS, but prefer the supratentorial structures. Clinical features are related to seizures or less frequently to an acute hemorrhage.

IMAGING. On CT CMs present with calcifications, whereas on MRI they show a quite typical appearance with mixed signal intensity in the central portion and a hemosiderin rim of different sizes well evident on T2* GRE or SWI sequences (Fig. 8.4).

(c) Cerebral arteriovenous malformation (AVM) is a fast-flow vascular anomaly consisting of arteriovenous connections through a nidus or fistula of malformed instead of arteries and veins instead of a normal capillary bed.

AVMs can involve cortical or deep regions of the brain or meninges.

IMAGING. On CT they can present calcification and the malformed vessels and nidus strongly enhanced after contrast administra-tion. The diagnosis should be made with an angiographic study and MRI could be helpful in determining the presence of perimalformative brain damage (Fig. 8.5).

(d) Capillary telangiectasia is an aggregation of individually dispersed dilated capillary-type vessels with interposed normal brain parenchyma.

They can be found everywhere within the CNS, but are typically present in the pons.

IMAGING. Before contrast they can be detected only on SWI sequence, after contrast they present a slight enhancement (Fig. 8.6).

8.3.2 Hemangioblastoma

Definition. Hemangioblastoma is a highly vascular tumor containing neoplastic stromal cells that have clear to vacuolated cytoplasm and characteristic immunoistochemical features and molecular findings.

It is a WHO grade 1 neoplasm.

This tumor occurs in approximately 30% of cases in association with Von Hippel Lindau (VHL) syndrome and in the remaining cases as sporadic forms.

Epidemiology. VHL syndrome is an autosomal dominant disorder with an annual incidence of 1 case per 40.000 populations, caused by a germlike mutation of the VHL tumor suppressor gene located in chromosome 3p 25–26. VHL is

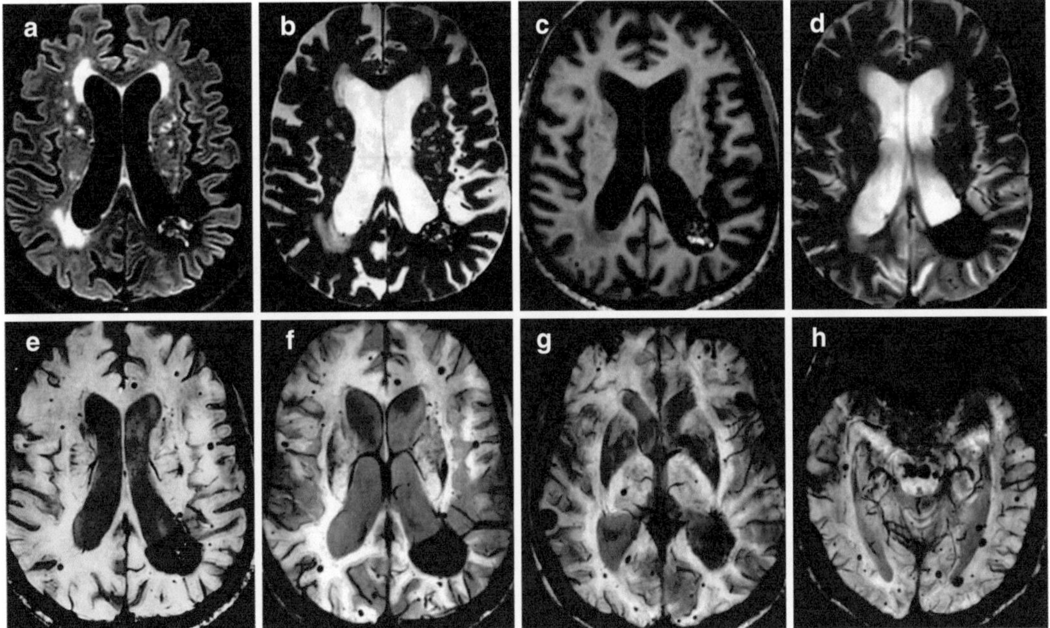

Fig. 8.4 Multiple cavernous hemangiomas in a patient with familial syndrome. MRI FLAIR (**a**), T2WI (**b**), T1WI (**c**), T2*GRE (**d**), SWI (**e**), SWI MinIP (**f–h**). A large hemangioma is visible in left peritrigonal white matter with some central hyperintense component on FLAIR and T1WI. On SWI and particularly on MinIP SWI reconstruction many tiny hypointense spots are visible, familial cases can present with a miliariform diffusion of hundreds of this vascular anomaly

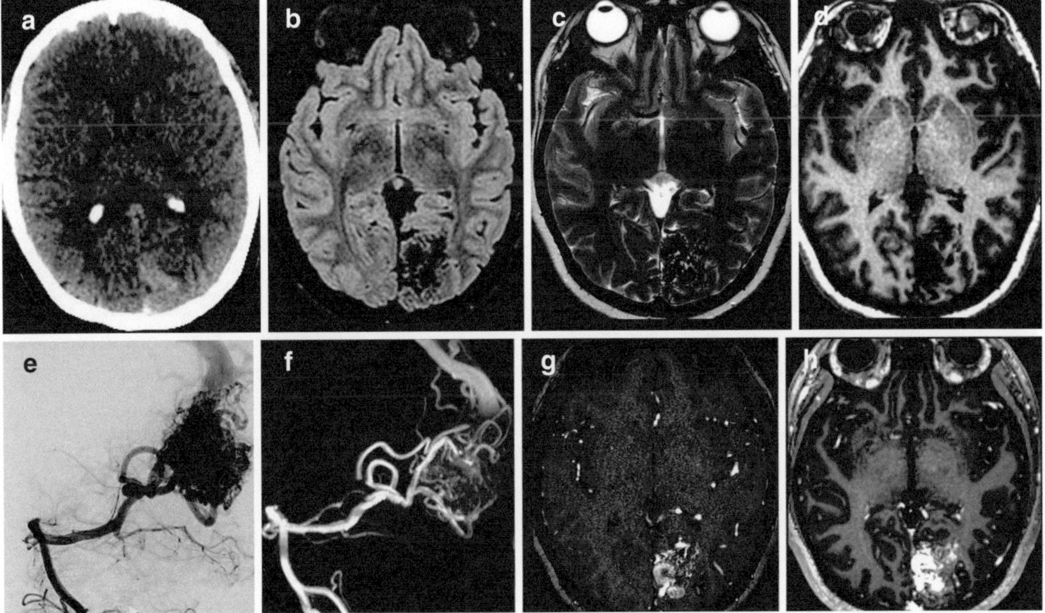

Fig. 8.5 Cerebral arteriovenous malformation. CT (**a**), MRI FLAIR (**b**), T2WI (**c**), T1WI (**d**), DSA (**e**), MR angio (**f**), partition of MR angio (**g**), post-contrast T1WI (**h**). A huge arteriovenous malformation is visible in the mesial aspect of left occipital lobe. The typical appearance of the AVM nidus with multiple irregular flow voids that enhance after contrast is visible on MR sequences (**b–d**, **h**). The anatomy of the AVM is well depicted on MR angio both in the single partition and in the MIP reconstruction; however, DSA study is mandatory to obtain a complete evaluation of arterial feeders and venous afferents

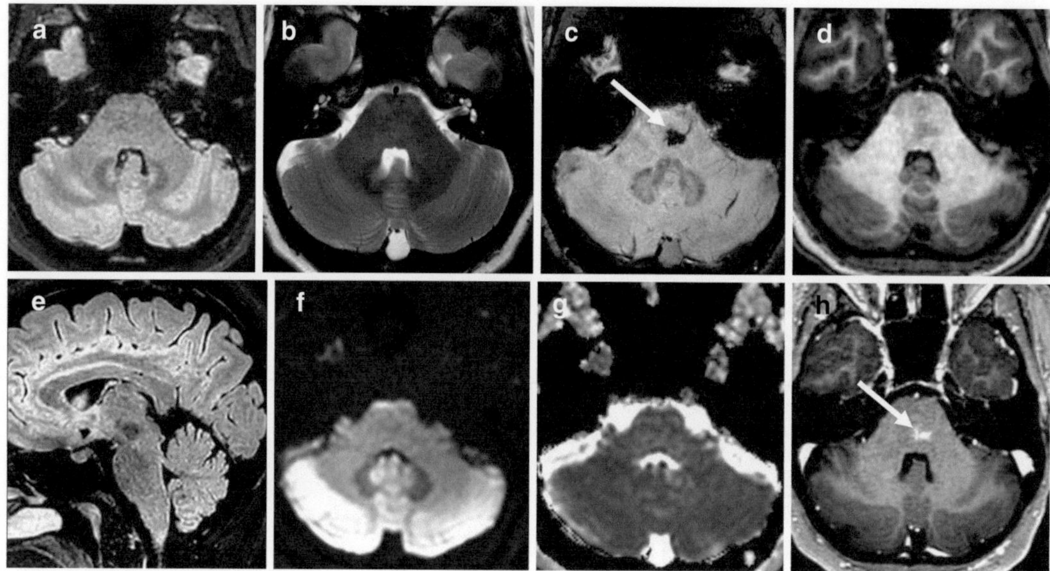

Fig. 8.6 Capillary teleangectasia. MRI FLAIR (**a**, **e**), T2WI (**b**), SWI (**c**), T1WI (**d**), DWI (**f**), ADC (**g**), post-contrast T1WI (**h**). A capillary teleangectasia in the typical pontine location. Before contrast administration it can be found only on SWI (arrow **c**) or on T2*GRE sequences, after contrast administration a mild enhancement is usually present (arrow **h**)

associated with haemangioblastomas of the brain and of the retina, endolymphatic sac cystic tumor of the ear, clear renal cell carcinoma, pheochromocytoma of the adrenal gland, and neuroendocrine islet cell pancreatic tumor.

The mean age of HB occurrence in VHL patients is around 30 years of age, from 10 to 20 years before the occurrence in sporadic forms.

Location. These tumors are typically located within the posterior fossa and the cerebellum is the more frequent location in particular in patients with sporadic forms. Patients with VHL showed frequently multiple HBs not only in cerebellum but also in the cervico-medullary junction or along the spinal cord. Supratentorial location is more rare.

Clinical features. Signs and symptoms vary according to location and to the presence of other manifestations of the syndrome in patients with VHL syndrome.

Prognosis. Loss of function of the VHL onco-suppressor gene is the central event in HB formation both in patients with VHL syndrome and in patients with sporadic forms. Patients with sporadic forms exhibit a good prognosis with no recurrence after surgical removal of the tumor. The prognosis is less favorble in VHL patients mostly due to the presence of multiple CNS tumors but also due to the presence of other extra CNS tumors.

8.3.2.1 Imaging

Hemangioblastoma presents typical features on both CT and MRI characterized by a mural nodule deeply enhancing after contrast media injection and a non-enhancing cyst of variable sizes. Mural nodule can be homogeneous or heterogeneous on both basal images and after contrast administration, it is iso-hyperdense on CT, slightly hyperintense on T2/FLAIR images, iso-hypointense on T1 weighted images (Figs. 8.7 and 8.8).

Diffusion, spectroscopy. Diffusion is increased (Figs. 8.7 and 8.8), whereas reports on spectroscopy are scarce, an almost absent NAA is reported together with the possible presence of a lipid peak.

Perfusion. Perfusion is increased (Fig. 8.8).

Being cerebellum the most frequent location a differential diagnosis with pilocytic astrocytoma must be considered in more young patients (Fig. 8.9). In pilocytic astrocytoma the satellite cysts can enhance or not after contrast administration, whereas in hemangioblastoma they do not. A more confident differential diagnosis can be however achieved by angiography that shows a striking tumor blush (Figs. 8.10 and 8.11).

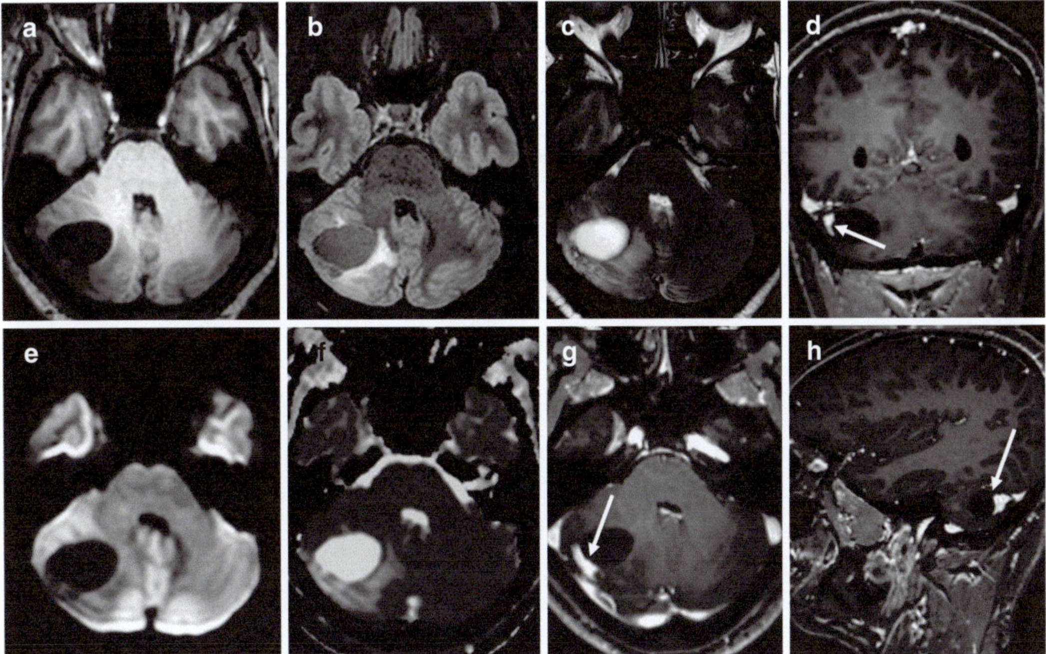

Fig. 8.7 Cerebellar hemangioblastoma in patient without Von Hippel Lindau syndrome. MRI T1WI (**a**), FLAIR (**b**), T2WI (**c**), post-contrast T!WI (**d, g, h**), DWI (**e**), ADC (**f**). The small deeply enhancing mural nodule is clearly visible after contrast administration (arrows **d, g, h**)

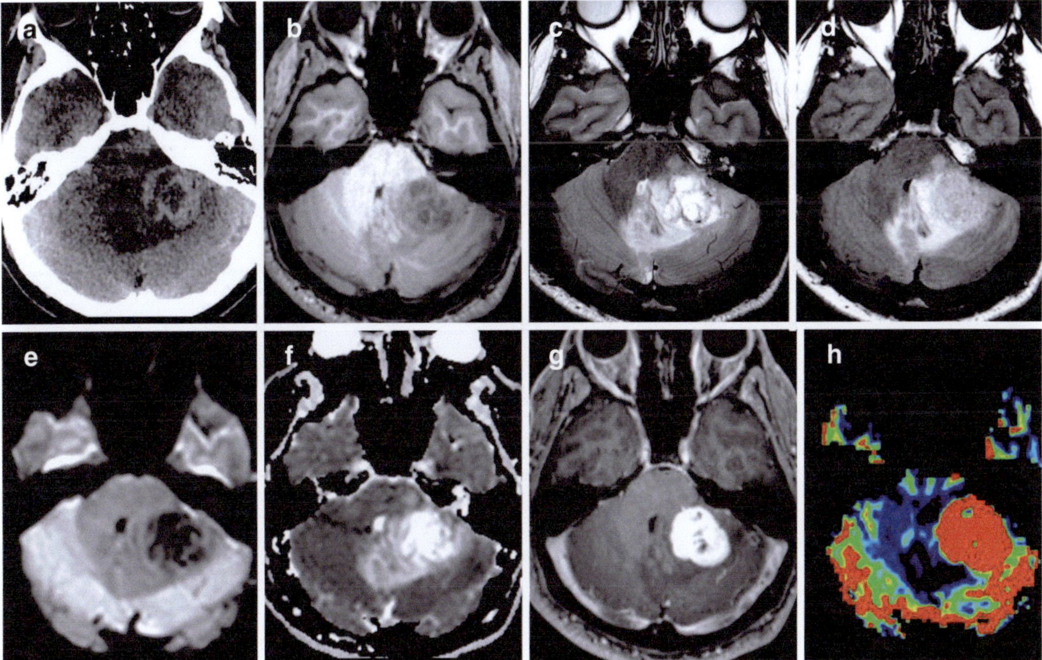

Fig. 8.8 Cerebellar haemangioblastoma. CT (**a**). MRI T1WI (**b**), T2WI (**c**), FLAIR (**d**), DWI (**e**), ADC (**f**), post-contrast T1WI (**g**), CBV (**h**). The satellite cyst is not clearly evident and the nodule is heterogeneous with strong enhancement and high CBV; however, hemangioblastoma is a WHO grade 1 tumor

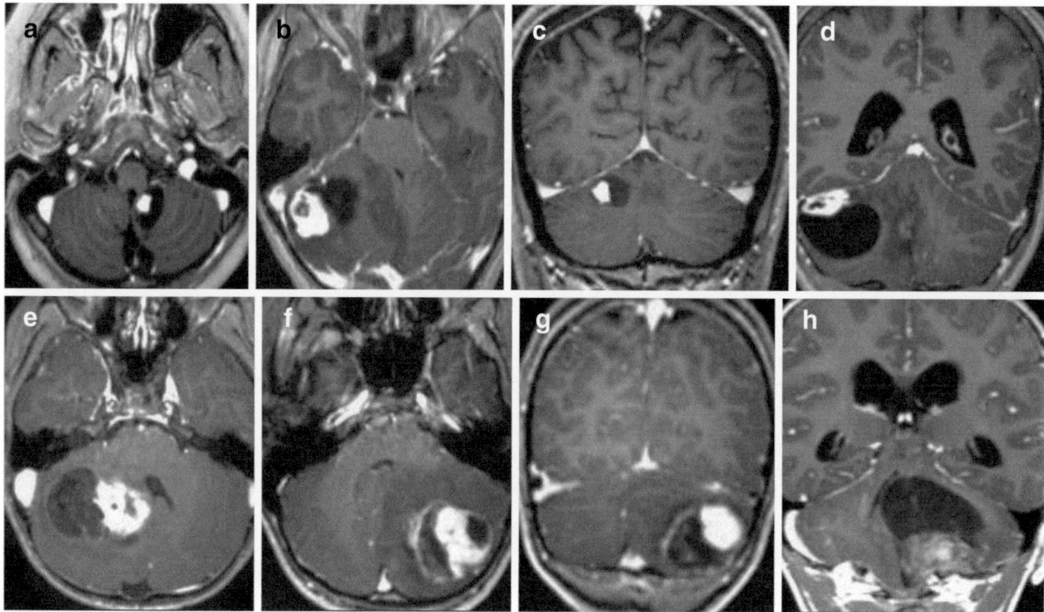

Fig. 8.9 Cerebellar hemangioblastoma vs. cerebellar pilocytic astrocytoma. MRI post-contrast T1WI in four different cases of cerebellar hemangioblastoma (**a–d**) and of four different cases of pilocytic astrocytoma (**e–h**). On post-contrast T1WI the tumors are very similar even though the satellite cyst of pilocytic astrocytoma can enhance (**f, g**)

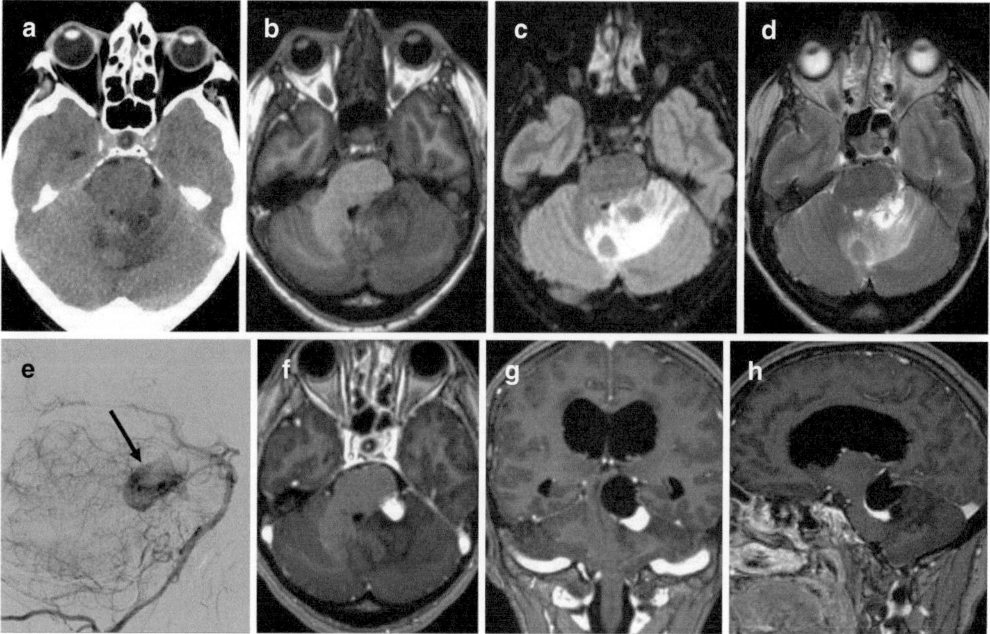

Fig. 8.10 Cerebellar hemangioblastoma. CT (**a**). MRI T1WI (**b**), FLAIR (**c**), T2WI (**d**), digital subtraction angiography with selective vertebral catheterization (**e**), post-contrast T1WI (**f–h**). The angiographic feature of HB is quite characteristic with an intense blush (arrow **e**)

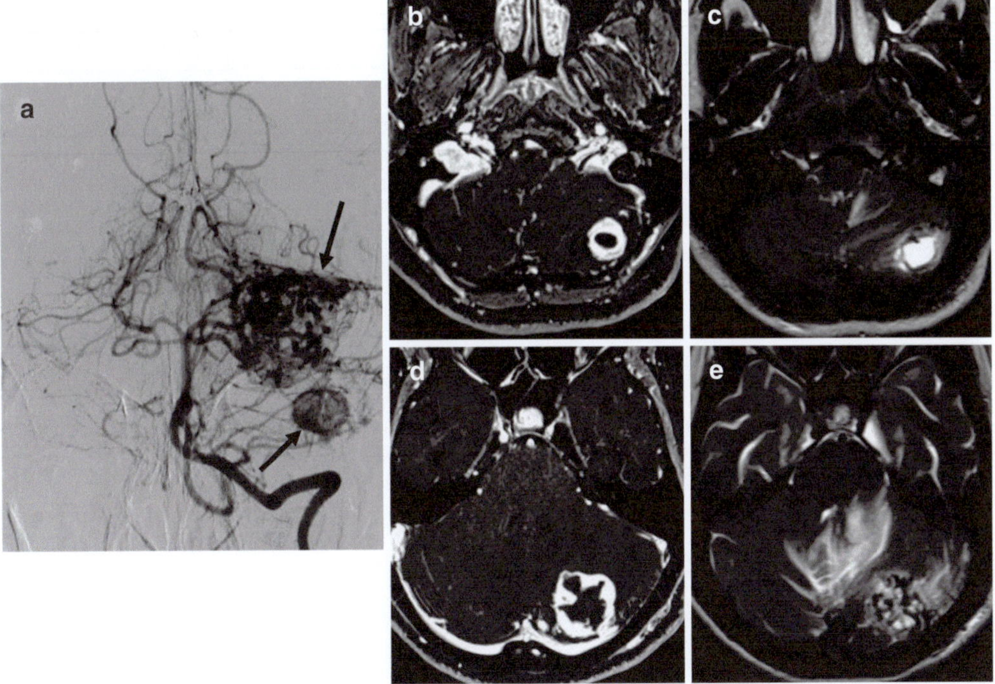

Fig. 8.11 Cerebellar hemangioblastomas in a patient with VHL syndrome. DSA with selective left vertebral artery catheterization (**a**). MRI post-contrast T1WI (**b**, **d**), T2WI (**c**, **e**). In this case two separate lesions are visible in left cerebellar hemisphere with apparently no cysts, the DSA confirmed the typical patter of HBs clearly identifying two separate areas of intense blush (arrows **a**)

Table 8.3 Hemangioblastoma imaging features

Mass effect	Edema	Inhomogeneity	Cysts	Necrosis	Hemorrhage	Calcifications
+/+++	0/++	0/++	0/+++	0	0/+	0

CT	T1	T2	FLAIR	DWI	ADC	T1 Gd	CBV	Spec
◯	●	◯	◯	◯	◯	++/+++	🔴	↓↓(absent)NAA ↑Lipids?

In some cases the satellite cyst is not clearly evident and hemangioblastoma can be more difficult to diagnose; moreover, the possible heterogeneity of the nodule and the high CBV can mimic a more aggressive tumor (Fig. 8.8). The typical angiographic pattern can be helpful also in these cases (Figs. 8.10 and 8.11).

The presence of multiple lesions can facilitate the diagnosis and suggest the presence of a VHL syndrome (Fig. 8.11). Imaging features of hemangioblastoma are summarized in Table 8.3.

8.4 Skeletal Muscle Tumors

8.4.1 Rhabdomyosarcoma

Definition. Rhabdomyosarcoma is a family of malignant primitive neoplasms that show at least focal, predominantly skeletal muscle differentiation and are rarely identified as a primary tumor in the CNS.

It is not currently staged because of the limited number of cases; however, it shows almost always aggressive behavior (grade 4).

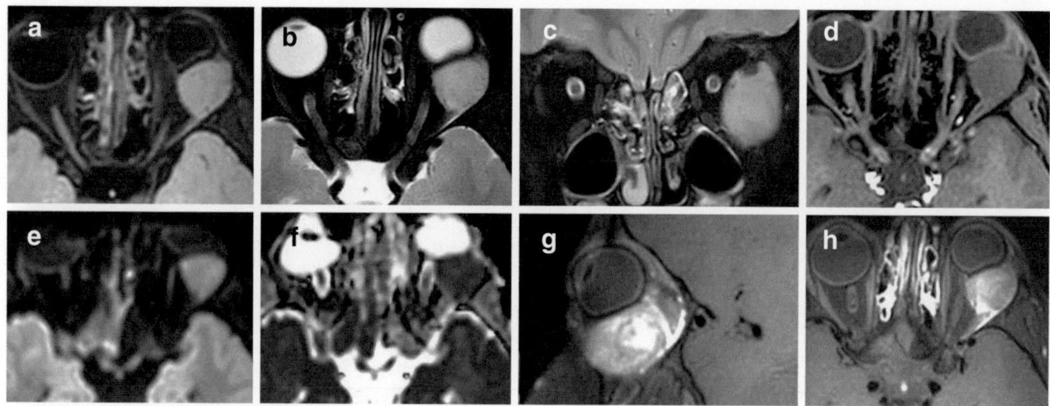

Fig. 8.12 Rhabdomyosarcoma in a 4-year-old girl. MRI FLAIR (**a**), T2WI (**b**, **c**), T1WI (**d**), DWI (**e**), ADC (**f**), post-contrast T1WI (**g**, **h**). A huge homogeneous left infraorbital mass is detectable. It is not dissociable from the external rectus muscle and from the postero-inferior aspect of the eye with left exophthalmos

Table 8.4 Rhabdomyosarcoma imaging features

Mass effect	Edema	Inhomogeneity	Cysts	Necrosis	Hemorrhage	Calcifications
+/+++	0/++	0	0/+	0	0/+	0

CT	T1	T2	FLAIR	DWI	ADC	T1 Gd	CBV	Spec
◐	●	○	○	○	●	+/+++	NA[a]	NA[a]

[a]*NA* incomplete or sporadic reports

Epidemiology. Children are most frequently affected, but some cases are reported also in adulthood.

Location. Infratentorial and/or skull base site is predominantly over supratentorial location.

Clinical features. They are related to the site of origin of the tumor.

Prognosis. It is an aggressive tumor with a survival rate at 24 months extremely low.

8.4.1.1 Imaging

It is a highly cellular tumor with a homogeneous T1, T2, and FLAIR isointensity with brain parenchyma or muscles, homogeneous enhancement after contrast, and diffusion restriction.

Orbital and skull base locations are quite typical (Fig. 8.12). Imaging features of rhabdomyosarcoma are summarized in Table 8.4).

8.5 Tumors of Uncertain Differentiation

8.5.1 Intracranial Mesenchymal Tumor, FET::CREB Fusion Positive

Definition. This is a provisional entity of an intracranial mesenchymal tumor with variable histomorphology and fusion of a FET RNA-binding protein family gene with a member of a CREB family of transcription factors.

Epidemiology. It is a rare intracranial tumor occurring mainly in children or young adults.

Location. This tumor can be both intra- and extra-axial and more commonly located in the supratentorial compartment, but it can be found everywhere intracranially.

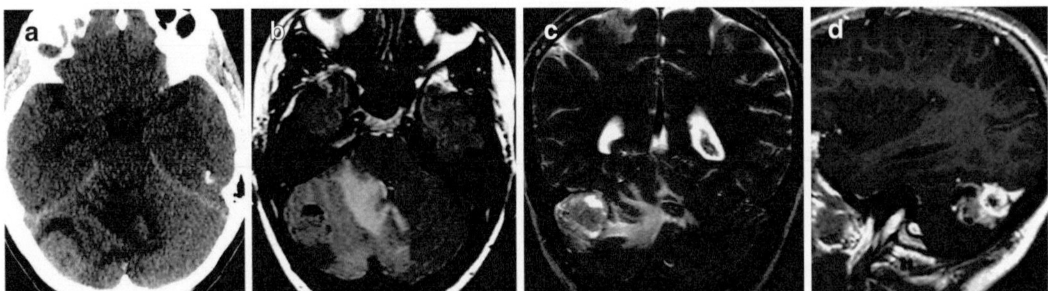

Fig. 8.13 Intracranial mesenchymal tumor, FET::CREB fusion positive in a 26-year-old woman. CT (**a**). MRI FLAIR (**b**), T2WI (**c**), post-contrast T1WI (**d**). A superficial apparently extra-axial tumor is visible in the left posterior fossa with a possible involvement of the tentorial dura. It is a lobulated inhomogeneous mass with clear enhancement, mass effect, and diffuse cerebellar edema. (Courtesy S. Colafati, Rome)

Clinical features. They are related to the site of origin of the tumor.

Prognosis. The prognosis of this tumor is variable, and it can range from slow growth to rapid recurrence.

8.5.1.1 Imaging

These tumors are reported more frequently extra-axially in the meninges with compression of the subjacent brain parenchyma. They are lobulated masses often with both solid and cystic components, avid enhancement after contrast administration, intratumoral blood products, and substantial peritumoral edema (Fig. 8.13). Some tumors showed a dural tail or bony involvement of the overlying skull mimicking meningioma. Diffuse leptomeningeal dissemination along the spinal cord has been reported [5].

8.5.2 *CIC*-Rearranged Sarcoma

Definition. This tumor is a high-grade poorly differentiated sarcoma defined by *CIC* fusion with different gene partners.

Epidemiology. It is a rare tumor more frequently found in adolescents or young adults.

Location. It is a sarcoma occurring usually in the deep soft tissue with about only 10% involving the viscera and even the brain.

Clinical features. They are related to the site of origin of the tumor.

Prognosis. The intracranial location is rare, but it is usually and aggressive tumor with an unfavorable clinical course.

8.5.2.1 Imaging

There are few cases reported in the literature, with aspecific pattern of aggressive neoplasm.

8.5.3 Primary Intracranial Sarcoma, *DICER1*-Mutant

Definition. It is a primary intracranial sarcoma composed of spindled or pleomorphic tumor cells, genetically defined by mutations in the *DICER1* gene.

Epidemiology. It is a rare intracranial tumor occurring mainly in childhood.

Location. The supratentorial location is more typical with a frequent involvement of the dura.

Clinical features. They are related to the site of origin of the tumor.

Prognosis. The prognosis remains still not known due to the rarity of the tumor, but the aggressive nature of this tumor seems related to an unfavorable course.

8.5.3.1 Imaging

Brain imaging demonstrated complex, solid and cystic, heterogeneously enhancing masses usually in the frontal or parietal lobes with frequent meningeal involvement, possible hemor-

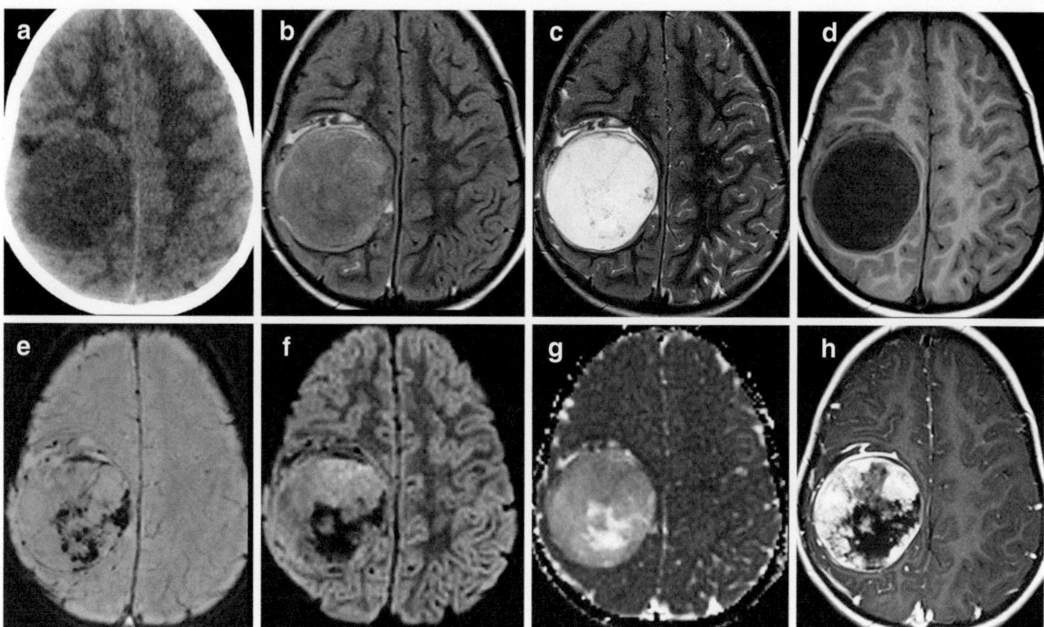

Fig. 8.14 Primary intracranial sarcoma, DICER1-mutant in a 3-year-old child. CT (**a**). MRI FLAIR (**b**), T2WI (**c**), T1WI (**d**), SWI (**e**), DWI (**f**), ADC (**g**), post-contrast T1WI (**h**). A large mass is evident in the superficial left fronto-parietal region. The lesion is homogeneously hypodense on CT and homogeneously hyperintense on T2WI and hypointense on T1WI. Microhemorrhagic components are visible on SWI, diffusion is not clearly reduced, the enhancement is evident but inhomogeneous. (Courtesy S. Colafati, Rome)

rhages, and peritumoral edema (Fig. 8.14). They can be associated with neurofibromatosis type 1 [6].

8.5.4 Ewing Sarcoma

Definition. Ewing sarcoma of the nervous system is an extraosseous small round cell sarcoma containing a fusion between one FET family gene and one ETS family gene.

Epidemiology. The intracranial Ewing sarcoma is an extremely rare tumor encountered mainly in children and young adolescent.

Location. A small subset of the extraosseous Ewing sarcoma involves the cranial spinal axis with a more frequent location in the meninges both intracranial and spinal.

Clinical features. They are related to the site of origin of the tumor and typically related to the mass effect of the lesion.

Prognosis. At present day due to the improvement of chemotherapy the estimated 5-year survival rate in patients with localized lesion is about 70–80%. The presence of metastases at the time of diagnosis is however a strong negative predictor for a good prognosis, and in this case the 5-year survival rate drops to 30%.

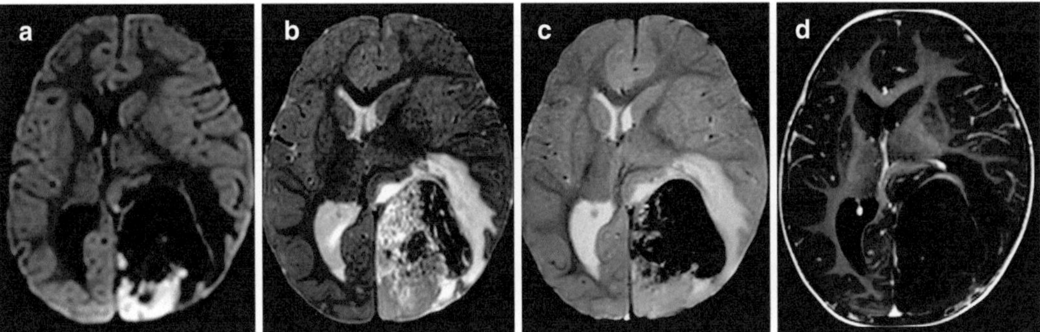

Fig. 8.15 Ewing sarcoma in a 1-year-old child. MRI FLAIR (**a**), T2WI (**b**), T2*GRE (**c**), post-contrast T1WI (**d**). A large apparently intraparenchymal but superficial mass is evident in the left occipital region with a huge mass effect and perilesional edema. The lesion shows diffuse microhemorrhagic components mostly visible on T2* GRE sequence, the enhancement is minimal and the meningeal involvement is doubtful. (Courtesy S. Colafati, Rome)

8.5.4.1 Imaging

Intracranial Ewing sarcomas mostly showed mixed isointense to hypointense signals on T1WI and isointense to hyperintense signals on T2WI. In a literature review of the few cases reported [7] an heterogeneous enhancement was present in about 40.0% cases, an intense enhancement in 52.5% cases, and a moderate enhancement in 7.5% of cases. A possible reason for such heterogeneous enhancement could be the characteristic presence of high density small round cells, and the large amount of protein-rich mucus in some areas, which was accompanied by hemorrhage and necrosis (Fig. 8.15).

Skull involvement was observed in few cases, whereas meningeal involvement was reported in 80.0% cases making the differential diagnosis with SFT or meningioma in adult patients complex if not possible.

8.6 Chondrogenic Tumors

8.6.1 Mesenchymal Chondrosarcoma. Chondrosarcoma

Definition. Mesenchymal chondrosarcoma is a rare, biphasic, malignant tumor composed of undifferentiated small cells and island of well-differentiated hyaline cartilage. The presence of a *HEY1::NCOA2* gene fusion is characteristic.

Chondrosarcomas are a family of malignant mesenchymal tumors with cartilaginous differentiation comprising conventional and dedifferentiated central, conventional and dedifferentiated peripheral, and clear cell chondrosarcomas.

Epidemiology. Mesenchymal chondrosarcoma is more frequent in the second and third decades of life.

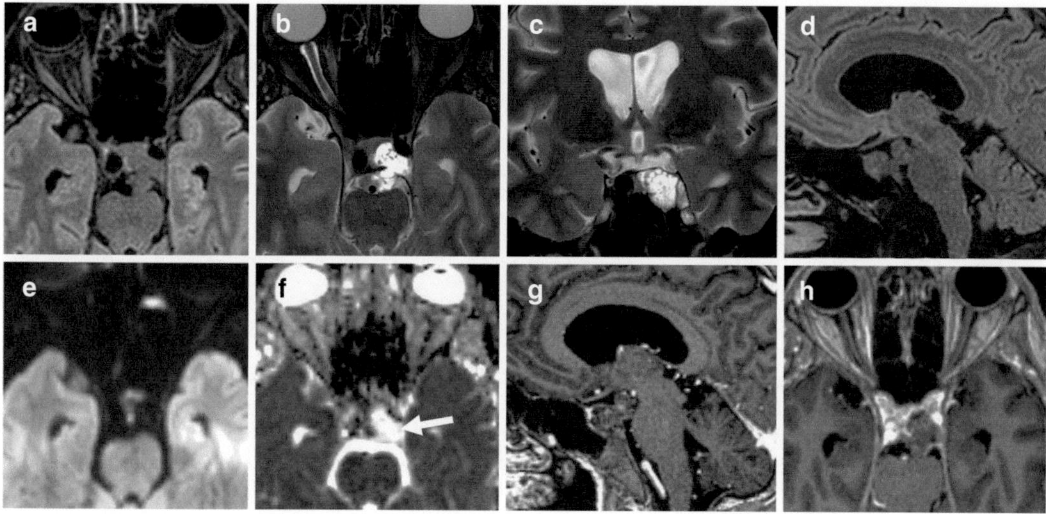

Fig. 8.16 Chondrosarcoma. MRI FLAIR (**a**, **d**), T2WI (**b**, **c**), DWI (**e**), ADC (**f**), post-contrast T1WI (**g**, **h**). The lesion is located in left parasellar region with an exophytic component directed toward the prepontine cistern. The lesion is highly hyperintense on T2WI (**b**, **c**) and isointense on FLAIR (**a**, **d**). ADC is clearly increased (arrow **f**), the post-contrast enhancement is scarce

Intracranial chondrosarcomas account for 1% of all chondrosarcomas, they are more frequent in young adults.

Location. In mesenchymal chondrosarcomas intracranial location is more frequent than spinal location.

Cranial chondrosarcomas are the most common tumors of the cranial bones, skull base is the most frequent location.

Clinical features. They are related to the site of origin of the tumor.

Prognosis. Mesenchymal chondrosarcoma is an aggressive tumor and recurrence after surgery is very frequent in particular for cranial location.

The prognosis of chondrosarcomas family tumor is variable, hystologically they can be classified from grade 1 to grade 3, accordingly the prognosis if completely resected could be favorable, whereas in more aggressive grade the recurrence rate can be relatively high.

8.6.1.1 Imaging

On CT chondrosarcoma is mainly isodense or hypodense relatively to brain parenchyma, even though a minority of case can be hyperdense. They can be both homogeneous and heterogeneous and present calcification in approximately 50% of cases.

On T1WI the great majority of the lesions are isointense or hypointense to brain parenchyma and 2/3 of cases show a homogenous signal.

On T2WI chondrosarcomas are hyperintense or strongly hyperintense in roughly 90% of cases. On FLAIR they can be either isointense (Fig. 8.16) or hyperintense (Fig. 8.17).

They enhance after contrast administration in 95% of cases even with different degrees [8].

Diffusion. On diffusion chondrosarcoma shows a marked increase of ADC, with a mean of 2.5. According to some authors this noticeable increase could help to differentiate chondrosarcoma from chordoma and metastases (Figs. 8.16 and 8.17) [9]. Imaging features of chondrosarcoma are summarized in Table 8.5.

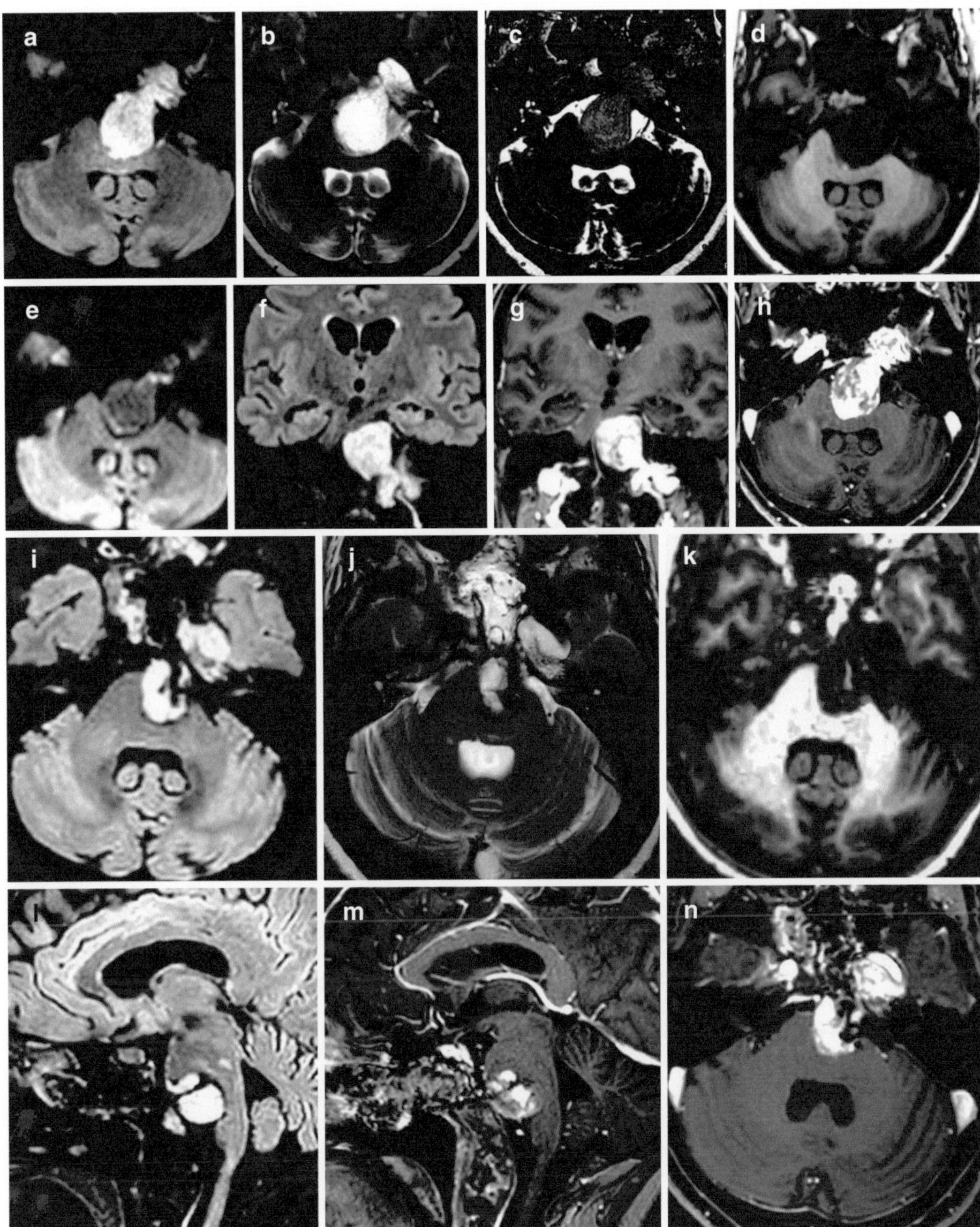

Fig. 8.17 Chondrosarcoma. MRI FLAIR (**a**, **f**), T2WI (**b**), T2 bSSFP (**c**), T1WI (**d**), DWI (**e**), post-contrast T1WI (**g**, **h**). The lesion is located between the left petrous apex and the lateral clivus region with a large exophytic component causing a marked mass effect on pons. The lesion is hyperintense on T2WI (**b**) but not on bSSFP, hyperintense on FLAIR and hypointense on T1WI (**d**). Diffusion is increased and the enhancement is diffuse and relatively strong. Post-operative findings. MRI FLAIR (**i**, **l**), T2WI (**j**), T1WI (**k**), post-contrast T1WI (**m**, **n**). A large biopsy with partly debulking of the exophytic mass was performed through a trans-sphenoidal approach

Table 8.5 Chondrosarcoma imaging features

Mass effect	Edema	Inhomogeneity	Cysts	Necrosis	Hemorrhage	Calcifications
+/+++	0	0/++	0	0	0	0/++

CT	T1	T2	FLAIR	DWI	ADC	T1 Gd	CBV	Spec
◕	●	○	◔	●	○	+/+++	NA[a]	NA[a]

[a]*NA* incomplete or sporadic reports

8.7 Notochordal Tumors

8.7.1 Chordoma

Definition. Chordomas are a family of primary malignant bone neoplasm demonstrating notochordal differentiation, comprising conventional, chondroid, poorly differentiated and dedifferentiated types.

Epidemiology. They represent 0.5% of all intracranial tumors. Conventional, chondroid, and dedifferentiated types are adult tumors with a median age between 45 and 60 years, whereas poorly differentiated chordoma SMARCB1-deficient is typically a pediatric tumor with a median age of around 7 years.

Location. It can occur anywhere in the axial skeleton but sacrococcygeal region is most frequently involved in the conventional and dedifferentiated types, whereas the skull base is the preferred location in chondroid and poorly differentiated types.

Clinical features. They are related to the site of origin of the tumor.

Prognosis. Dedifferentiated and poorly differentiated types have the worst prognosis with a median overall survival of 15 and 13 months and metastases in 1/3 of cases.

The other cases are less aggressive, but still with an unfavorable progression and a median survive of 4 years.

8.7.1.1 Imaging

The imaging characteristic is quite similar to chondrosarcoma, even though the location is on midline, they are lytic and destructive lesion mainly hypointense on T1WI and hyperintense on T2WI with a variable enhancement after contrast.

Diffusion is however lower than in chondrosarcoma [9], with a value that is however similar to the ADC value of metastases (Figs. 8.18 and 8.19). Imaging features of chordoma are summarized in Table 8.6.

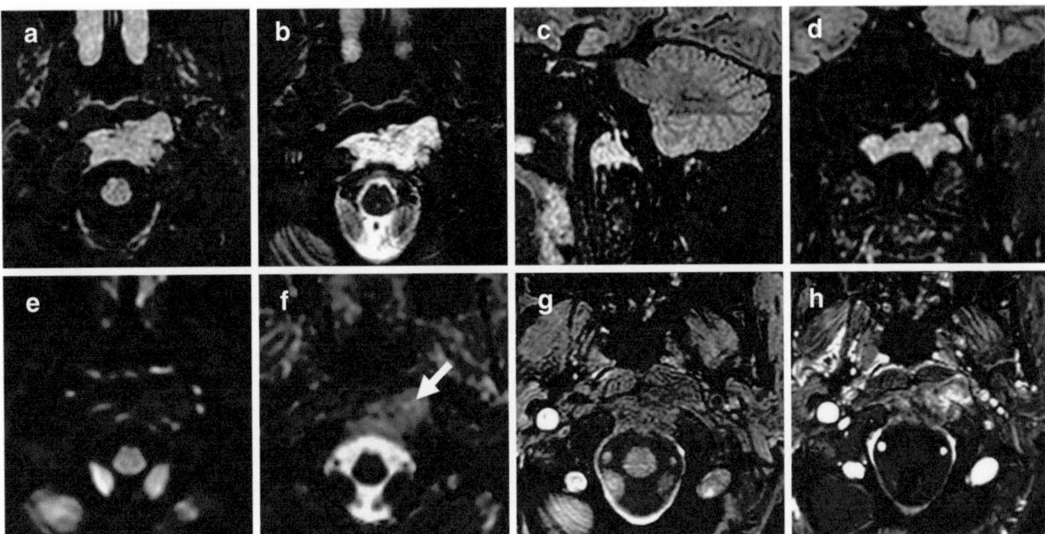

Fig. 8.18 Chordoma of the inferior clivus in a 49-year-old female. MRI FLAIR (**a, c, d**), T2WI (**b**), DWI (**e**), ADC (**f**), T1WI (**g**), post-contrast T1WI (**h**). The lesion is clearly hyperintense on T2WI, but mainly isointense on FLAIR, the enhancement is inhomogeneous and scarce, the ADC is not clearly increased (arrow **f**)

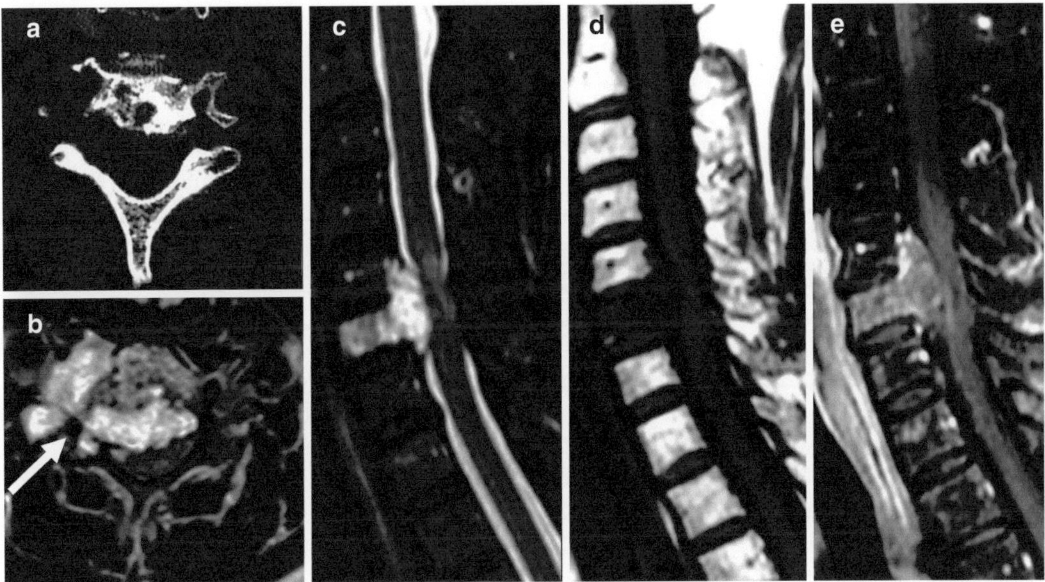

Fig. 8.19 Chordoma of the cervical spine in a 57-year-old female. CT (**a**). MRI post-contrast T1WI (**b**), T2WI (**c**), T1WI (**d**), post-contrast fat-suppressed T1WI (**e**). There is a lytic lesion of C6 vertebral body and of the right transverse process of the vertebra involving vertebral artery that is displaced posteriorly (arrow **b**). The lesion is clearly hyperintense on T2WI and hypointense on T1WI with a diffuse homogeneous enhancement after contrast injection. Cervical spinal cord is compressed but without any signal abnormalities

Table 8.6 Chordoma imaging features

Mass effect	Edema	Inhomogeneity	Cysts	Necrosis	Hemorrhage	Calcifications
+/+++	0	0/++	0	0	0	0/++

CT	T1	T2	FLAIR	DWI	ADC	T1 Gd	CBV	Spec
◐	●	○	○	◐	○	+/+++	NA[a]	NA[a]

[a]*NA* incomplete or sporadic reports

8.8 Melanocytic Tumors

8.8.1 Diffuse Meningeal Melanocytic Neoplasm

8.8.1.1 Meningeal Melanocytosis and Melanomatosis

Definition. Meningeal melanocytosis is a diffuse or multifocal meningeal proliferation of cytologically bland melanocytic cells that arises from leptomeningeal melanocytes.

Meningeal melanomatosis is a diffuse or multifocal meningeal proliferation of melanoma cells that arises from leptomeningeal melanocytes and often shows CNS invasion.

Epidemiology. Diffuse meningeal melanocytic neoplasms are extremely rare, they can occur in both adults and children, in particular melanocytosis may affect pediatric population with neurocutaneus melanosis (Fig. 8.20).

Location. This tumor can spread everywhere in the meninges often involving the Virchow-Robin spaces and large areas of leptomeninges with sparse nodularity.

Clinical features. Symptoms and signs related to increased intracranial pressure are the most frequent clinical feature.

Prognosis. Prognosis is generally poor for both conditions, with melanomatosis presenting with a very aggressive behavior.

Imaging

These tumors present with a thickening of the leptomeninges and the most typical feature is the presence of a spontaneous hyperintensity on T1WI (Fig. 8.20). However this hyperintensity depends on melanin content and could be not always present. In case of high melanin content the leptomeningesal thickening shows a hypointense signal on T2WI.

The lesion clearly enhances after contrast administration. Imaging features of meningeal melanocytosis and melanomatosis are summarized in Table 8.7.

8.8.2 Circumscribed Meningeal Melanocytic Neoplasm

8.8.2.1 Meningeal Melanocytoma and Melanoma

Definition. Circumscribed meningeal melanocytic neoplasms are tumors that arise from leptomeningeal melanocytes and ranged histologically from well-differentiated tumors (meningeal melanocytoma) to frankly malignant neoplasms with aggressive growth properties (meningeal melanoma).

Epidemiology. These are extremely rare tumors with a peak incidence estimated around the fourth and fifth decade of life.

Location. They occur more frequently in cervical or dorsal spine or more rarely in posterior fossa.

Clinical features. Clinical signs and symptoms are related to the location of the tumor.

Prognosis. The prognosis correlated with the histopathological features.

Imaging

These tumors are nonspecific extra-parenchymal masses that in case of spinal origin can be easily confounded with spinal neurinomas. The lesion can be slightly hyperintense on T1WI, but this aspect can be extremely slight and could be of little help in differential diagnosis.

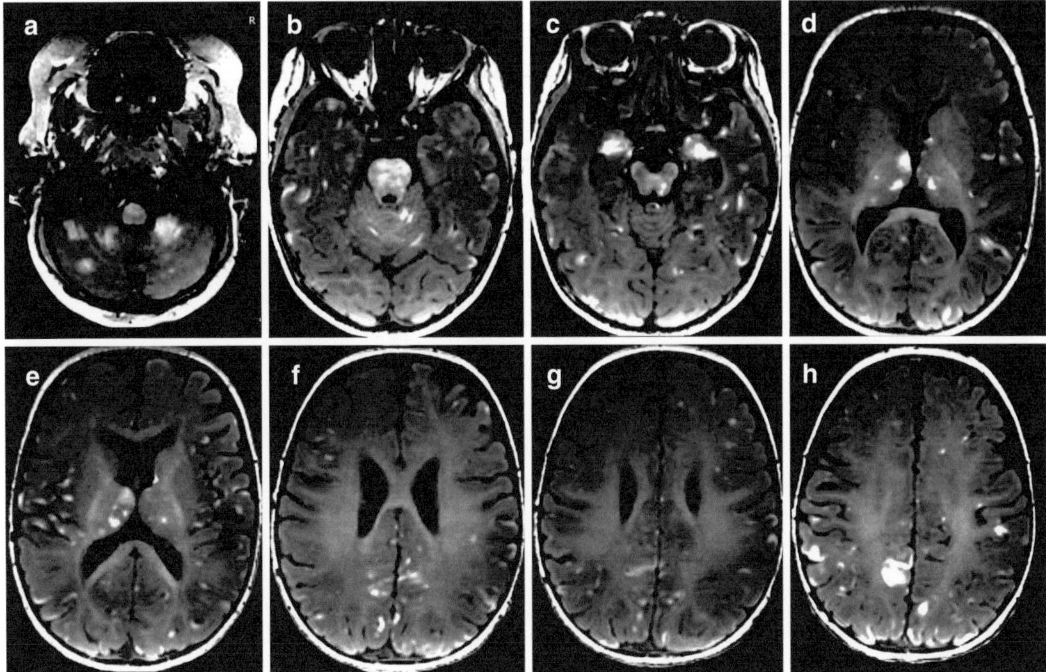

Fig. 8.20 Neurocutaneous melanosis in a 7-month-old boy. MRI T1WI (**a–h**). A severe form of neurocutaneous melanosis with diffuse multifocal proliferation of spontaneous T1 hyperintense melanocytic cells and initial involvement of pia mater predominantly in parieto-occipital region

Table 8.7 Meningeal melanocytosis and melanomatosis imaging features

Mass effect	Edema	Inhomogeneity	Cysts	Necrosis	Hemorrhage	Calcifications
+/+++	0/+	0	0	0	0	0

CT	T1	T2	FLAIR	DWI	ADC	T1 Gd	CBV	Spec
◯	◯	●	◯	◯	●	+/+++	NA[a]	NA[a]

[a]*NA* incomplete or sporadic reports

In case of nevus of Ota primary meningeal melanocytic neoplasm can be found in the ipsilateral trigeminal cave or middle cranial fossa [10].

References

1. Ratneswaren T, Avila Hogg FR, Gallagher MJ, Ashkan K. Surveillance for metastatic haemangiopericytoma-solitary fibrous tumor systematic litarature review of incidence, predictors and diagnosis of extracranial disease. J Neurooncol. 2018;138:447–67.
2. Wang XQ, Zhou Q, Li ST, Liao CL, Zhang H, Zhang BY. Solitary fibrous tumors of the central nervous system: clinical features and imaging findings in 22 patients. J Comput Assist Tomogr. 2013;37:658–65.
3. Chourmouzi D, Potsi S, Moumtzouoglou A, Papadopoulou E, Drevelegas K, Zaraboukas T, Drevelegas A. Dural lesions mimicking meningiomas: a pictorial essay. World J Radiol. 2012;4(3):75–82.
4. Liu G, Chen ZY, Ma L, Lou X, Li SJ, Wang YL. Intracranial hemangiopericytoma: MR imaging findings and diagnostic usefulness of minimum ADC values. J Magn Reson Imaging. 2013;38:1146–51.
5. Sloan EA, Chiang J, Villanueva-Meyer JE, et al. Intracranial mesenchymal tumor with FET-CREB fusion. A unifying diagnosis for the spectrum of intracranial myxoid mesenchymal tumors and angiomatoid fibrous histiocytoma-like neoplasms. Brain Pathol. 2021;31(4):e12918.

6. Lee JC, Villanueva-Meyer JE, Ferris SP, et al. Primary intracranial sarcomas with DICER1 mutation often contain prominent eosinophilic cytoplasmic globules and can occur in the setting of neurofibromatosis type I. Acta Neuropathol. 2019;137:521–5.

7. Jiang Y, Zhao L, Wang Y, Liu X, Wu X, Li Y. Primary intracranial Ewing sarcoma/peripheral primitive neuroectodermal tumor mimicking meningioma: a case report and literature review. Front Oncol. 2020;10:528073.

8. Pamir MN, Ozduman K. Analysis of radiological features relative to histopathology in 42 skull base chordomas and chondrosarcomas. Eur J Radiol. 2006;58:461–70.

9. Ota Y, Liao E, Capizzano AA, Baba A, Kurokawa R, Kurokawa M, Srinivasan A. Differentiation of skull base chondrosarcomas, chordomas, and metastases: utility of DWI and dynamic contrast-enhanced perfusion MR imaging. AJNR Am J Neuroradiol. 2022;43:1325–32.

10. LiangKuo K, LungLin C, HsinWu C, et al. Meningeal melanocytoma associated with nevus of ota: analysis of twelve reported cases. World Neurosurg. 2019;127:e311–20.

9.1 Hematolymphoid Tumors Involving the CNS

9.1.1 CNS Lymphoma

Primary CNS lymphoma (PCNSL) is in their vast majority referred to diffuse large B-cell lymphoma confined to the CNS at presentation. Other CNS lymphomas such as intravascular B-cell lymphoma, primary T-cell lymphoma or lymphomas with systemic involvement or with secondary involvement of the CNS are extremely rare.

9.1.2 Primary Diffuse Large B-Cell Lymphoma of the CNS

WHO definition. Diffuse large B-cell lymphoma of the CNS (CNS-DLBCL) is large B-cell lymphoma confined to the CNS at presentation. Its cytological features correspond to those of its systemic counterpart.

Epidemiology. The incidence rate of DLBCL is 0.46 cases per 100,000 population and accounts for approximately 3% of all brain tumors with a peak incidence between 55 and 65 years and a male/female ratio of 3:2.

Location. DLBCLs preferentially involved the supratentorial compartment. The neoplasm can affect any lobe and frequently the basal ganglia and the periventricular regions. Leptomeninges can be involved as well but unusually as a single location. Meningeal dissemination from the primitive tumor is reported in 15% of cases.

Parenchymal localizations can be single or multiple. Ocular involvement is reported in 20% of cases, whereas extra CNS dissemintion is exceedingly rare even though not impossible.

Clinical features. Signs and symptoms vary according to location, but other than possible focal neurological deficits or cranial nerve palsies, lymphomas can be typically associated with cognitive dysfunction and psychomotor slowing.

Prognosis. In immunocompetent patients genetic predisposition to DLBCL has not been demonstrated. DLBCL shows worst prognosis in comparison with systemic lymphoma, in particular in elderly patients. The mean overall survival is estimated at approximately 3 years.

9.1.2.1 Imaging

Similarly to glioblastoma or even diffuse astrocytoma, DLBCL is an infiltrative tumor with ill-defined margins in nature; nevertheless, it frequently appears as an homogeneous enhancing mass usually in the deep part of the cerebral hemisphere or in a periventricular location (Figs. 9.1, 9.2, 9.3, and 9.4).

The high cellularity of this tumor is responsible for the typical slight hyperdensity on CT and to the relative iso to slight hyperintensity on T2WI/FLAIR sequences.

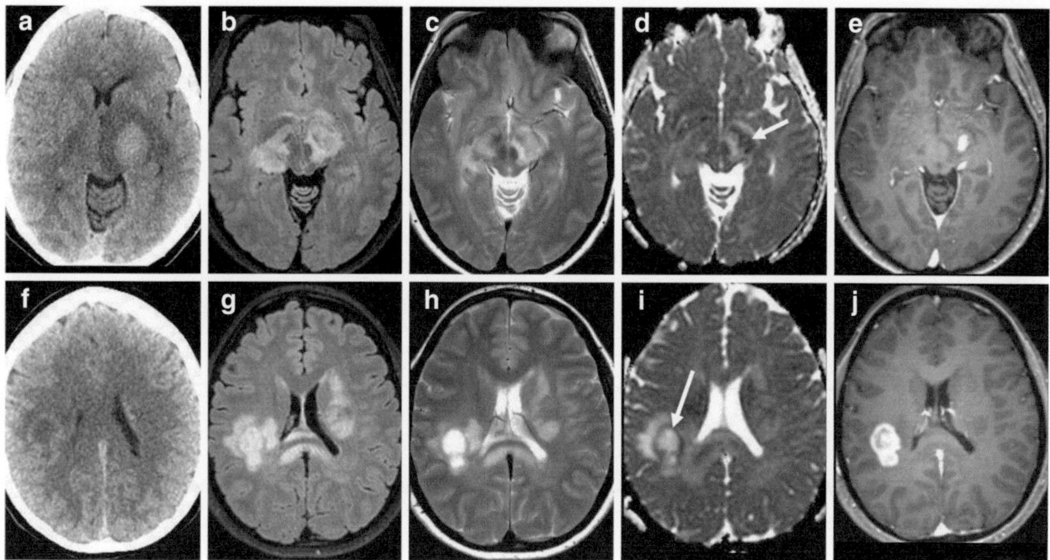

Fig. 9.1 DLBCL in a 29-year-old female with slight right hemiparesis and psychomotor slowing. CT (**a**, **f**), MRI FLAIR (**b**, **g**), T2WI (**c**, **h**), ADC (**d**, **i**), post-contrast T1WI (**e**, **j**). The lesion is clearly hyperdense on CT and exhibits a diffusion restriction (arrows **d**, **i**) in the enhancing portion

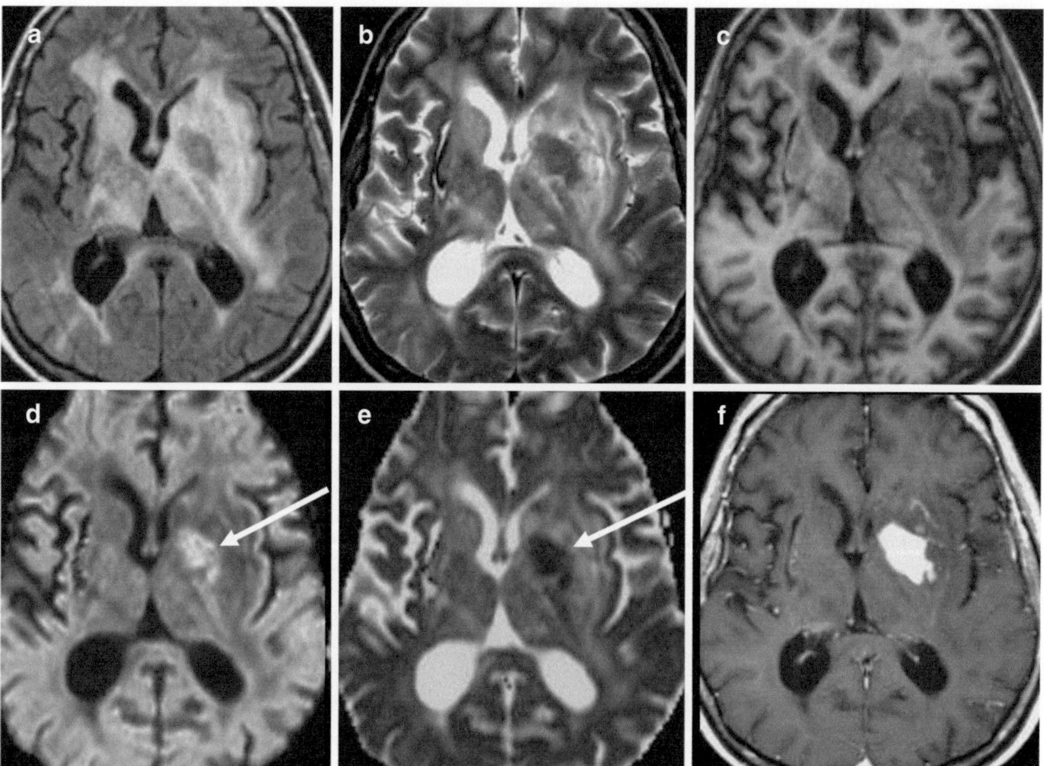

Fig. 9.2 DLBCL in a 62-year-old male with right hemiparesis and psychomotor slowing. MRI FLAIR (**a**), T2WI (**b**), T1WI (**c**), DWI (**d**), ADC (**e**), post-contrast T1WI (**f**). As in the previous case the core of the neoplasm shows a clear diffusion restriction (arrow **d**, **e**) and enhancement after contrast (**f**). A diffuse signal intensity abnormality (more evident in **a** and **b**) is visible all around ventricles and in basal ganglia demonstrates a more diffuse infiltrating lesion

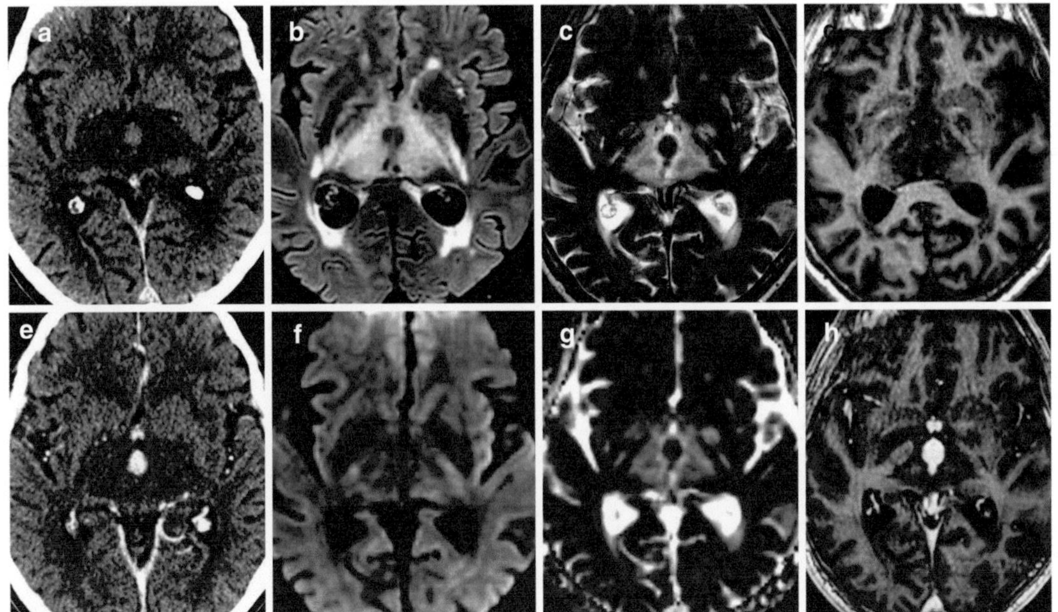

Fig. 9.3 DLBCL in a 76-year-old male with psychomotor slowing. CT (**a**), post-contrast CT (**e**). MRI FLAIR (**b**), T2WI (**c**), T1WI (**d**), DWI (**f**), ADC (**g**), post-contrast T1WI (**h**). The lesion is localized in the lateral walls of the third ventricle and in the hypothalamic region with abundant perilesional edema, diffusion restriction, and marked enhancement after contrast administration

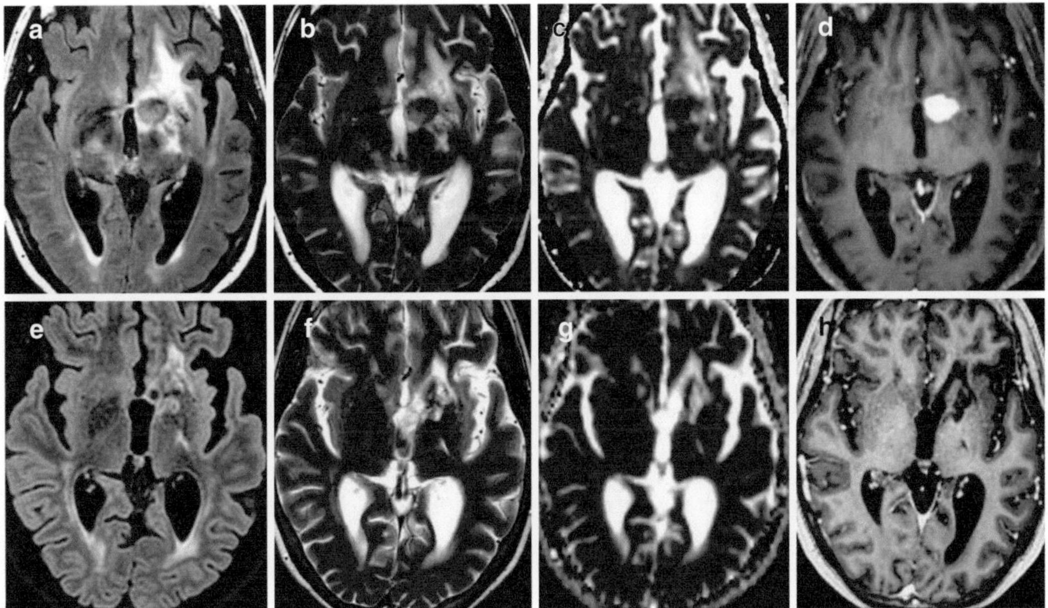

Fig. 9.4 DLBCL in a 37-year-old male, first MR study and 4 years follow-up after chemotherapy. MRI FLAIR (**a, e**), T2WI (**b, f**), ADC (**c, g**), post-contrast T1WI (**d, h**). Clinical signs are similar to those of the previous cases, but with a more circumscribed lesion involving only the left cerebral deep structures (**a–d**). The 4 years follow-up does not show any residual enhancing lesion (**e–h**)

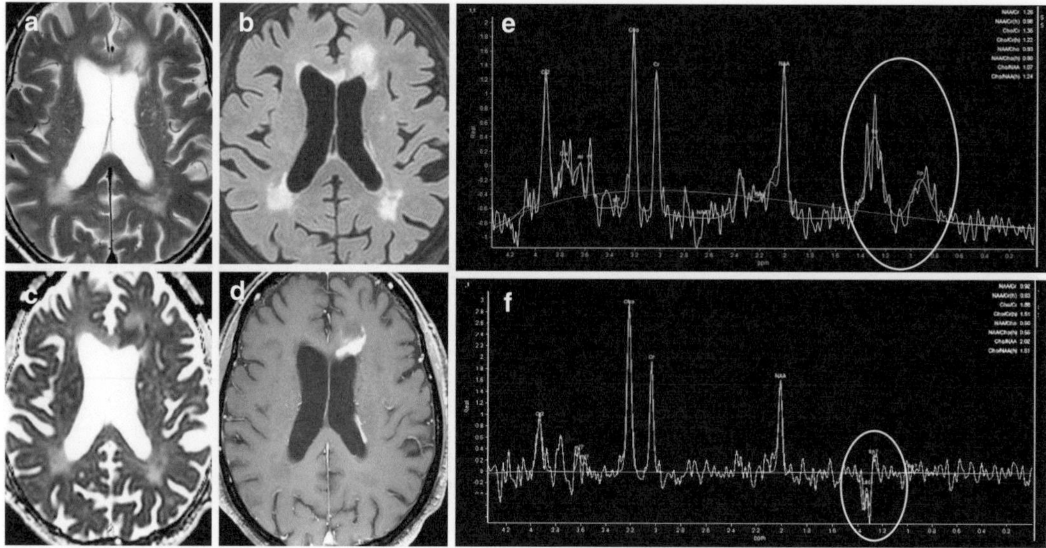

Fig. 9.5 DLBCL. MRI T2WI (**a**), FLAIR (**b**), ADC (**c**), post-contrast T1WI (**d**), short TE spectroscopy (**e**), intermediate TE spectroscopy (**f**). The left periventricular lymphoma shows a clear increase in Cho/Cr and Cho/NAA ratio as well as the presence of lipids (oval **e**) and lactate (oval **f**) peaks

Peritumoral edema is in general less evident than in gliomas and in particular in comparison with metastases, and necrotic areas are rare in immunocompetent patients.

Diffusion. The high cellularity of this tumor is also responsible for the typical diffusion restriction of DLBCL.

Spectroscopy. The homogeneous enhancement of lymphoma may disappear in few days (if not hours) after steroid therapy, this behavior could mimic an acute pseudotumoral inflammatory demyelinating lesion. MR spectroscopy can however help in differentiate these two conditions, in particular lymphoma can be suggested when the Cho/Cr ratio and the Cho/NAA ratio were particularly high (more than 2.5 and 1.7, respectively), and a high lipid and/or lactate peak was seen (Fig. 9.5).

As previously noted lymphoma can be found in leptomeninges, but usually with a contemporary parenchymal localization as shown in Fig. 9.6.

Perfusion, permeability. Brain perfusion and permeability have been reported with variable values. They can be reduced such in the case of Fig. 9.6 but even increased mimicking a glioblastoma behavior. For the differential diagnosis of malignant glioma (Fig. 9.7) it has been reported

that the most reliable value remains the diffusion restriction usually more pronounced in lymphomas. Image features of DLBCL are summarized in Table 9.1.

9.1.3 Immunodeficiency-Associated CNS Lymphoma

WHO definition. Immunodeficiency-associated CNS lymphomas comprise a family of CNS lymphomas arising in patients with inherited or acquired immunodeficiency (AIDS and iatrogenic diseases).

Epidemiology. This tumor can occur in patients with rare congenital immunodeficiency or more frequently in patients with iatrogenic immunodeficiency. AIDS-related lymphomas have become less frequent after the introduction of HAART therapy.

Location. The locations are similar to those of CNS lymphoma in immunocompetent patients, even multifocal location is more frequent in immunodeficient patients.

Clinical features. Even clinical features are quite similar to those of immunocompetent patients.

Prognosis. Prognosis is usually poor.

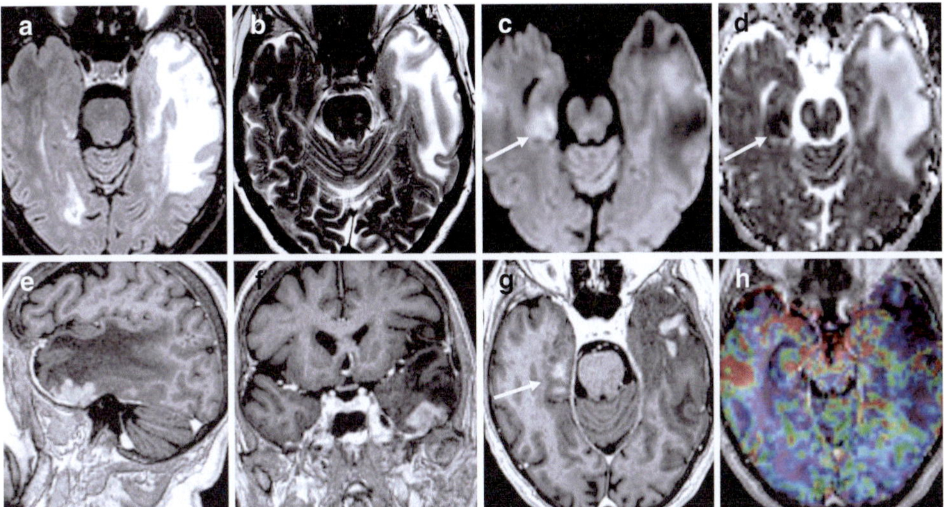

Fig. 9.6 DLBCL. MRI FLAIR (**a**), T2WI (**b**), DWI (**c**), ADC (**d**), post-contrast T1WI (**e**, **f**, **g**), CBV (**h**). In this case cortical temporal lymphoma localization is present on both sides with a leptomeningeal involvement. The left temporal lesion shows an unusually marked perilesional edema, whereas perilesional edema is almost absent in the right location where the diffusion restriction is well evident (arrow **c**, **d**) in a region of post-contrast enhancement (**g**). CBV is decreased

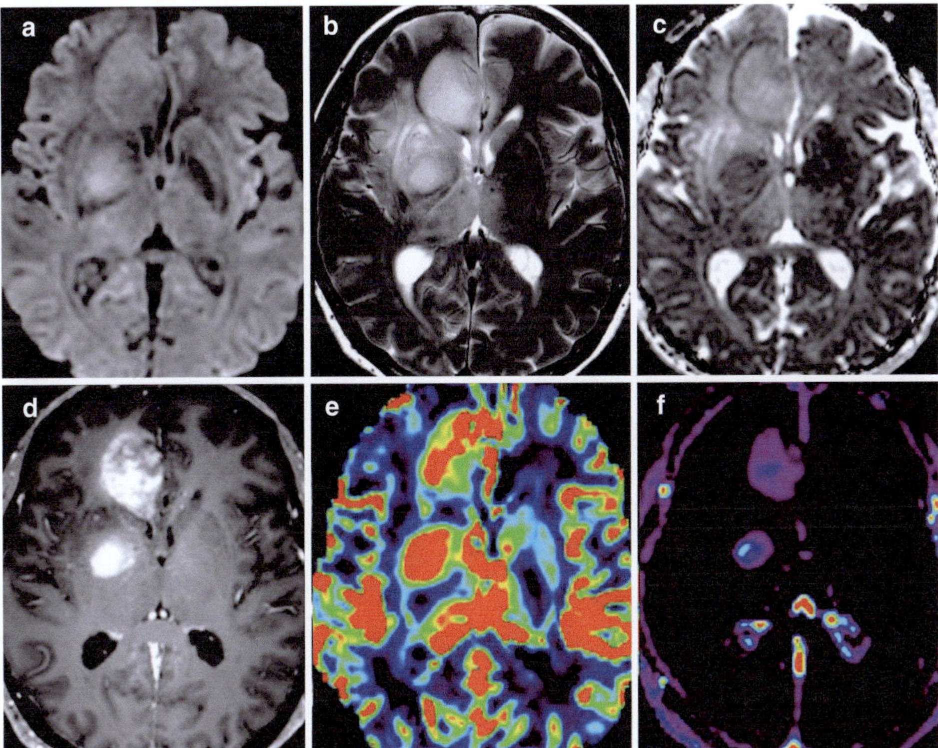

Fig. 9.7 Glioblastoma. MRI FLAIR (**a**), T2WI (**b**), ADC (**c**), post-contrast T1WI (**d**), CBV (**e**), permeability Ktrans (**f**). The location and post-contrast characteristic of this glioblastoma can mimic a DLBCL. However diffusion is apparently only slightly reduced (**c**) and also the T2WI aspect of the enhancing tumor (**c**) is not hypo-isointense as expected in case of DLCBL

Table 9.1 DLBCL imaging features

Mass effect	Edema	Inhomogeneity	Cysts	Necrosis	Hemorrhage	Calcifications
+/++	+/++	0/+	0	0	0	0

CT	T1	T2	FLAIR	DWI	ADC	T1 Gd	CBV	Spec
○	●	○	○	○	●	+/+++	○ ●	↑Cho/NAA, ↑Lipids, ↑Lac

9.1.3.1 Imaging

The main difference with DLCBL in immunocompetent patients is the inhomogeneity of the lesions that very frequently display a ring-like pattern, similar to abscess or secondary lesions (Fig. 9.8).

In a series of 23 cases lesions are single in roughly half of cases with a huge edema in all cases. The ring like pattern was present in 80% of cases, with diffusion slightly reduced at the periphery of the lesions and increased in the center and a clear ring enhancement [1].

9.1.4 Lymphomatoid Granulomatosis

Lymphomatoid granulomatosis is an angiocentric and angiodestructive lymphoproliferative disorder characterized by polymorphous lymphoid infiltrates composed of EBV-positive atypical B cells in a T-cell rich inflammatory background.

In the previous 2016 WHO classification of CNS tumors it is considered one of the immunodeficiency-associated CNS lymphomas.

From an imaging point of view, it could be confused with angiocentric lymphoma due to the presence of multiple punctate lesions along the perivascular spaces or it could occur as a solid mass everywhere in the CNS like DLBCL.

9.2 Miscellaneous Rare Lymphomas of the CNS

Apart from DLBCL other lymphoid neoplasms rarely arise primarily in the CNS. In the 2021 WHO classification these different types of rare primary lymphomas of the CNS are reported.

1. **Intravascular large B-cell.** This rare large B-cell lymphoma is characterized by an apparently exclusive intravascular growth. Usually this lymphoma mimics vascular lesions from multiple infarcts to vasculitis. Lesion can affect frequently the pons and a meningeal thickening was reported; however, a differential diagnosis with cerebrovascular disease is often impossible.

2. **MALT lymphoma of the dura.** Lymphoma primarily affecting the dura are rare, but among them MALT lymphoma is the most frequent. This typically presents a focal thickening of the dura with evident enhancement and a characteristic diffusion restriction which can be useful in the differential diagnosis of meningiomas even if this is often difficult if not impossible also considering the prevalence in both these tumors of female gender and of the same gender age range. The prognosis could be however favorable [2].

3. **Other low-grade B-cell lymphoma of the CNS.** These tumors show a less aggressive prognosis than DLBCL but they are exceedingly rare. The imaging pattern is similar to DLBCL.

4. **Anaplastic large cell lymphoma (ALK+/ALK−).** This rare variant is the most aggressive one with a poor prognosis and no substantial imaging pattern differeces with DLBCL.

5. **T-cell and NK/T-cell lymphoma.** Also the primary CNS variant of T-cell and NK/T-cell lymphomas is rare. For primary T-cell lymphoma the differential diagnosis includes an inflammatory process due to the small size of the tumor, whereas primary NK/T-cell lymphomas aer usually confounded with DLBCL or angiocentric lymphoma due to its angiocentric growth.

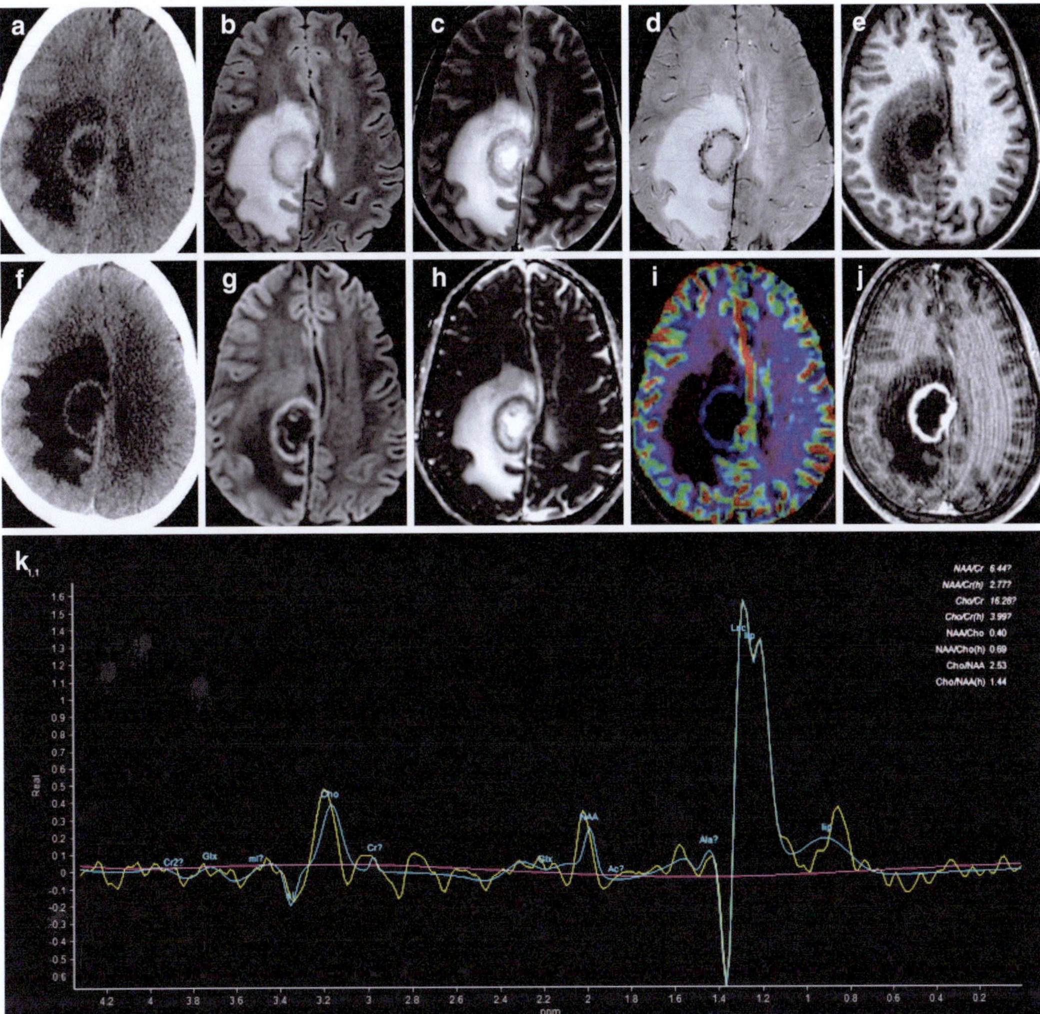

Fig. 9.8 DLBCL in a 28-year-old female with immuno-suppressive therapy for scleroderma. CT (**a, f**). MRI FLAIR (**b**), T2WI (**c**), SWI (**d**), T1WI (**e**), DWI (**g**), ADC (**h**), CBV (**i**), post-contrast T1WI (**j**), spectroscopy (**k**). The lesion shows the typical aspect of a ring-enhancing lesion with a peripheral rim of enhancement (**j**). Differently from a typical pyogenic abscess the center of the lesion shows a diffusion increase, whereas diffusion is slightly reduced at the periphery (**g, h**). SWI shows an increased susceptibility in the ring, but mainly of apparent vascular nature (**d**). The ring is slightly hyperdense on CT (**a, f**) and CBV is only slightly increased (**i**). MRI spectroscopy single voxel TE 144 ms (**k**) center in the central part of the lesions shows a huge lipidic peak with a possible lactate component, the other peaks are all depressed

9.3 Secondary CNS Lymphomas

In the 2016 WHO classification of CNS tumor, secondary CNS lymphomas were reported in the section of CNS lymphomas instead of in the metastases section. From an imaging perspective given the similarity between primary and secondary lymphomas of the CNS, it might make sense to place this section at the end, of the CNS lymphoma chapter.

Secondary involvement of CNS is a rare complication of systemic lymphoma almost always fatal. Different types of systemic lymphoma can spread to CNS, the most frequent being diffuse large B-cell lymphoma. Burkitt lymphoma, T-cell lymphoma (Fig. 9.9), and chronic lymphocytic

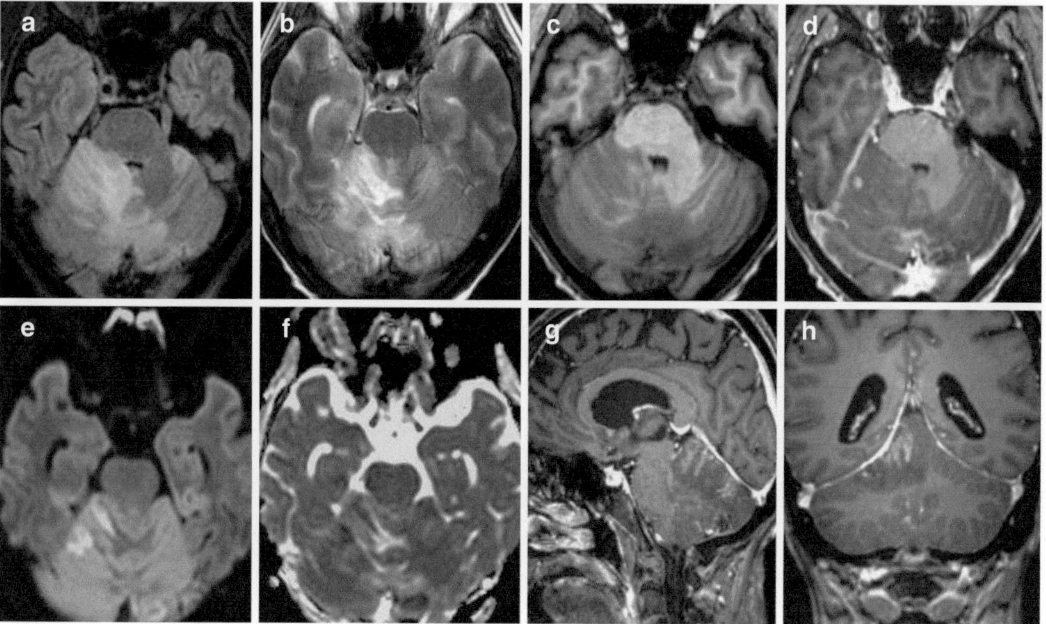

Fig. 9.9 Secondary CNS lymphoma. MRI FLAIR (**a**), T2WI (**b**), T1WI (**c**), post-contrast T1WI (**d, g, h**), DWI (**e**), ADC (**f**). Secondary CNS location from a systemic T-cell lymphoma. Neoplasm is localized within leptomeninges and subarachnoid spaces in left cerebellar region

leukemia with lymphomatous transformation (Richter syndrome, Fig. 9.10) can very rarely spread to CNS. The secondary CNS involvement is predominantly at the level of the leptomeninges, but secondary parenchymal involvement was reported as well.

9.4 Histiocytic Tumors

9.4.1 Langherans Cells Histiocytosis

WHO definition. Langerhans cells histiocytosis of the CNS or the meninges is a clonal proliferation of Langerhans-type cells manifesting in the CNS or the meninges, with or without systemic lesions, which pathologically corresponds to its counterparts occurring elsewhere.

Epidemiology. Most cases occurred in childhood even though it can be found at any age.

Location. There are different patterns of localization, the more frequent is the involvement of the cranial vault or of the skull base and, intracranially, the involvement of the pituitary-hypothalamic axis. Another pattern causes leukoencephalopathy with possible involvement of the basal ganglia and neurodegeneration.

Clinical features. The involvement of pituitary-hypothalamic axis can typically cause a diabetes insipidus, whereas patients with leukoencephalopathy and/or basal ganglia degeneration can present with cerebellar signs, pyramidal tract signs, or even neuropsychiatric symptoms.

Prognosis. Chemotherapy is usually efficacious if neurodegenerative lesions are not present.

9.4.1.1 Imaging

The bone lesions are nonspecific lytic lesion with enhancement after contrast. In children, the lesions are usually found in the skull vault (Fig. 9.11) or at the level of vertebral body that eventually collapsed with the so-called features of *vertebra-plana* (Fig. 9.12).

Intracranial histiocytosis can be frequently localized at the level of the hypothalamic-pituitary axis with a typical thickening of the pituitary stalk. In this case diabetes insipidus is often the only clinical sign and consequently the T1 spontaneous hyperintensity of the neurohypophysis on T!WI is not visible (Fig. 9.13).

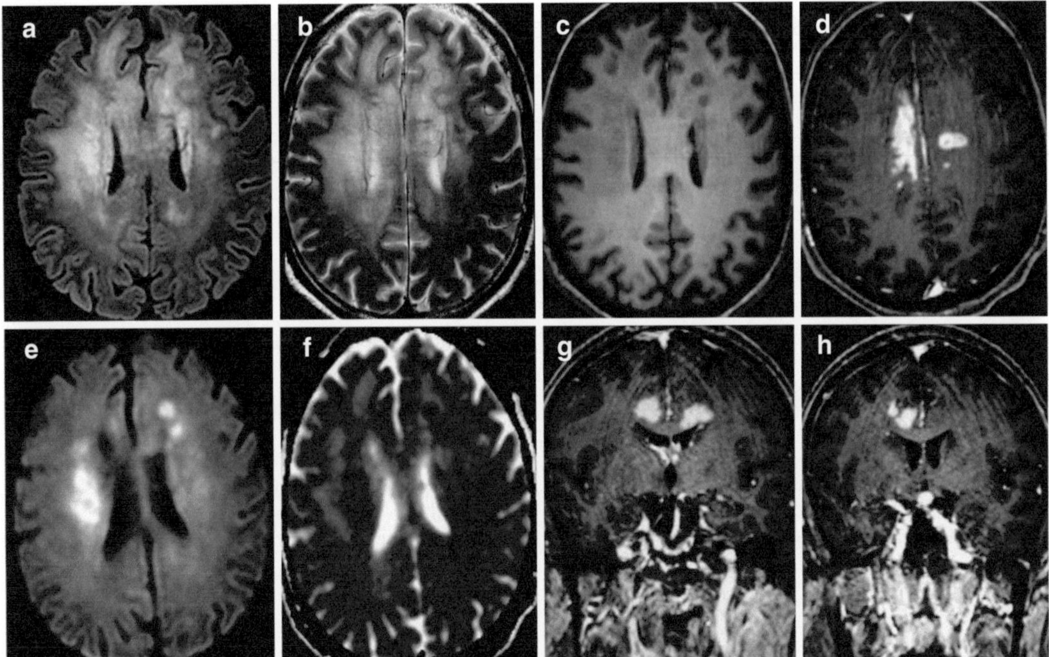

Fig. 9.10 Secondary CNS lymphoma. MRI FLAIR (**a**), T2WI (**b**), T1WI (**c**), post-contrast T1WI (**d, g, h**), DWI (**e**), ADC (**f**). In this case the CNS localization comes from a large B-cell systemic lymphoma secondary to a transformation from chronic lymphatic leukemia (Richter syndrome) with diffuse parenchymal lesions in both parasagittal mesial regions, with typical diffusion restriction (**e, f**) and contrast enhancement (**d, g, h**)

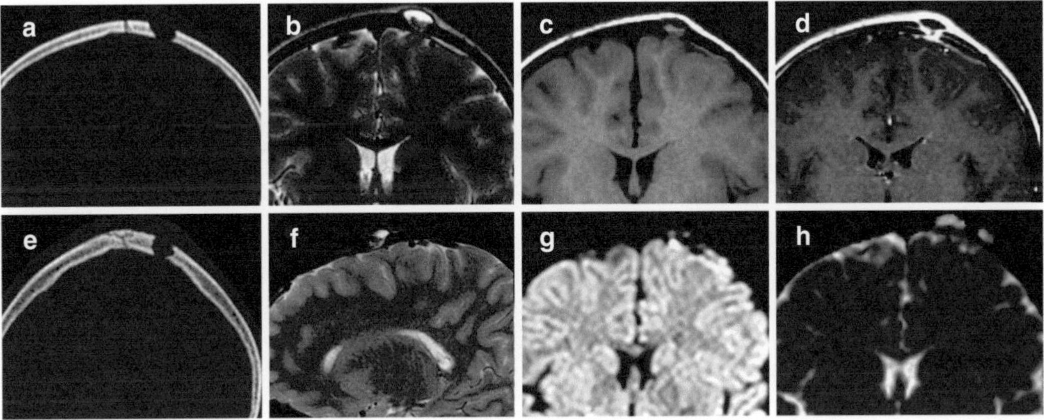

Fig. 9.11 Langherans cell histiocytosis, skull lesion in a 9-year-old boy. CT (**a, e**). MRI T2WI (**b, f**), T1WI (**c**), post-contrast T1WI (**d**), DWI (**g**), ADC (**h**). The lytic lesion is predominantly hyperintense on T2WI and hypointense on T1WI, with increased diffusion and partial enhancement after contrast administration

A third pattern of intracranial Langerhans cell histiocytosis is the so-called neurodegenerative pattern with specific involvement of cerebellar dentate nuclei, dorsal pons, and lentiform nuclei. These alterations can be found in asymptomatic patients, but more frequently in patients with symptoms suggestive of neurodegenerative disease such as gait disturbance, ataxia, behavioral disturbances, or psychiatric disease. The dentate lesions appear to be hyperintense on T2/FLAIR sequences and with variable signal intensity on T1WI from hypointense to slight hyperintense,

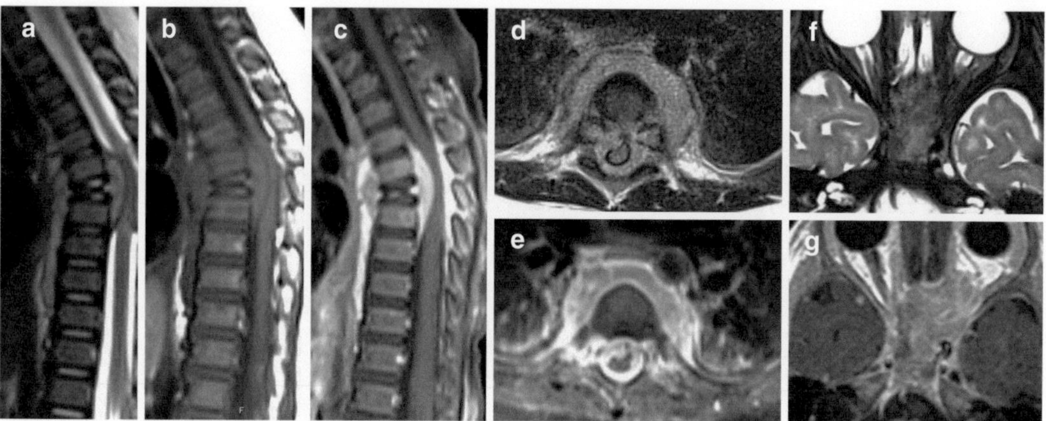

Fig. 9.12 Langherans cell histiocytosis, multiple bone lesions in a 1-year-old girl. MRI T2WI (**a, d, f**), T1WI (**b**), post-contrast T1WI (**c, e, g**). A huge lytic lesion involves the D6 vertebral body that is completely collapsed (vertebra-plana) with pathological tissue involving the anterior epidural space and compressing the spinal cord. Another huge bone lesion is localized in the upper sphenoid bone with initial involvement of the left orbital apex (**f, g**)

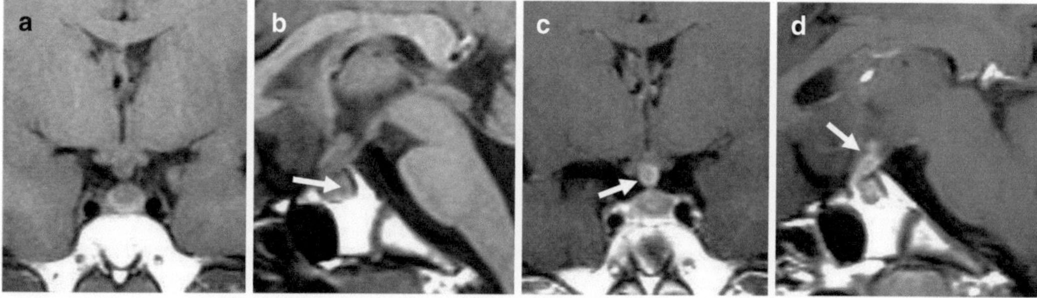

Fig. 9.13 Langherans cell histiocytosis of the hypothalamic-pituitary axis. MRI T1WI (**a, b**), post-contrast T1WI (**c, d**). A thickening of the pituitary stalk is visible on both pre- and post-contrast studies with an homogeneous enhancement after contrast injection (arrows **c, d**). On pre-contrast study the spontaneous hyperintensity of the neurohypophysis is not visible (arrow **b**)

post-contrast enhancement is rare (Figs. 9.14 and 9.15) [3].

9.4.2 Rare Histiocytic Tumors

1. **Erdheim-Chester disease.** Erdheim-Chester disease of the CNS or the meninges with or without systemic lesions pathologically corresponds to its counterparts. Lesions can involve the dura or the brain including the ponto-cerebellar structures. They are nonspecific enhancing masses.
2. **Rosai-Dorfman disease.** Rosai-Dorfman disease of the CNS or the meninges with or without systemic lesionsn pathologically corresponds to its counterparts. The lesions are usually located at the level of the dura with a typical differential diagnosis with meningiomas or solitary fibrous tumor.
3. **Juvenile xanthogranuloma.** Juvenile xanthogranuloma involving the CNS or the meninges, with or without systemic lesions, pathologically correspond to its counterparts. Like the other histiocytic tumor can be localized in the dura but also in the brain with enhancing masses occurring mainly in pediatric patients.
4. **Histiocytic sarcoma.** It is a malignant proliferation of cells showing morphological and immunophenotypic features of tissue histiocytes and exhibiting no other lines of

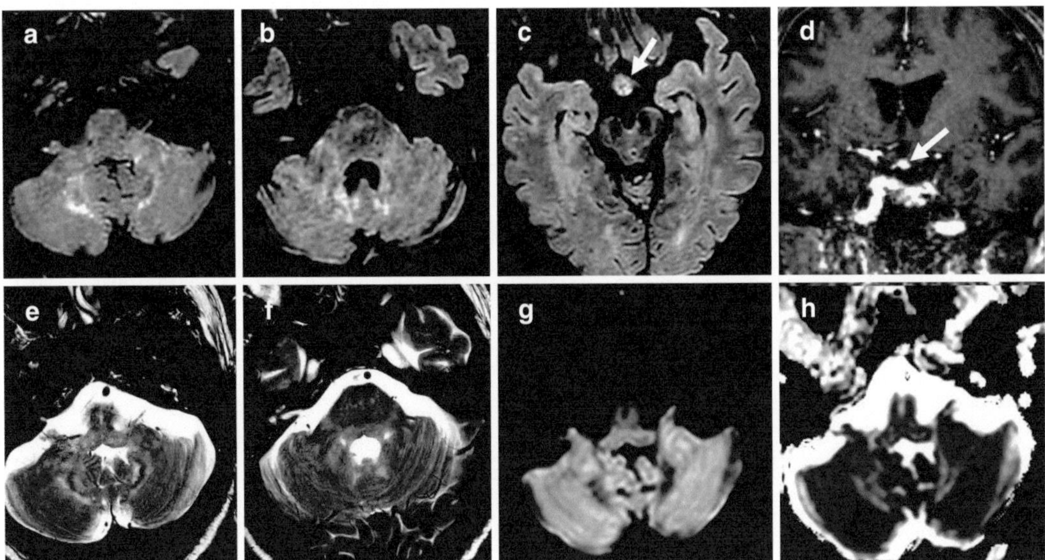

Fig. 9.14 Langherans cell histiocytosis, neurodegenerative pattern in a 64-year-old man. MRI FLAIR (**a–c**), post-contrast T1WI (**d**), T2WI (**e, f**), DWI (**g**), ADC (**h**). The typical T2/FLAIR symmetrical lesions of the dentate nuclei are visible as well as an hypothalamic localization of the disease (arrows **c, d**). Dentate lesions exhibit an increased diffusion (**g, h**)

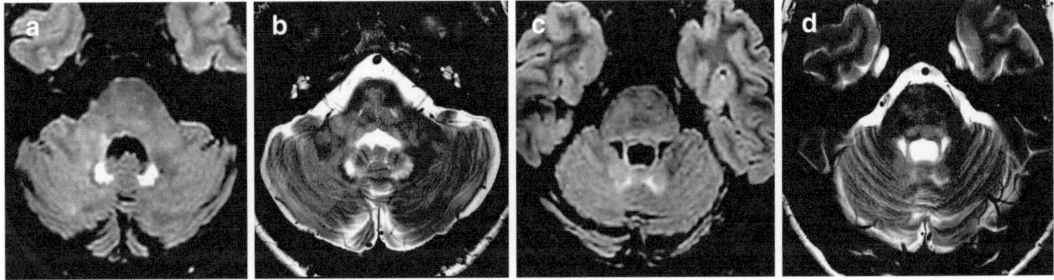

Fig. 9.15 Langherans cell histiocytosis, neurodegenerative pattern in a 42-year-old man. MRI FLAIR (**a–c**), T2WI (**b, d**). Another typical involvement of dentate nuclei in the neurodegenerative pattern of intracranial Langherans cell histiocytosis

differentiation. This is a nonspecific aggressive tumor similar to other sarcomas of the CNS.

9.5   Germ Cell Tumors

Germ cell tumors of the CNS are a family of morphological and immunophenotypic homologous of gonadal and other extra-neuraxial germ cell neoplasms sharing certain generic features (Table 9.2).

Epidemiology. Germ cell tumors are rare tumors affecting mainly pediatric population and are extremely uncommon in the adult. They can be found also in fetuses or as a congenital mass (Fig. 9.16). The annual incidence is greater in the far-east countries (Korea, Japan, Taiwan) than in Europe or America. Males are more typically affected in the case of pineal tumor location, whereas no sex prevalence is present for suprasellar location.

Location. Germ cell tumors are predominantly found in the midline brain structures being pineal region and suprasellar region the most typically affected. There are some differences among the different subtypes. Pineal region is the most fre-

Table 9.2 Germ cell tumor definitions

1. Teratoma	Mature teratoma	A germ cell tumor composed solely of fully differentiated adult-type somatic tissue components that recapitulate the differentiating potential of the ectoderm, endoderm, and mesoderm
	Immature teratoma	A germ cell tumor containing incompletely differentiated fetal-like somatic tissue components that recapitulate the differentiating potential of the ectoderm, endoderm, and mesoderm
	Teratoma with somatic-type malignancy	A germ cell tumor containing mature or immature teratomatous type that develops a distinct secondary component resembling a somatic-type malignant neoplasm
2. Germinoma	A malignant germ cell tumor composed of cells resembling primordial germ cells	
3. Embryonal carcinoma	A malignant germ cell tumor composed of large epithelioid cells resembling those of the embryonic germ disc	
4. Yolk sac tumor	A malignant germ cell tumor that differentiates to resemble extraembryonic structures, including the yolk sac, allantois, and extraembryonic mesenchyme	
5. Choriocarcinoma	A malignant germ cell tumor that differentiates to resemble the trophoblastic cells of the extraembryonic chorion, including syncytiotrophoblastic and cytotrophoblastic elements	
6. Mixed germ cell tumors	Malignant germ cell tumor with at least two germ cell tumor subtypes in any combination	

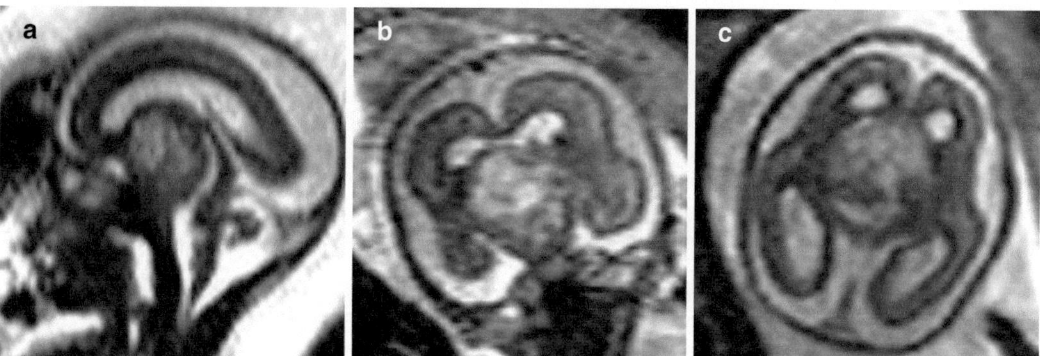

Fig. 9.16 Immature suprasellar teratoma in a 20 gestational weeks fetus. MRI SSFSE T2WI (**a–c**). A huge inhomogeneous mass is clearly visible in the diencephalic-hypothalamic region with a marked mass effect on the deep brain structures

quent location for non-germinoma subtypes (70%), whereas germinomas are located in this region in roughly 25% of cases. The sellar/suprasellar region accounts for 1/3 of germinoma, and for only 13% of non-germinoma cases. Another relatively frequent location is the basal ganglia accounting for 27% of germinoma cases and 13% of non-germinoma cases.

Germinomas could typically present as a double location in both pineal and suprasellar regions.

Clinical features. In case of pineal region involvement an aqueduct compression with subsequent hydrocephalus and/or Parinaud syndrome can ensue. Suprasellar involvement can be associated with visual disturbances, diabetes insipidus, or endocrines disturbances. Germ cell tumors can express different tumor markers the most diffuse is human chorionic gonadotropin (HGC) mainly present in germinoma and choriocarcinoma, and alpha fetoprotein (AFP), mostly present in yolk sac tumors and in some types of teratoma.

Prognosis. The prognosis is related to the histologic subtypes. Congenital teratomas usually carried an unfavorable prognosis, but mature teratomas in older children present with a more favorable course and radio-chemotherapy is usually highly effective in germinomas.

9.5.1 Imaging

Apart from different locations some structural differences are visible between germinomas and non-germinoma germ cell tumors. Germinomas are more frequently solid homogeneous masses, whereas non-germinoma germ cell tumors are often nonhomogeneous lesions and in 2/3 of cases exhibited some spontaneous T1 hyperintensities and present a more conspicuous enhancement after contrast administration (Figs. 9.16, 9.17, and 9.18). T2/FLAIR images show in germinomas an iso to slight hyperintense aspect. In non-germinoma tumors T2/FLAIR is inhomogeneous with frequent hyperintense components. Germinomas may present as slightly hyperdense on CT.

Diffusion. Diffusion restriction is a typical feature of germinomas with a mean value of approximately 1.1×10^{-3} mm²/s. In non-germinoma germ cell tumors the diffusion value is usually greater with a mean value of roughly $1.5\ 1 \times 10^{-3}$ mm²/s [4].

Spectroscopy. Spectroscopy is nonspecific with a decrease of NAA, increase of Cho, and a variable lipid peak [5]. Imaging features of germinoma are reported in Table 9.3.

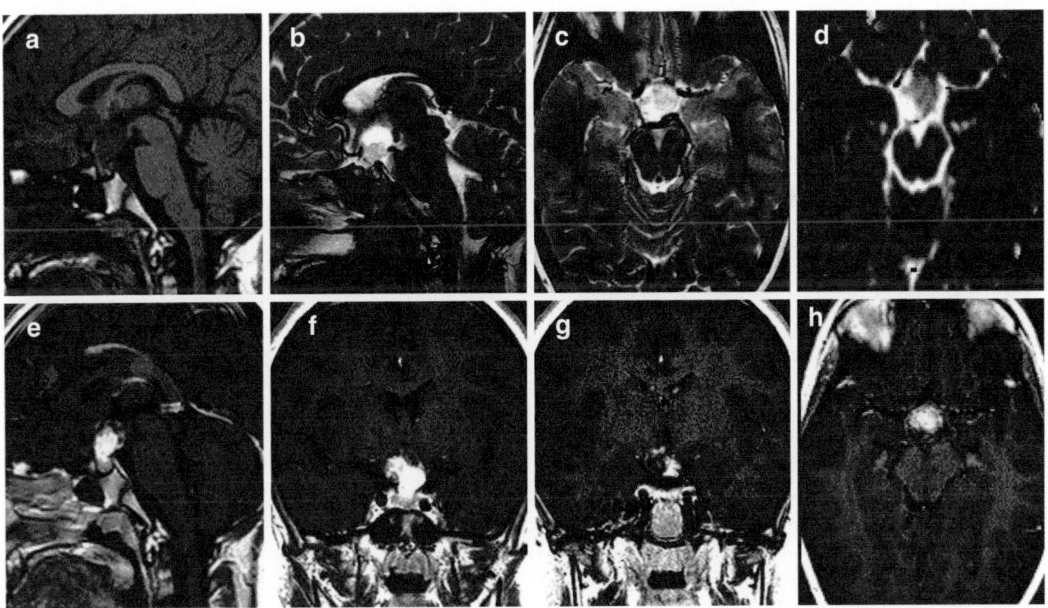

Fig. 9.17 Suprasellar germinoma in an 8-year-old boy with diabetes insipidus. MRI T1WI (**a**), T2WI (**b, c**), ADC (**d**), post-contrast T1WI (**e–h**). A large, partly inhomogeneous, mass is present at the level of the hypothalamus and pituitary stalk, the spontaneous T1 hyperintensity of the neurohypophysis is not visible (**a**), the enhancement is irregular but marked. (Courtesy C. Baldoli, Milan)

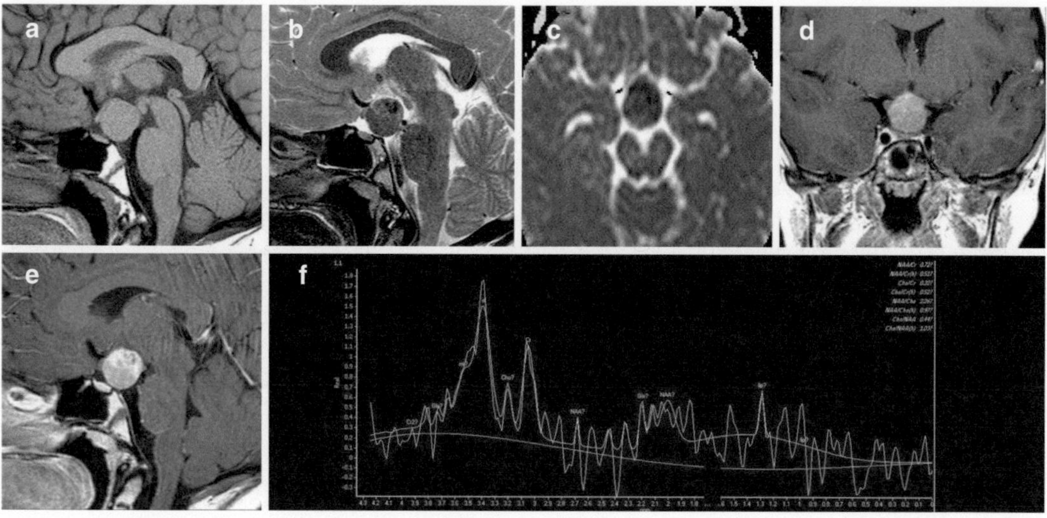

Fig. 9.18 Suprasellar germinoma in a 13-year-old boy with visual disturbances. MRI T1WI (**a**), T2WI (**b**), ADC (**c**), post-contrast T1WI (**d**, **e**), spectroscopy (**f**). The lesion is in this case quite homogeneous with a diffusion restriction and moderate enhancement. The spectroscopy study shows an almost absent NAA peak with some lipids. (Courtesy C. Baldoli, Milan)

Table 9.3 Germinoma imaging features

Mass effect	Edema	Inhomogeneity	Cysts	Necrosis	Hemorrhage	Calcifications
+/++	+/++	0/+	0	0	0	0/+ *(pineal)*

CT	T1	T2	FLAIR	DWI	ADC	T1 Gd	CBV	Spec
◯	◉	◯	◯	◯	⬤	+/+++	NA[a]	↑Cho/NAA, ↑Lipids

[a]NA (not available) incomplete or sporadic reports

References

1. Kaulen LD, Galluzzo D, Hui P, et al. Prognostic markers for immunodeficiency-associated primary central nervous system lymphoma. J Neurooncol. 2019;144:107–15.
2. Smith AB, Horkanyne-Szakaly I, Schroeder JW, et al. From the radiologic pathology archives: mass lesions of the dura: beyond meningioma-radiologic-pathologic correlation. Radiographics. 2014;34:295–312.
3. Prosch H, Grois N, Wnorowski M, Steiner M, Prayer D. Long-term MR imaging course of neurodegenerative Langerhans cell Histiocytosis. AJNR Am J Neuroradiol. 2007;28:281022–8.
4. Wu CC, Guo WY, Chang FC, et al. MRI features of pediatric intracranial germ cell tumor subtypes. J Neurooncol. 2017;134:221–30.
5. Gavrilovic S, Lavrnic S, Thurnher M, Macvanski M, Grujicic D, Stosic-Opincal T. Proton MR spectroscopy and diffusion-weighted imaging of intracranial germ cell tumors: implications for differentiation from other lesions. Eur J Radiol Extra. 2011;79:e59–64.

10.1 Adamantinomatous Craniopharyngioma

WHO definition. Adamantinomatous craniopharyngioma is a mixed solid and cystic squamous epithelial tumor with stellate reticulum and wet keratin, usually localized to the hypothalamic-pituitary axis and characterized by activating *CTNNB1* mutation.

Epidemiology. Adamantinomatous craniopharyngioma exhibits a bimodal age distribution with a double incidence peak in childhood and in adult (45–60 years). In childhood it accounts for 5–11% of all intracranial tumor. The adamantinous variant is almost the only variant present in children and accounts for 80% of all craniopharyngiomas in adults.

Location. This tumor can theoretically arise everywhere along the craniopharyngeal canal (Fig. 10.1), but it occurs in the majority of case in the infudibulo-tuberal region.

Clinical features. Adamantinomatous craniopharyngiomas grow slowly, and sometimes the diagnosis can be made only when the tumor causes an important mass effect with increased intracranial pressure. The most common signs in any age group are visual imbalance and diabetes insipidus with or without endocrine disturbance. In children GH deficiency can be present with reduced growth rate. More rarely symptomatology involves hypothalamus with obesity, cognitive impairment, and psychiatric symptoms.

Prognosis. The prognosis is closely related to the possibility of complete removal of the tumor. However, some sort of hypothalamic infundibular damage is difficult to avoid with any type of surgery. Local invasiveness is a crucial variable in defining prognosis, and this tumor, even if WHO grade I, has often a relatively worse prognosis.

10.1.1 Imaging

Imaging features of adamantinomatous craniopharyngioma are quite characteristic. It is a sellar suprasellar inhomogeneous mass composed usually by three components: a solid enhancing portion, a cystic component, and variable calcifications.

The solid portion is frequently smaller than the cystic component with a variable signal intensity on MRI and density on CT. The enhancement of the solid portion is almost always present. The cystic component can be formed by a single, sometimes huge cyst, or by multiple cysts with variable signal intensity. The presence of spontaneous T1WI hyperintensity is a peculiar feature of the cyst (Figs. 10.1, 10.2, and 10.3), but it can show a CSF-like signal or a slight T1WI hypointensity and an hyperintense signal on both T2WI and FLAIR images (Figs. 10.4, 10.5, and 10.6). The cystic wall may or may not enhance.

© The Author(s), under exclusive license to Springer Nature Switzerland AG 2023
F. M. Triulzi, *Neuroradiology of Brain Tumors*, https://doi.org/10.1007/978-3-031-38153-9_10

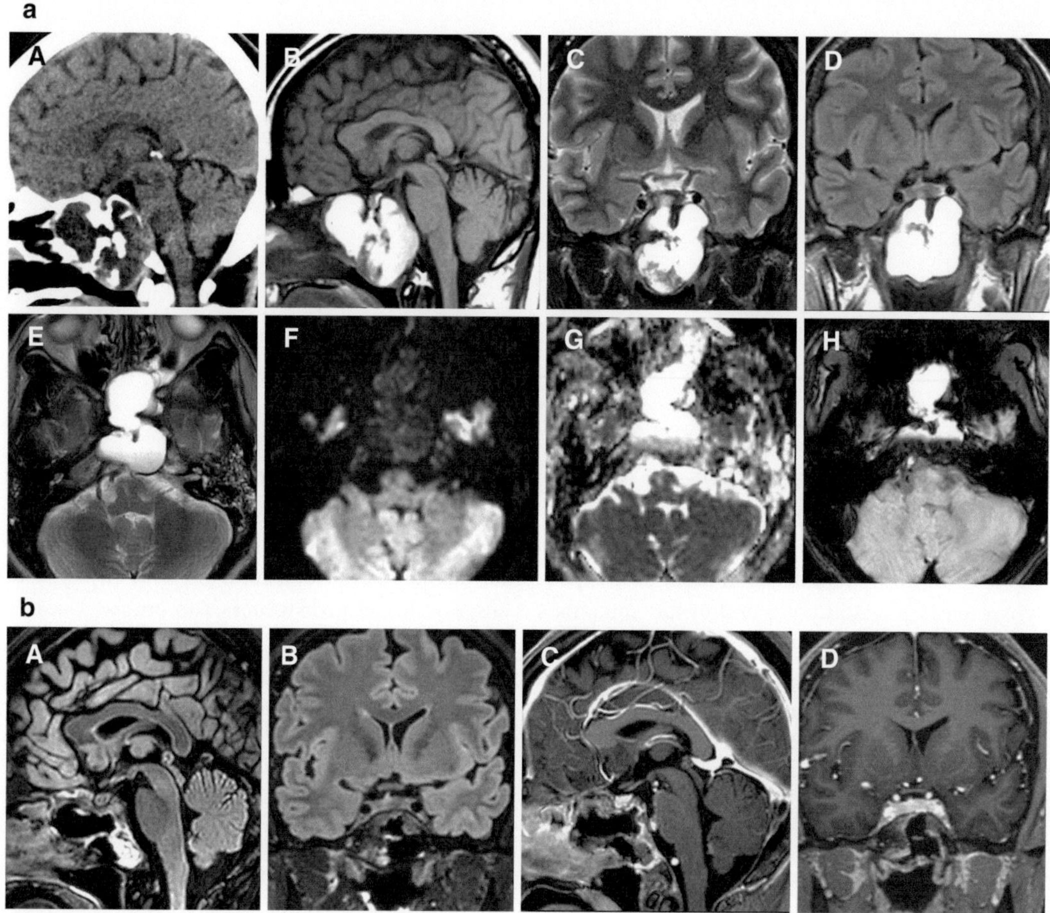

Fig. 10.1 (**a**) Extracranial adamantinomatous craniopharyngioma in a 41-year-old female with nasal obstruction. CT (**a**). MRI T1WI (**b**), T2WI (**c, e**), FLAIR (**d**), DWI (**f**), ADC (**g**), SWI (**h**). Extracranial locations are rare, but craniopharyngioma may be located anywhere along the craniopharyngeal canal. In this case it occupies the sphenoid bone with progressive bone erosion, the cyst shows spontaneous hyperintensity on T1WI. (**b**) Extracranial adamantinomatous craniopharyngioma in a 41-year-old female with nasal obstruction (cont.). A total removal is obtained via a trans-sphenoidal approach. MRI FLAIR (**a, b**), post-contrast T1WI (**c, d**).

Calcifications are very frequent with different sizes and morphology (Figs. 10.2, 10.3, 10.4, and 10.6).

The presence of the solid portion and of the calcification can differentiate craniopharyngioma from the Rathke cleft cyst that is simple cyst and not a neoplastic lesion, located along the craniopharyngeal canal without solid portion and calcification.

Diffusion. On diffusion images the cyst shows a CSF-like signal. The *shine trought* artifact can affect DWI with an hyperintense aspect not due to a diffusion restriction. The artifacts from calcifications and skull base prevent usually the evaluation of diffusion in the solid portion.

Spectroscopy. When the spectra are not affected by calcifications a lipid peak can be detected in the cyst. Imaging features of adamantinous craniopharyngioma are summarized in Table 10.1.

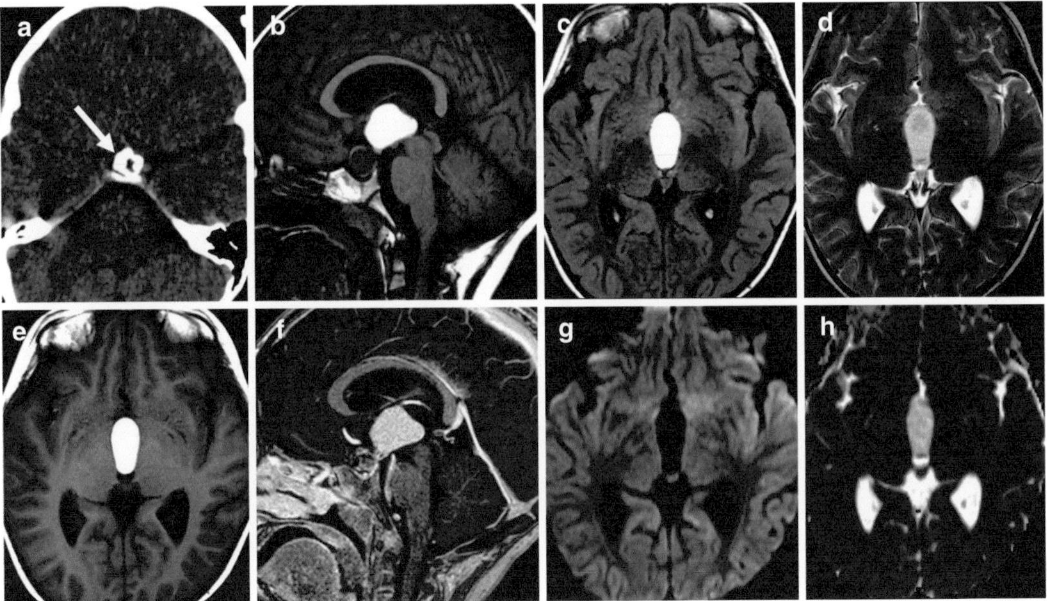

Fig. 10.2 Sellar and suprasellar adamantinomatous craniopharyngioma in a 4-year-old male with diabetes insipidus. CT (**a**). MRI T1WI (**b, e**), FLAIR (**c**), T2WI (**d**), post-contrast T1WI (**f**), DWI (**g**), ADC (**h**). The lesion presents an infundibular calcification (arrow **a**) and a cystic component in the anterior part of the third ventricle with a spontaneous hyperintensity on T1WI

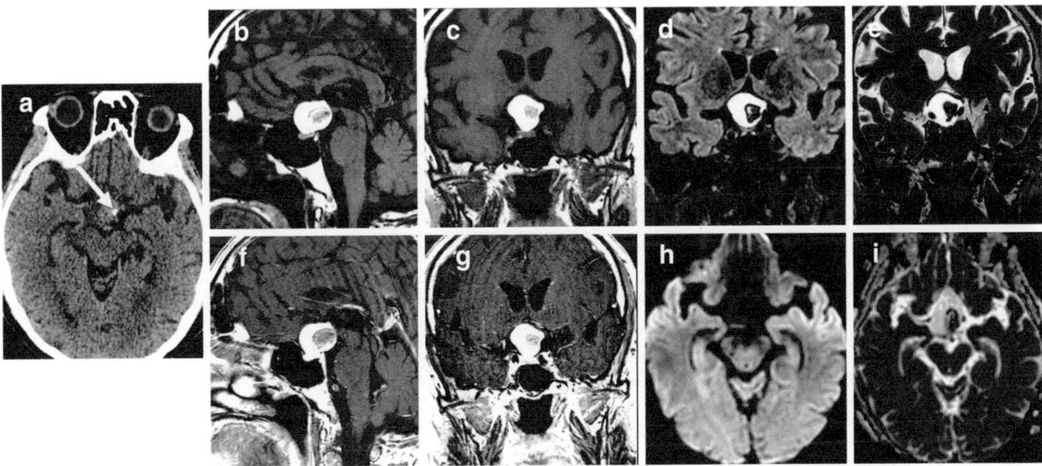

Fig. 10.3 Suprasellar and infundibular adamantinomatous craniopharyngioma in a 62-year-old male with visual disturbances. CT (**a**). MRI T1WI (**b, c**), FLAIR (**d**), T2WI (**e**), post-contrast T1WI (**f, g**), DWI (**h**), ADC (**i**). In this adult case the calcification is relatively small (arrow **a**) and the cyst is centered on the infundibular region with a spontaneous T1WI hyperintensity

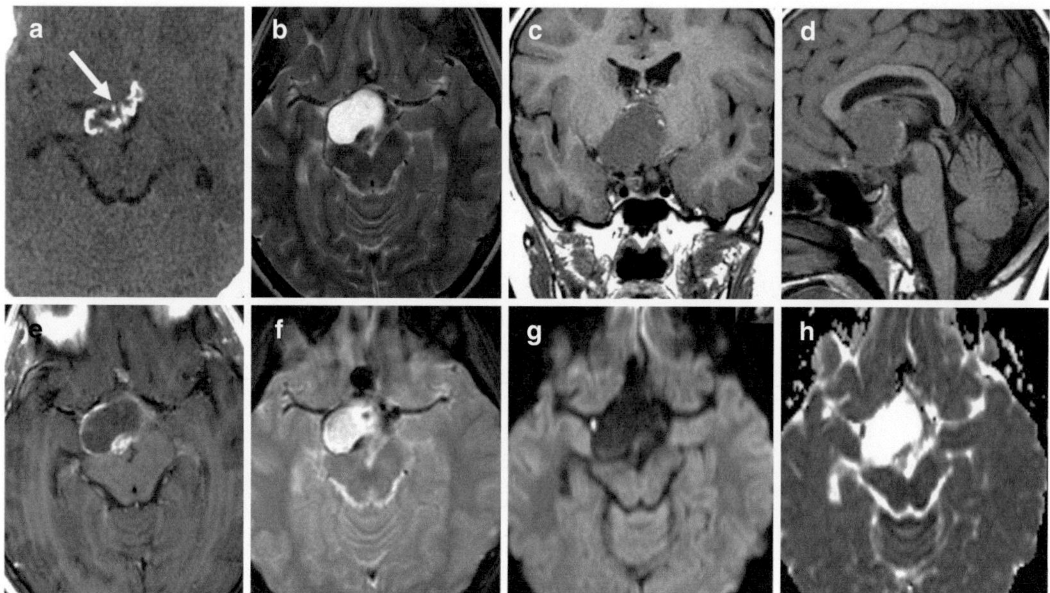

Fig. 10.4 Suprasellar and infundibular adamantinomatous craniopharyngioma in a 9-year-old female with hypothalamic syndrome. CT (**a**). MRI T2WI (**b**), T1WI (**c, d**), post-contrast T1WI (**e**), T2*GRE (**f**), DWI (**g**), ADC (**h**). The calcification is larger than in the previous case (arrow **a**), the cyst growth in the third ventricle but without a spontaneous T1WI hyperintensity. The cystic wall enhances after contrast administration (**e**)

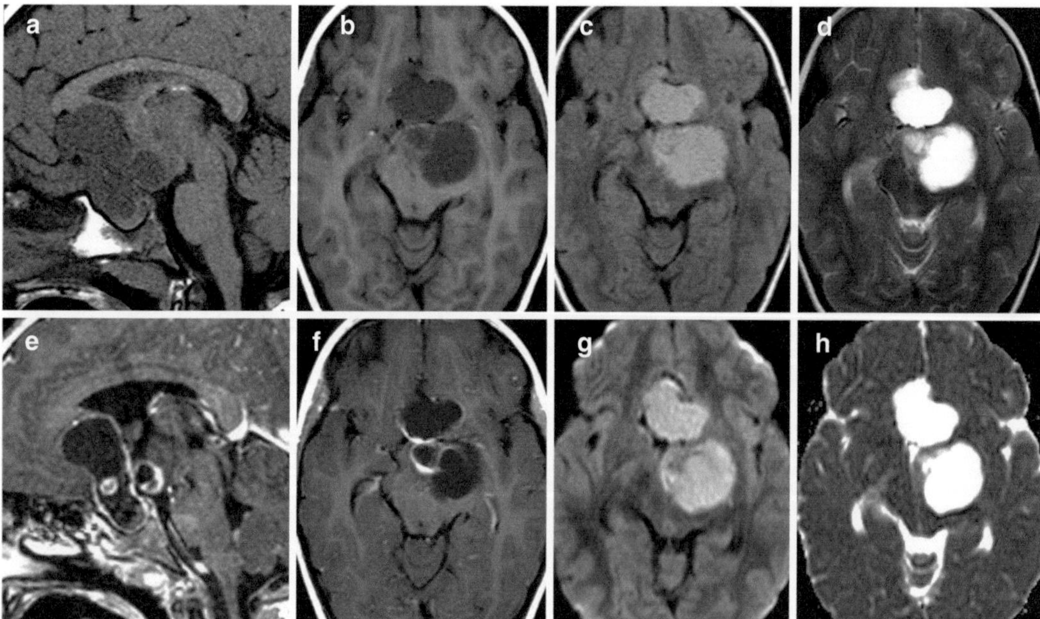

Fig. 10.5 Sellar and suprasellar infundibular adamantinomatous craniopharyngioma in a 4-year-old female with diabetes insipidus and visual disturbances. MRI T1WI (**a, b**), FLAIR (**c**), T2WI (**d**), post-contrast T1WI (**e, f**), DWI (**g**), ADC (**h**). There is a multiloculated huge cyst occupying the suprasellar space and the anterior part of the third ventricle

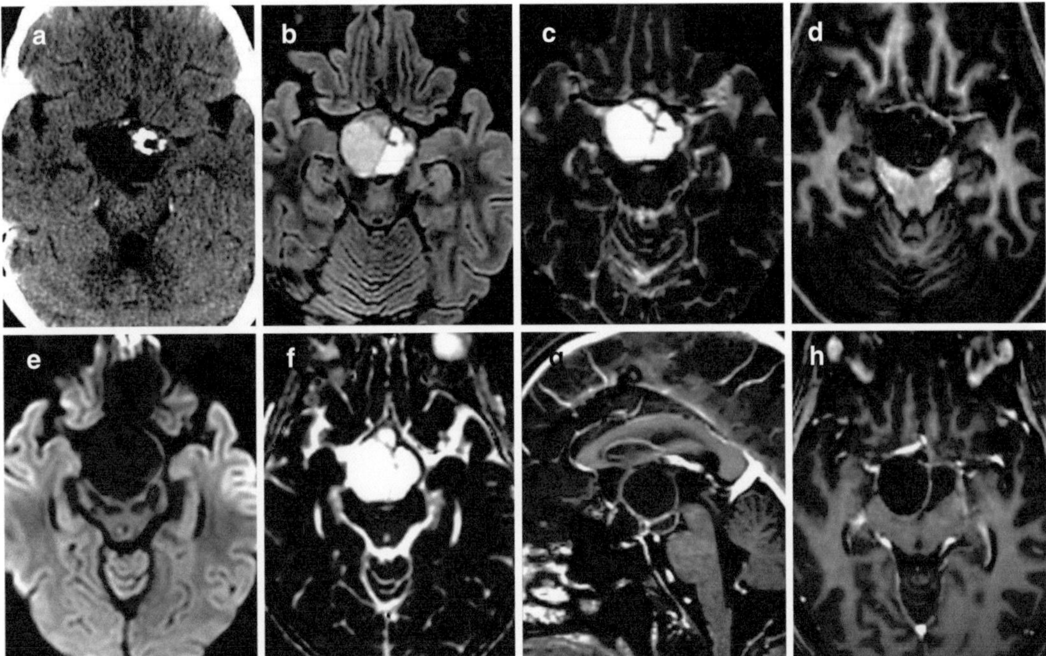

Fig. 10.6 Suprasellar and infundibular adamantinomatous craniopharyngioma in a 51-year-old female with visual disturbances. CT (**a**). MRI FLAIR (**b**), T2WI (**c**), T1WI (**d**), DWI (**e**), ADC (**f**), post-contrast T1WI (**g**, **h**). There is a huge multiloculated cyst with hypointense aspect on T1WI

Table 10.1 Adamantinomatous craniopharyngioma imaging features

Mass effect	Edema	Inhomogeneity	Cysts	Necrosis	Hemorrhage	Calcifications
+/++	+/++	+/+++	+/+++	0	0/+	+/+++

CT	T1	T2	FLAIR	DWI	ADC	T1 Gd	CBV	Spec
◯	⬤ ◯	◯	◯	⬤	◯	+/++	NA[a]	↑Lipids

[a]*NA* incomplete or sporadic reports

10.2 Papillary Craniopharyngioma

WHO definition. Papillary craniopharyngioma is a solid or partially cystic non-keratinizing squamous epithelial tumor that develops in the infundibulotuberal region of the third ventricle floor, most often in adults, and is characterized by *BRAF* p.V600E mutations.

Epidemiology. This tumor accounts for approximately 10% of all craniopharyngiomas in adults. It is extremely rare in children.

Location. This tumor is usually located on the floor of the third ventricle and in the region of the infundibulum and tuber cinereum.

Clinical features. Clinical features include endocrine disturbances, hypothalamic syndrome, and diabetes insipidus.

Prognosis. The prognosis is strictly related to the resectability of the tumor such as for adamantinomatous variant.

10.2.1 Imaging

This craniopharyngioma is usually located in the anterior portion of the third ventricle with a solid portion usually more evident than the adamantinomatous variant and a cystic component that presents an hypointense aspect on T1WI and a slight hyperintense signal on T2/FLAIR sequences. Spontaneous T1WI hyperintensity of the cyst is extremely rare. Even calcification is quite rare in papillary craniopharyngiomas (Fig. 10.7) [1].

Spectroscopy. The lipid peak of the cystic portion of the adamantinomatous craniopharyngioma is not present in the spectroscopy profile of

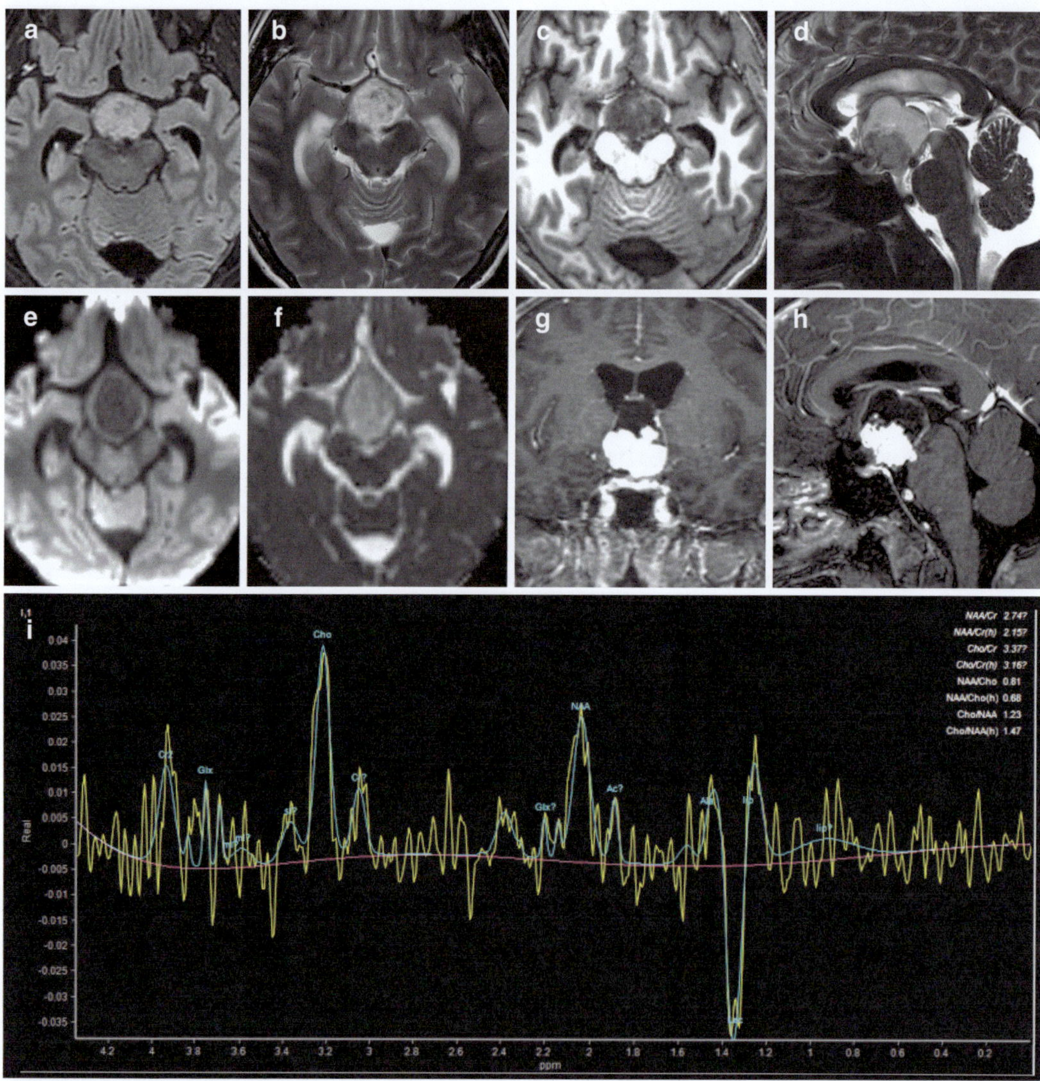

Fig. 10.7 (a) Suprasellar papillary craniopharyngioma in a 45-year-old male. MRI FLAIR (**a**), T2WI (**b**), T1WI (**c**), bSSFP (**d**), DWI (**e**), ADC (**f**), post-contrast T1WI (**g, h**), spctroscopy with 144 ms TE (**i**). The lesion is located in the anterior part of the third ventricle without an apparent involvement of the sellar and suprasellar structures. There is a solid portion and a cystic component hypointense on T1WI and slightly hyperintense on T2/FLAIR images. There is an increase in Cho/NAA ratio and a huge doublet peak of lactate

Table 10.2 Papillary craniopharyngioma imaging features

Mass effect	Edema	Inhomogeneity	Cysts	Necrosis	Hemorrhage	Calcifications
+/++	+/++	+/++	+/++	0	0/+	0

CT	T1	T2	FLAIR	DWI	ADC	T1 Gd	CBV	Spec
○	●	○	○	●	○	+/++	NA	↑Lactate

papillary craniopharyngioma where a lactate peak can be found (Fig. 10.7). Imaging features of papillary craniopharyngioma are summarized in Table 10.2.

10.3 Pituicytoma, Granular Cell Tumor of the Sellar Region, Spindle Cell Oncocytoma

WHO definition. These tumors constitute a distinct family of low-grade neoplasms that arise from pituicytes of the posterior pituitary or infundibulum, most likely representing a spectrum of a single nosological entity.

Epidemiology. Epidemiological data are scarce due to the rarity of these tumors. They are tumors occurring meanly in adult between the fifth and sixth decade of life.

Location. These tumors are located in the region of the pituitary stalk with a possible hypothalamic diffusion.

Clinical features. Clinical signs are similar to other lesion of sellar and suprasellar region; however, diabetes insipidus is rare.

Prognosis. These are benign slow growing tumor, the prognosis is related to the possibility of a complete surgical removal.

10.3.1 Imaging

These tumors are often similar to the other more common tumors of the sellar and suprasellar region. From the small series reported up to now [2] granular cell tumor appears as a iso- or slight hyperdense suprasellar mass on CT with a peculiar hypointense aspect on T2WI/FLAIR images. Calcifications are absent.

There is a homogeneous enhancement after contrast administration and a possibile slight diffusion restriction (Fig. 10.8). Imaging features of granulae cell tumor of the sellar region are summarized in Table 10.3.

10.4 Pituitary Adenoma, Pituitary Neuroendocrine Tumor

WHO definition. Pituitary adenoma/pituitary neuroendocrine tumor (PitNET) is a clonal neoplastic proliferation of anterio-pituitary hormone-producing cells.

Epidemiology. Pituitary adenomas are among the most frequent tumors found in humans, and they are reported in about 20% of all autopsies. Their incidence increases with age and according to CBTRUS they account for 16.5% of all surgically treated brain tumors. Prolactin secreting adenomas are the more frequent pituitary adenomas in female patients, whereas non-secreting adenomas are more frequently found in male patients.

Location. These tumors originate in the pituitary gland with centrifugal growth most often upward into the suprasellar region or laterally into the cavernous sinus, but in a minority of cases they may grow downward toward the sphenoid sinus. An ectopic growth is rare although possible.

Clinical features. Clinical signs and symptoms are related to the presence of an excessive hormone secreting adenoma leading to hyperprolactin syndrome, acromegaly, Cushing disease, or hyperthyroidism. In non-secreting adenomas clinical symptoms are related to the mass effect with visual disturbances or signs of pituitary-hypothalamic disconnection.

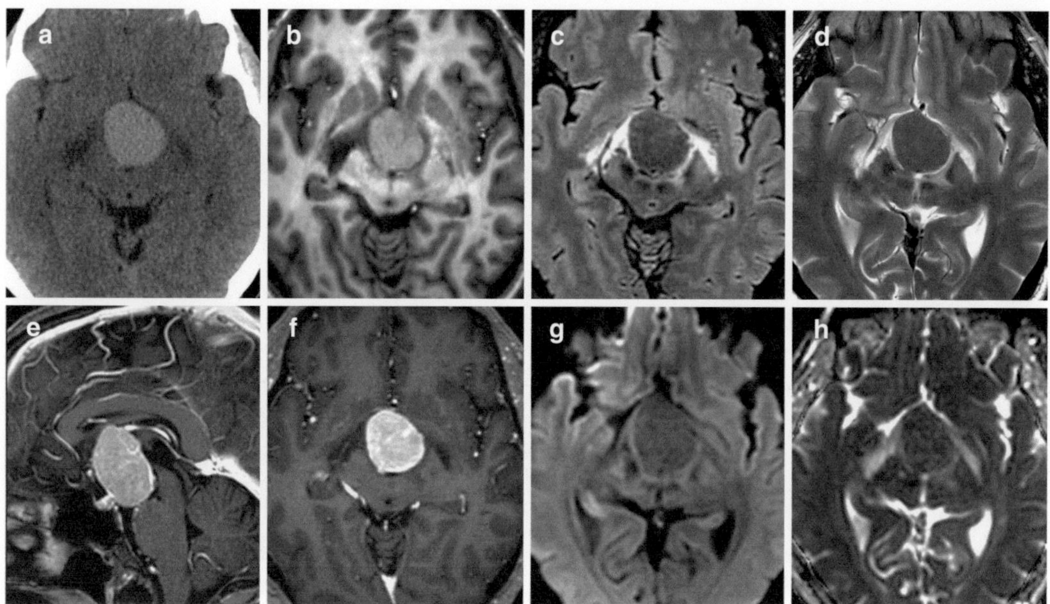

Fig. 10.8 Granular cell tumor of the sellar origin in a 54-year-old male. CT (**a**). MRI T1WI (**b**), FLAIR (**c**), T2WI (**d**), post-contrast T1WI (**e**, **f**), DWI (**g**), ADC (**h**). There is a large homogeneous suprasellar infundibular mass with a slight hypodensity on CT and an hypointense aspect on T2WI/FLAIR images. Diffusion is similar to brain parenchyma or slightly decreased. The post-contrast enhancement is homogeneous

Table 10.3 Granular cell tumor of the sellar region imaging features

Mass effect	Edema	Inhomogeneity	Cysts	Necrosis	Hemorrhage	Calcifications
+/++	0/++	0	0	0	0	0

CT	T1	T2	FLAIR	DWI	ADC	T1 Gd	CBV	Spec
◯	◯	●	◯	◯	◯	++	NA[a]	NA[a]

[a]*NA* incomplete or sporadic report

Prognosis. Pituitary adenomas are usually benign slow growing tumors even though in a very small percentage of case carcinoma variant is reported. Therapy is related to the size of the tumor and to the presence of secreting hormone tumor.

10.4.1 Imaging

Pituitary adenomas are classically subdivided into microadenoma (<10 mm) or macroadenoma (>10 mm).

Microadenoma is better diagnosed on T1WI as a slight hypointense area before contrast administration or as an area with less contrast after contrast administration (Fig. 10.9). On T2WI they can result in isointense with normal parenchyma or sometimes slightly hyperintense. The use of dynamic sequence during contrast administration can increase the diagnostic accuracy due to different curves in contrast enhancement between normal parenchyma and adenoma. Imaging features of pituitary microadenoma are summarized in Table 10.4.

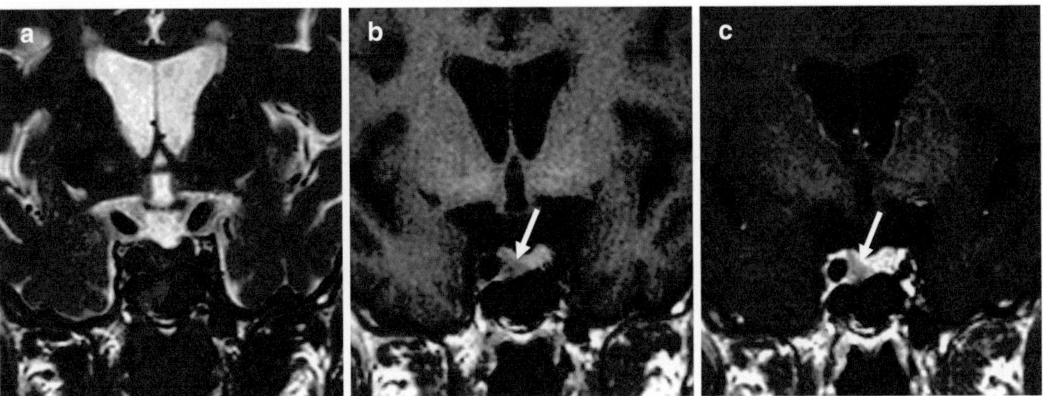

Fig. 10.9 GH-secreting pituitary microadenoma. MRI T2WI (**a**), T1WI (**b**), post-contrast T1WI (**c**). The microadenoma is visible on T1WI as a slightly hypointense area in the right lateral portion of the pituitary gland (arrow **b**). After contrast administration the adenoma shows less enhancement than the normal parenchyma (**c**). The adenoma causes a slight erosion of the corresponding sellar floor

Table 10.4 Pituitary microadenoma imaging features

Mass effect	Edema	Inhomogeneity	Cysts	Necrosis	Hemorrhage	Calcifications
0/+	0	0	0/+	0	0/+	0

CT	T1	T2	FLAIR	DWI	ADC	T1 Gd	CBV	Spec
○	◐	●	○	NA[a]	NA[a]	–	NA[a]	NA[a]

[a]*NA (not available)* incomplete or sporadic reports

Macroadenomas are more typically non-functioning adenomas that can grow in the suprasellar cistern and eventually compress the chiasm with typical bitemporal hemianopsia. They are more frequently homogeneous with signal intensity on T1WI quite similar to normal brain parenchyma, on T2WI they can be isointense or slightly hyperintense. Large adenomas may exhibit hemorrhages or may partially collapsed do to ischemic event. Calcifications are rare (Fig. 10.10).

Diffusion. Diffusion is usually isointese with brain parenchyma (Fig. 10.11), even though diffusion restriction has been reported [3].

Spectroscopy. Reports on spectroscopy are scarce, an increase of Cho/NAA ratio as well as presence of a lipid peak has been reported [3].

Perfusion. Even for perfusion data are scarce; however, an increase of CBV has been reported [4].

Macroadenomas can grow extensively before they become clinically evident. A diffuse invasion of the hypothalamic region and also of the sphenoid bone can be found at diagnosis. In this very large tumor hemorrhagic component is very frequent (Fig. 10.11). Imaging features of pituitary macroadenoma are summarized in Table 10.5.

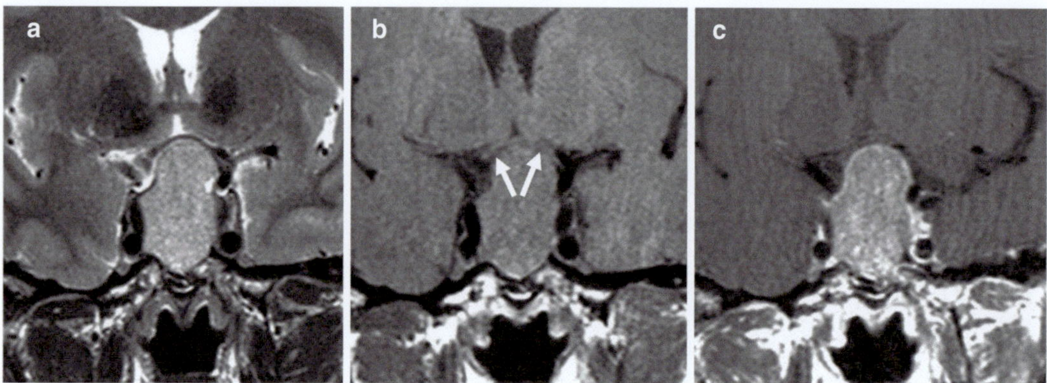

Fig. 10.10 Nonfunctioning macroadenoma in a 45-year-old female, disclosed occasionally after a head trauma. MRI T2WI (**a**), T1WI (**b**), post-contrast T1WI (**c**). The macroadenoma grows upward and compresses the optic chiasm (arrow **b**). It is an homogeneous mass with a moderate enhancement

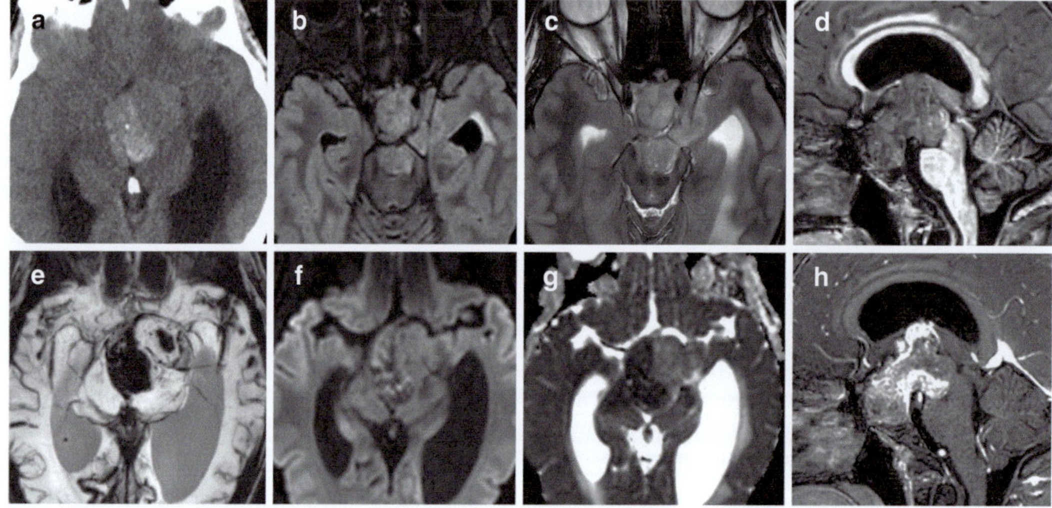

Fig. 10.11 Nonfunctioning macroadenoma in a 23-year-old male, with visual disturbances. CT (**a**). MRI FLAIR (**b**), T2WI (**c**), T1WI (**d**), SWI (**e**, DWI (**f**), ADC (**g**), post-contrast T1WI (**h**). This huge adenoma invades extensively the anterior third ventricle region, whereas inferiorly causes a diffuse erosion of the sellar floor and sphenoid bone. The lesion is diffusely inhomogeneous and microhemorrhagic components are visible on both CT (**a**) and SWI (**e**)

Table 10.5 Pituitary macroadenoma imaging features

Mass effect	Edema	Inhomogeneity	Cysts	Necrosis	Hemorrhage	Calcifications
+/+++	0/+	0/++	0/++	0/+	0/++	0/+

CT	T1	T2	FLAIR	DWI	ADC	T1 Gd	CBV	Spec
○	◔	○	○	○	◔	+	●	↑ Cho/NAA ↑Lipids

References

1. Lee IH, Zan EW, Bell WR, Burger PC, Sung H, Yousem DM. Craniopharyngiomas: radiological differentiation of two types. J Korean Neurosurg Soc. 2016;59:466–70.
2. Kusakawa A, Inoue A, Nakamura Y, et al. Clinical features and endoscopic findings of granular cell tumor of the sellar region: a case report and review of the literature. Surg Neurol Int. 2020;11:101.
3. Mohammad FF, Hasan DI, Ammar MG. MR spectroscopy and diffusion MR imaging in characterization of common sellar and supra-sellar neoplastic lesions. Egypt J Radiol Nucl Med. 2014;45:859–67.
4. Bladowska J, Zimny A, Guzinski M, et al. Usefulness of perfusion weighted magnetic resonance imaging with signal-intensity curves analysis in the differential diagnosis of sellar and parasellar tumors: preliminary report. Eur J Radiol. 2013;82:1292–8.

11.1 Metastases to the CNS

WHO definition. Metastases to the brain, spinal cord and meninges are tumors that originate outside the CNS and spread into these areas via hematogenous route or directly from adjacent anatomical structures.

Epidemiology. Metastases from extra CNS tumors are the most frequent CNS neoplasms in the adult and it is calculated that 30% of adult with cancer develop brain metastases.

The incidence rate is 14 cases for 100.000 population every year.

Of course the higher the incidence of the primitive tumor, the higher the probability of having a brain metastases, but other factors may contribute to their frequency as for instance the provenience from the lung for the direct access to the brain via the left heart.

Tables 11.1 and 11.2 reported the relative frequencies of primary tumor and brain metastases in male and female [1].

In the general population lung neoplasm accounts for more than the 40% of all brain metastases. In female metastases from breast neoplasm are close to 1/3 of the total, whereas the second most common metastases in male are from unknown origin. Notably the most common neoplasm in men, prostate carcinoma has almost no brain metastases. Despite its relatively low frequency, melanoma proportionally accounts for a relatively high frequency of brain metastases.

Table 11.1 Relative frequencies of primary tumor and brain metastases in male

Neoplasm	Brain MTS	Primary NPL
Lung	50%	15%
Unknown origin	14%	
Gastrointestinal	11,4%	30%
Melanoma	10%	3%
Kidney	6,9%	5%
Other	5,6%	9%
Bladder	1,4%	8%
Prostate	0,6%	30%

Table 11.2 Relative frequencies of primary tumor and brain metastases in female

Neoplasm	Brain MTS	Primary NPL
Lung	31,6%	8%
Breast	28,4%	30%
Unknown origin	8,4%	
Gastrointestinal	8,3%	25%
Melanoma	7,1%	5%
Kidney	6,1%	4%
Ovary	3,5%	5%
Other	3,5%	15%
Uterus	3,1%	8%

Location. Brain metastases are typically located at cortico-sucortical junction of the cerebal hemispheres (in the arterial border zone) and only 20% are found infratentorially. A single brain metastasis is frequent and accounts for 53% of all brain metastases, but a single brain metastasis without any other metastases in the whole body is not frequent. Leptomeninges are another frequent location for brain metastases.

F. M. Triulzi, *Neuroradiology of Brain Tumors*, https://doi.org/10.1007/978-3-031-38153-9_11

Clinical features. Brain metastases can present with different signs and symptoms related to their location and size. Frequently being at the cortico-subcortical junction, seizures are one of the most frequent signs at presentation. Headache is another frequent sign as well as a sign of intracranial hypertension, although infrequent focal neurologic deficits may sometimes be present.

Metastases to the leptomeninges may present with various clinical symptoms such as headache, mental disturbances, cranial nerve dysfunction, or radiculopathy.

11.1.1 Imaging

Brain metastases exhibit an extreme variety of presentations on neuroimaging. The first diagnostic clue is the presence of a <u>single versus multiple</u> lesion. Single lesion is frequently a diagnostic challenge because it can mimic any potential aggressive primitive CNS tumor or sometimes even non-neoplastic lesions such as a brain abscess. A relatively constant aspect is the presence of a conspicuous perilesional edema usually more prominent than in aggressive primary tumor. Single lesion presents as a nodular or multinodular mass with an irregular contour, cystic necrotic center with possible hemorrhagic component and irregular peripheral enhancement. CT density and MR signal intensity are heterogeneous with the solid component that can show a hyperdense aspect on CT and a slight hypointensity on T2WI (Figs. 11.1, 11.2, 11.3 and 11.4).

Diffusion. Diffusion can be restricted in the nodular part of metastasis, but frequently the diffusion aspect is quite inhomogeneous.

Perfusion. Perfusion and permeability are increased (Fig. 11.5), but differently from glial aggressive tumor metastases that exhibit a slow

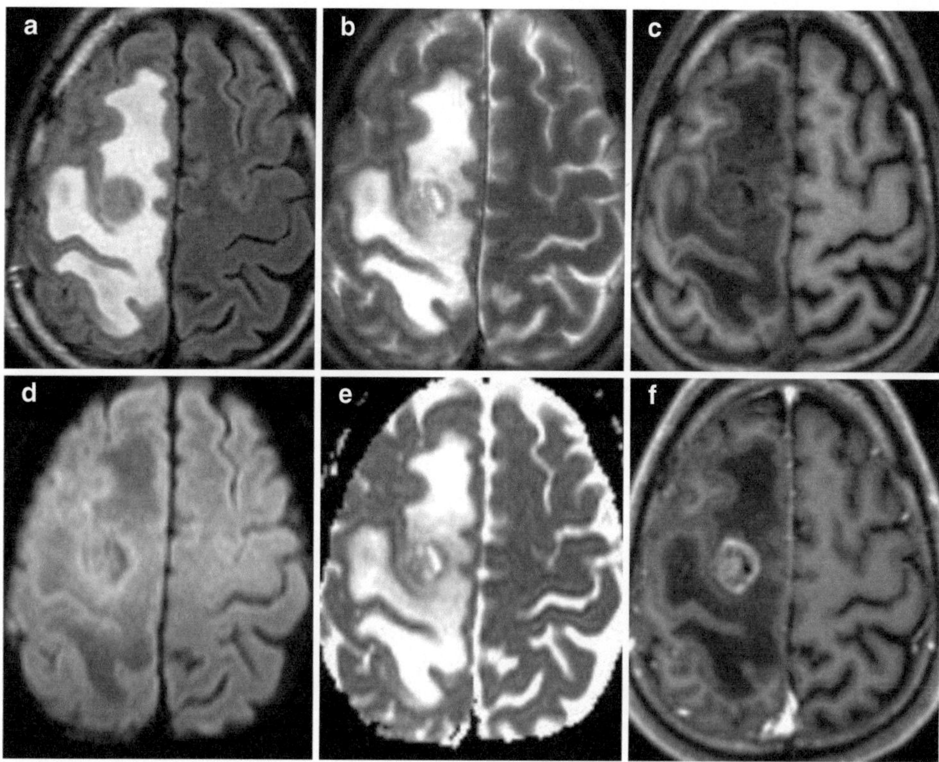

Fig. 11.1 Single metastasis. MRI FLAIR (**a**), T2WI (**b**), T1WI (**c**), DWI (**d**), ADC (**e**), post-contrast T1WI (**f**). Single metastasis in posterior aspect of the right superior frontal gyrus. The lesion is heterogeneous with an irregular enhancing rim and conspicuous perilesional edema

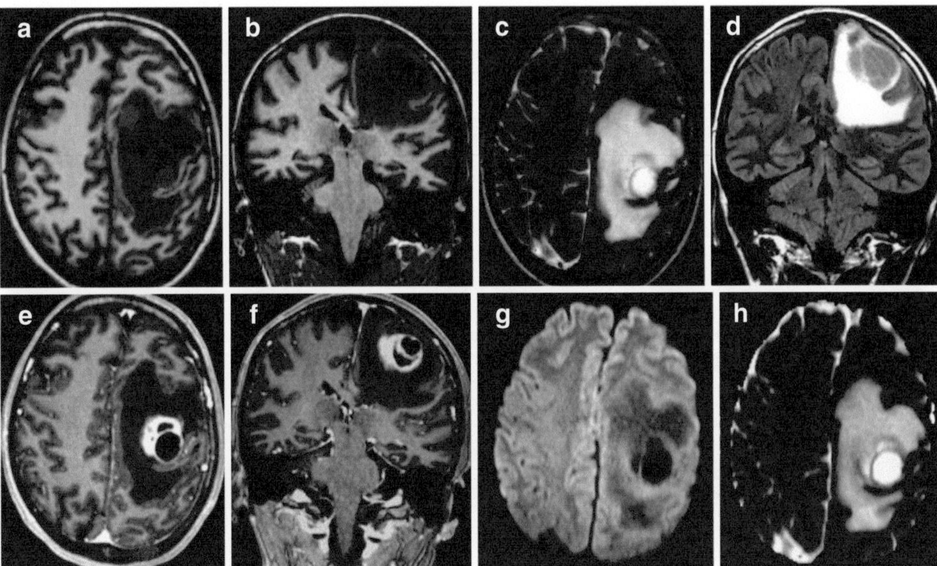

Fig. 11.2 Single metastasis. MRI T1WI (**a, b**), T2WI (**c**), FLAIR (**d**), post-contrast T1WI (**e, f**), DWI (**g**), ADC (**h**). Single metastasis in the left pre-rolandic area, quite similar to the case of Fig. 11.1 with an irregularly enhancing nodule and huge perilesional edema

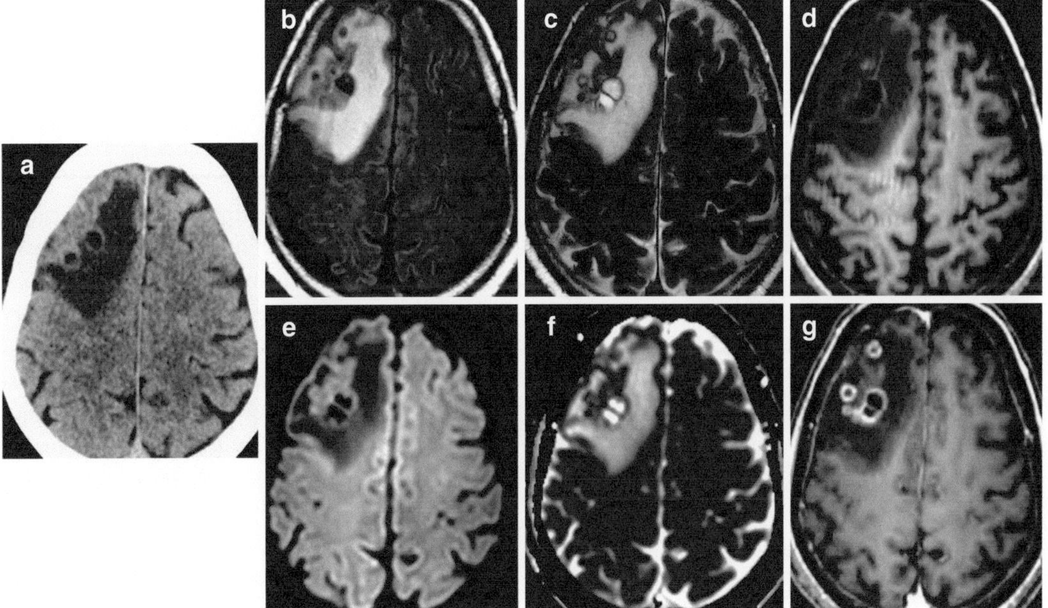

Fig. 11.3 Single multinodular metastasis. CT (**a**) MRI T1WI (**b**), T2WI (**c**), FLAIR (**d**), post-contrast T1WI (**e**), ADC (**f**), DWI (**g**). Single multinodular metastasis in the right frontal lobe. Multinodular lesions can be complex and irregular and may mimic multiple separate lesions

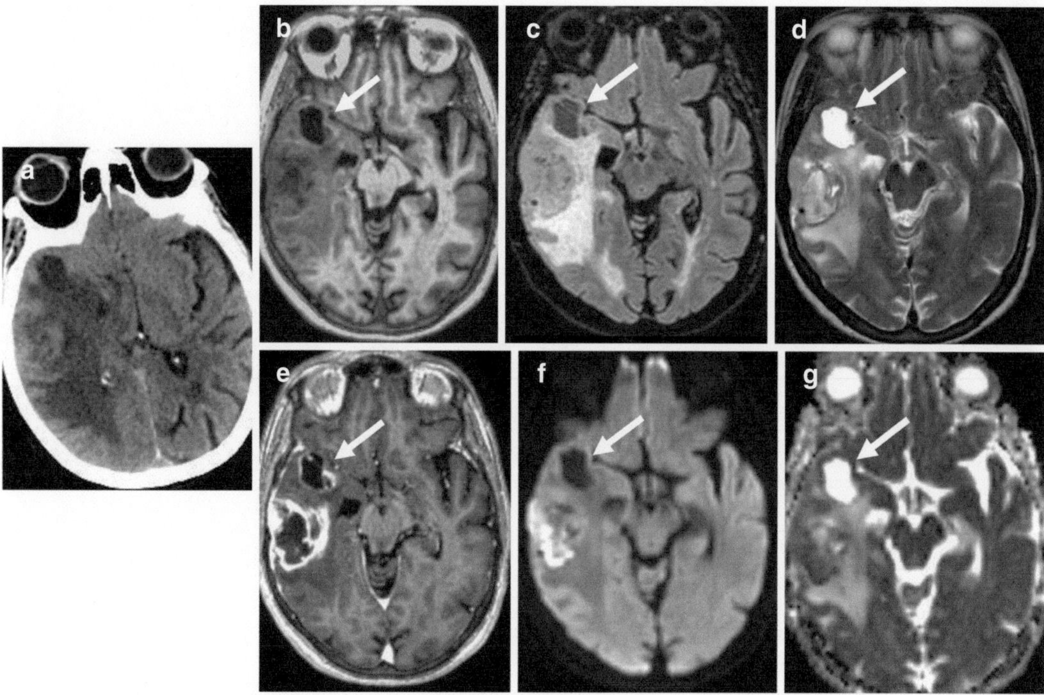

Fig. 11.4 Single vs. multiple metastases. CT (**a**) MRI T1WI (**b**), FLAIR (**c**), T2WI (**d**), post-contrast T1WI (**e**), DWI (**f**), ADC (**g**). Large right temporal lesion with a close cystic smaller lesion in the ipsilateral temporal pole (arrow **b**–**g**). In this case it is difficult to establish if the lesion is a huge single multinodular lesion rather than multiple close lesions

washout curve. Normal or even reduced CBV was reported in perilesional edema, on the contrary in case of primitive glial tumors CBV in perilesional edema was usually increased.

Spectroscopy. Spectroscopy usually shows an evident lipid peak in both short and intermediate echoes. Normal brain metabolites are markedly reduced with a relatively high Cho peak. Of course the spectra profile can change significantly according to the position of the volume of interest and due to partial volume effect. If the volume is centered within the necrotic portion of a metastasis a lactate peak can be evident as well. The amount of normal metabolite can depend on partial volume effect with normal brain in case of small parenchymal lesions (Figs. 11.5 and 11.6).

The presence of multiple metastases can of course facilitate the diagnosis, even some possible differential diagnosis still remains possible, in particular with infectious or inflammatory diseases.

As for single metastasis, even multiple metastases are usually extremely heterogeneous lesions with cystic necrotic or hemorrhagic component, diffuse restriction, and irregular enhancement after contrast (Fig. 11.7).

Lung and breast cancer are the most frequent neoplasms associated with multiple metastasis.

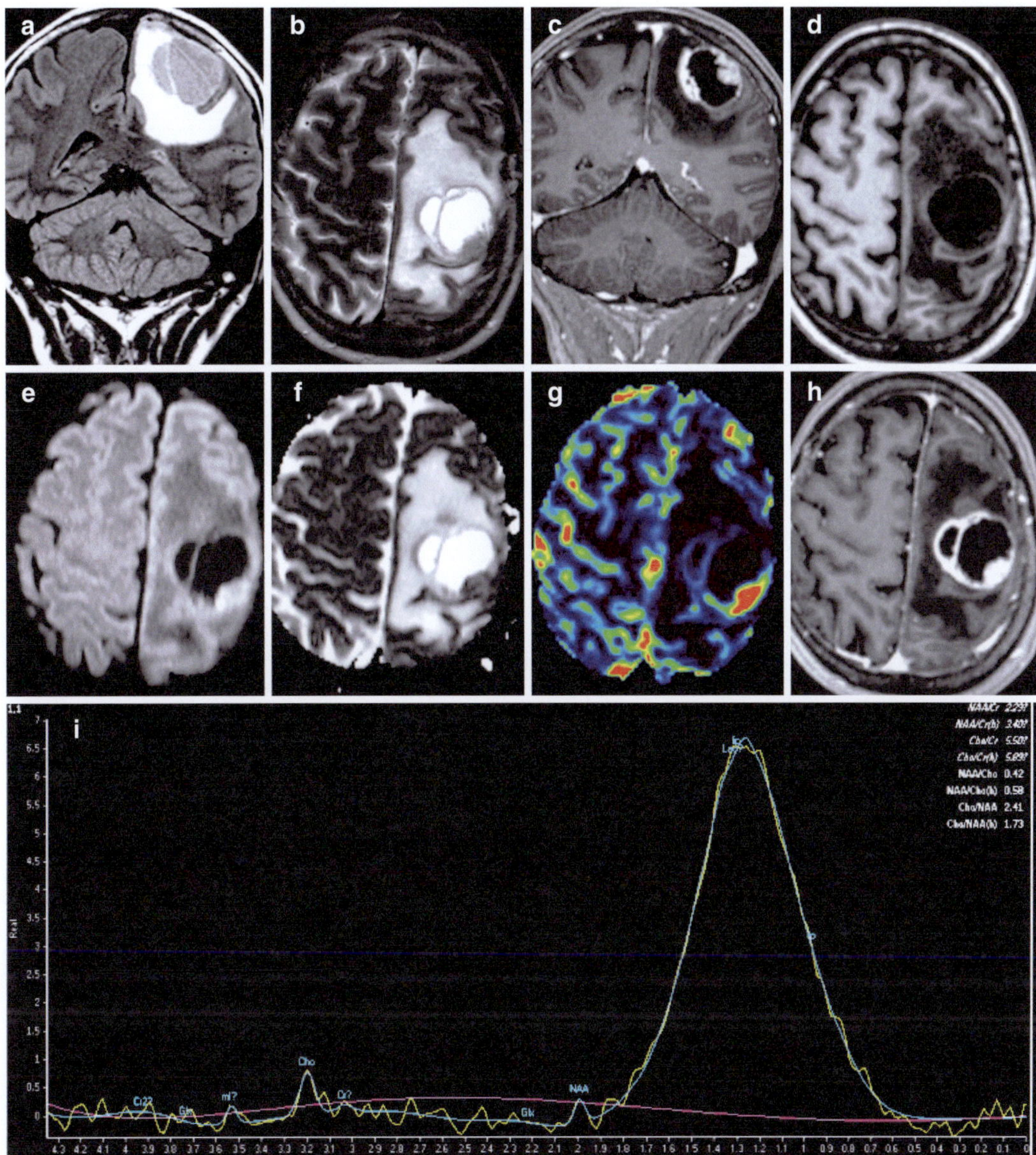

Fig. 11.5 Single metastasis. MRI FLAIR (**a**), T2WI (**b**), post-contrast T1WI (**c, h**), TY1WI (**d**), DWI (**e**), ADC (**f**), CBV (**g**), spectroscopy intermediate echo (**i**). A 36-year-old patient with ovarian carcinoma and diffuse body metastases with an apparently single metastasis in the left peri-rolandic region. The solid portion of the metastasis shows a diffuse restriction (**e, f**) and a CBV increase (**g**). MR spectroscopy intermediate echo (**i**) shows a huge lipid peak. Normal brain metabolites are almost undetectable

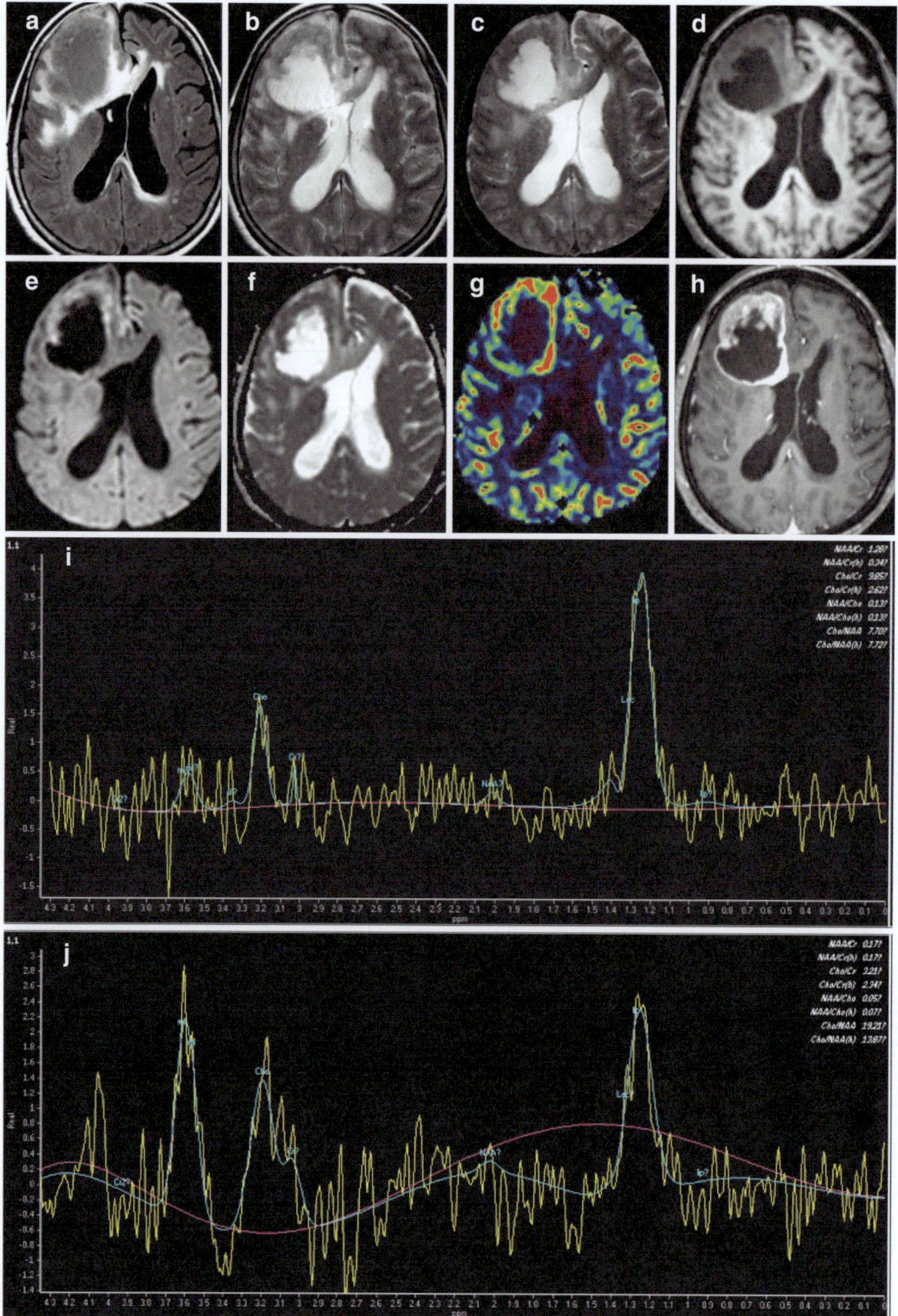

Fig. 11.6 Single metastasis. MRI FLAIR (**a**), T2WI (**b**), T2* GE (**c**), T1WI (**d**), DWI (**e**), ADC (**f**), CBV (**g**), post-contrast T1WI (**h**), spectroscopy (**i**, **j**). A 75-year-old patient with endometrial carcinoma and diffuse body metastases with an apparently single metastasis in the right anterior frontal region. The solid portion of the metastasis shows a diffuse diffusion restriction (**e**, **f**) and a CBV increase (**g**), but no hemorrhages (**C**). Even with artifacts due to the small volume MR spectroscopy shows a huge lipid peak on both intermediate (**I**) and short (**J**) echoes. Normal metabolites are reduced or not visible

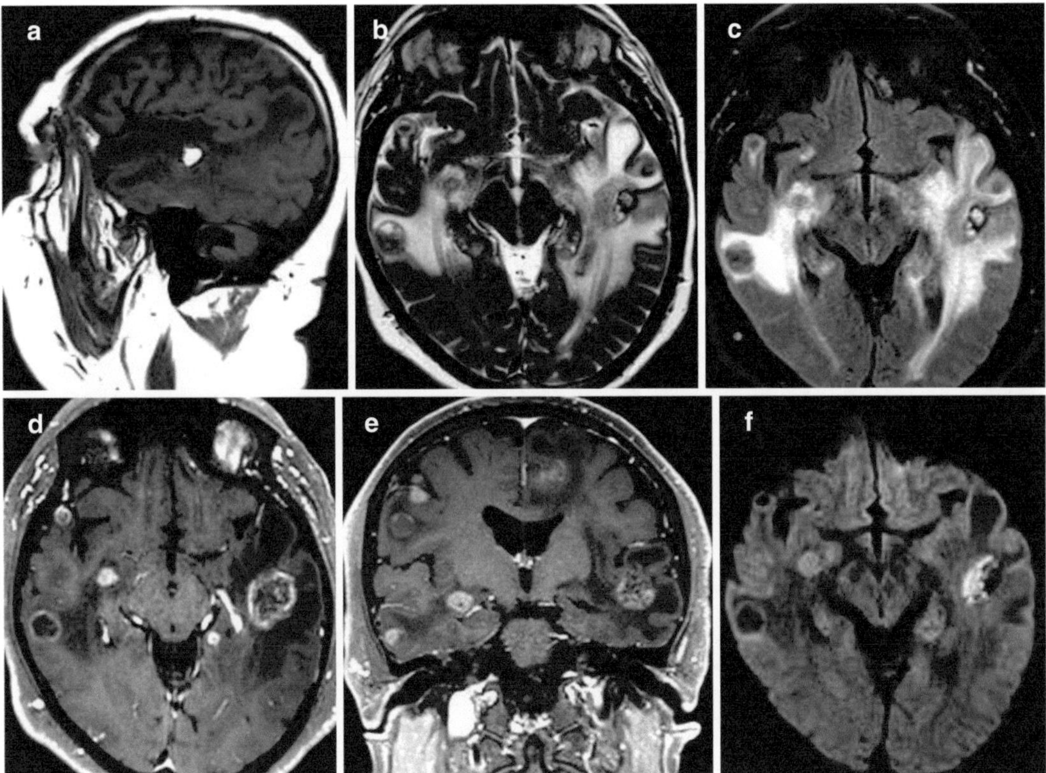

Fig. 11.7 Multiple metastases. MRI T1WI (**a**), T2WI (**b**), FLAIR (**c**), post-contrast T1 WI (**d, e**), DWI (**f**). Multiple metastases from breast carcinoma show an extremely heterogeneous pattern and abundant perile-sional edema with cystic necrotic and even haemorrhagic (**a**) components and irregular enhancement of the solid component

On both post-contrast CT and MRI an extreme accurate evaluation of the entire brain should be performed. In the standard oncologic total body follow-up multiple metastases may present as diffuse extremely small nodules barely visible only on post-contrast studies (Fig. 11.8).

In rare cases metastases can be present as a calcified lesion (Fig. 11.9). The real incidence of calcified brain metastases at diagnosis in unclear, but according to some authors they can be more frequent than previously suspected [2]. Primary tumors more frequently responsible of brain calcified metastases are lung and breast tumor.

Brain metastases calcification is however a frequent consequence of radiotheraphy.

Leptomeningeal metastases are relatively common in breast and lung cancer (other than in hematologic malignancies) (Fig. 11.10), but they can be found also in prostate cancer due to the dural spread from osseous metastases (Fig. 11.11). Image features of brain metastases are summarized in Table 11.3.

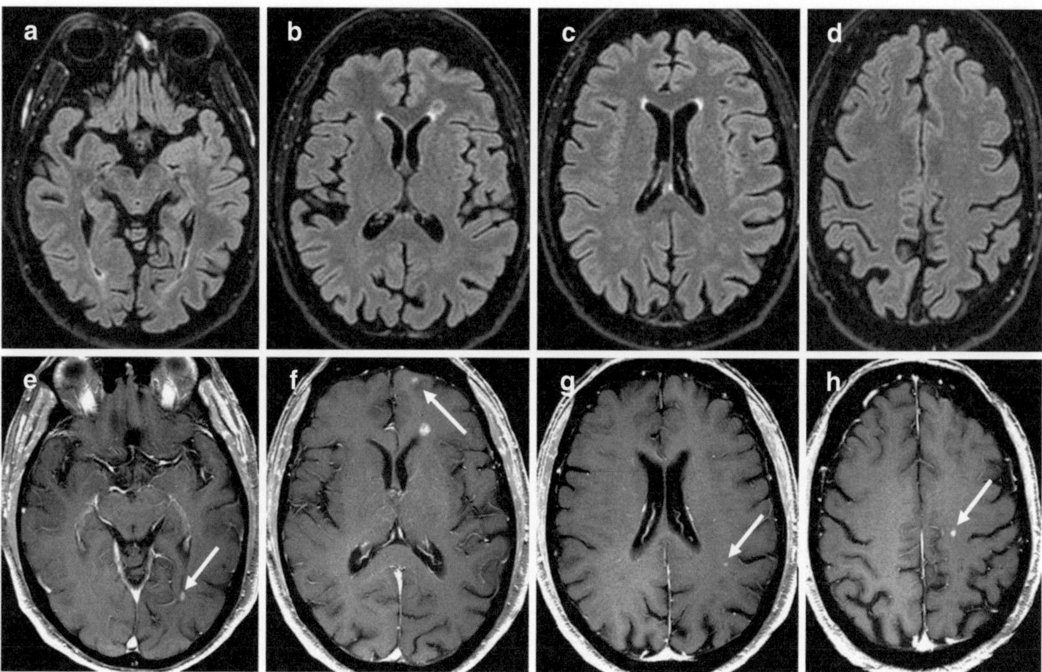

Fig. 11.8 Multiple metastasis. MRI FLAIR (**a–d**), post-contrast T1 WI (**e–h**). Multiple extremely small (miliari-form) metastases from lung carcinoma. On the pre-contrast FLAIR only one nonspecific periventricular left frontal lesion is visible, after contrast administration multiple tiny enhancing lesions are detectable (arrows)

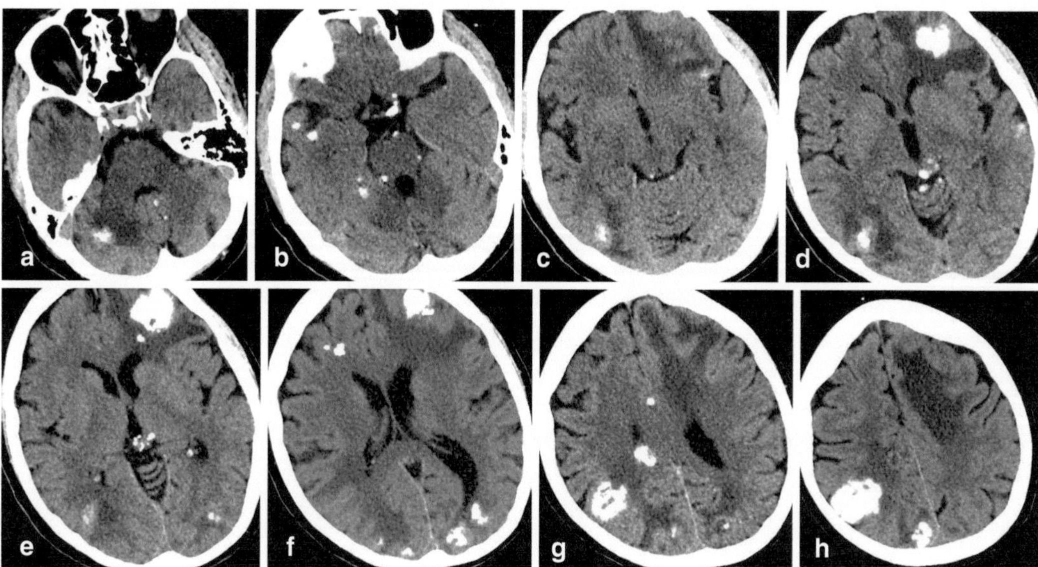

Fig. 11.9 Multiple calcified metastasis in a 75-year-old female with breast cancer. CT (**a–h**). Almost all lesions present huge calcifications at time of diagnosis

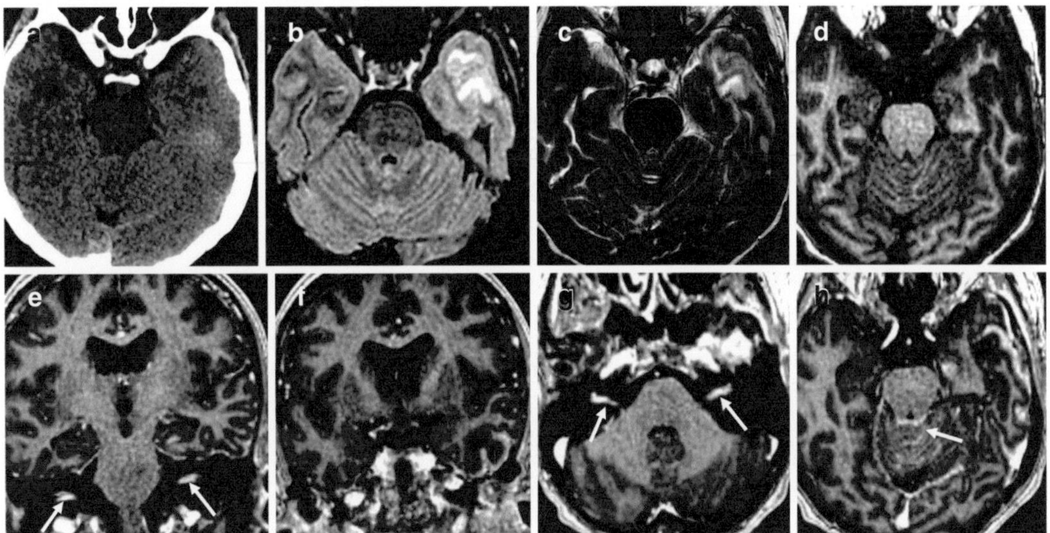

Fig. 11.10 Leptomeningeal metastases in a 56-year-old female with breast cancer. CT (**a**). MRI FLAIR (**b**). T2WI (**c**), T1WI (**d**), post-contrast T1WI (**e–h**). A diffuse leptomeningeal involvement with marked enhancement is visible in left temporal region with initial involvement of surrounding brain structures. Leptomeningeal spreading is however visible even around eighth cranial nerves bilaterally (**e, g** arrows) and in the quadrigeminal cistern and superior vermis (**h** arrow)

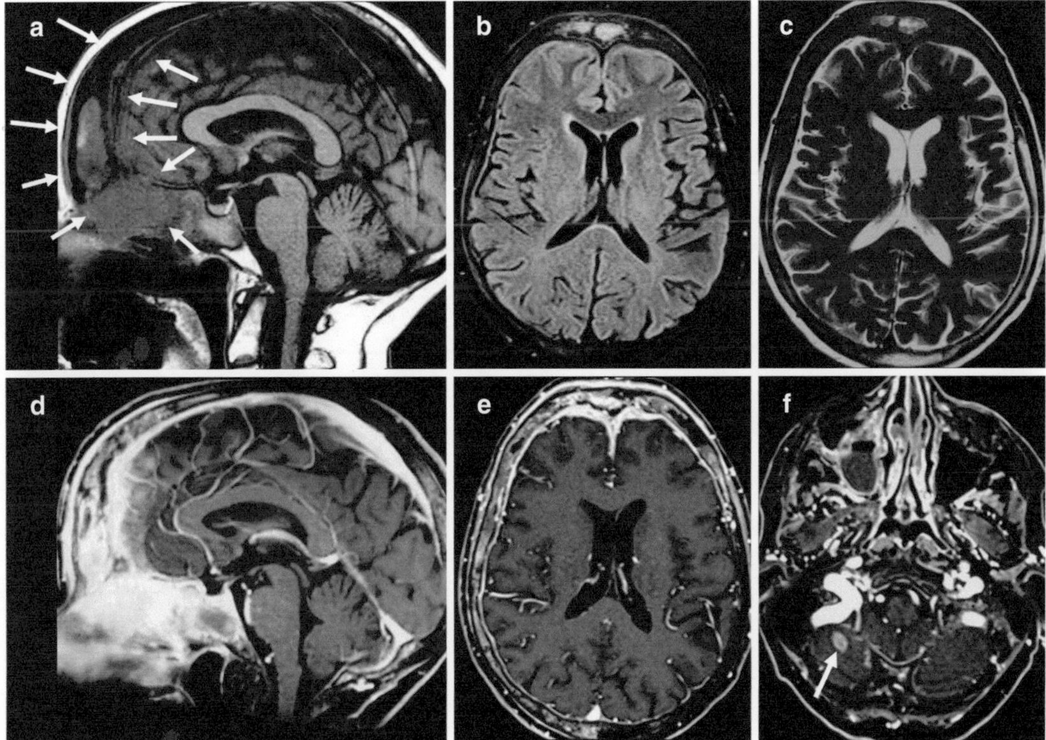

Fig. 11.11 Diffuse leptomeningeal spreading from a huge frontal bone metastasis. MRI T1WI (**a**), FLAIR (**b**), T2WI (**c**), post-contrast T1 WI (**d–f**). There is a large metastatic tumor (primitive unknown) spread through the frontal bone and anterior basicranium (arrows **a**). After contrast a diffuse leptomeningeal enhancement is visible corresponding to the dural invasion from the bone localization. A small superficial enhancing nodule (probably in a cortico-pial location) is visible in the inferiori aspect of left cerebellar hemisphere (arrow F)

Table 11.3 Brain metastases imaging features

Mass effect	Edema	Inhomogeneity	Cysts	Necrosis	Hemorrhage	Calcifications
+/+++	+/+++	+/+++	++	++	+	0/++

CT	T1	T2	FLAIR	DWI	ADC	T1 Gd	CBV	Spec
						+/+++		$\uparrow\uparrow$lipids,$\uparrow$lac $\downarrow\downarrow$NAA

References

1. Preusser M, Capper D, Ilhan-Mutlu A, et al. Brain metastases: pathobiology and emerging targeted therapies. Acta Neuropathol. 2012;123:205–22.

2. Rebella G, Romano N, Silvestri G, et al. Calcified brain metastases can be more frequent than normally considered. Eur Radiol. 2021;31:650–7.

Correction to: Neuroradiology of Brain Tumors: Practical Guide based on the 5th Edition of WHO Classification

Correction to:
F. M. Triulzi, *Neuroradiology of Brain Tumors* https://doi.org/10.1007/978-3-031-38153-9

The unit name in the author affiliation was initially published with an error as 'Nueoradiololgy', which has now been corrected.

The updated version of the book can be found at
https://doi.org/10.1007/978-3-031-38153-9